Disorders
of Hemostasis
and Thrombosis

A Clinical Guide

NOTICE

Medicine is an ever-changing science. As new research and clinical experience broaden our knowledge, changes in treatment and drug therapy are required. The editors and the publisher of this work have checked with sources believed to be reliable in their efforts to provide information that is complete and generally in accord with the standards accepted at the time of publication. However, in view of the possibility of human error or changes in medical sciences, neither the editors nor the publisher nor any other party who has been involved in the preparation or publication of this work warrants that the information contained herein is in every respect accurate or complete, and they are not responsible for any errors or omissions or for the results obtained from use of such information. Readers are encouraged to confirm the information contained herein with other sources. For example and in particular, readers are advised to check the product information sheet included in the package of each drug they plan to administer to be certain that the information contained in this book is accurate and that changes have not been made in the recommended dose or in the contraindications for administration. This recommendation is of particular importance in connection with new or infrequently used drugs.

Disorders

of Hemostasis

and Thrombosis

A Clinical Guide

William E. Hathaway, M.D.

Professor Emeritus of Pediatrics
University of Colorado School of Medicine
Denver, Colorado

Scott H. Goodnight, Jr., M.D.

Professor of Medicine and Clinical Pathology
Oregon Health Sciences University
Portland, Oregon

McGRAW-HILL, INC.

Health Professions Division

New York St. Louis San Francisco Auckland Bogotá Caracas Lisbon
London Madrid Mexico Milan Montreal New Delhi Paris San Juan
Singapore Sydney Tokyo Toronto

1234567890   DOC DOC   9876543

ISBN 0-07-027015-5

This book was set in Times Roman by Northeastern Graphic Services, Inc.
The editors were Jane Pennington and Susan Finn.
The production supervisor was Richard Ruzycka.
The cover and text were designed by José Fonfrias.
The index was prepared by Philip James.
R.R. Donnelly & Sons Company was printer and binder.

Library of Congress Cataloging-in-Publication Data

Hathaway, William E. (William Ellison),
    Disorders of hemostasis and thrombosis : a clinical guide   /
William Ellison Hathaway. Scott H. Goodnight, Jr.
      p.   cm.
    Includes bibliographical references and index.
    ISBN 0-07-027015-5
    1. Blood—Diseases—Handbooks, manuals, etc. 2. Hemostasis—
Handbooks, manuals, etc. 3. Thrombosis—Handbooks, manuals, etc.
I. Goodnight, Scott H. II. Title.
    [DNLM: 1. Hemostasis—handbooks. 2. Thrombosis—handbooks.
3. Blood Coagulation Disorders—handbooks.   WH 39 H363d 1993]
RC636.H37   1993
616. 1′5—dc20
DNLM/DLC
for Library of Congress   93-2121
                                                                        CIP

To the students, technologists, residents, fellows,
and colleagues who asked the critical questions

Contents

SECTION III

Thrombotic Disorders *305*

SECTION IV

Treatment Modalities *437*

Preface

During many years as teachers, researchers, clinicians, consultants, and directors of coagulation laboratories, the authors have been asked many questions regarding various aspects of hemostasis and thrombosis. These questions and the resulting dialogues have involved medical students, medical technologists, residents, and fellows oriented to hematology and oncology, academic and clinical colleagues and, most frequently, members of the practicing medical community. As a result of these conversations we realized that a need existed for organized and concise information which could be understood and assimilated by the questioners, who were not always experts in the field of platelet and clotting factor disorders. Indeed, during the academic careers of the authors, the field has exploded with new information, both basic and clinical, which has made it necessary for even the so-called "experts" to constantly review and place the new findings in perspective.

This book, therefore, is the result of the collaborative efforts of the authors, who attempt to combine their collective experience and interests from the disciplines of pediatrics, internal medicine, hematology, and laboratory medicine in order to present the hemostatic and thrombotic disorders as they affect humans from the newborn to the elderly. Each chapter is the result of much planning and discussion and involved the viewpoints of both authors.

The attempt to be comprehensive but still remain current and concise has resulted in a selection of examples of particular defects and modes of therapy rather than an exhaustive review. For the same reason, a limited number of key references have been included for each topic. We hope these references will allow and stimulate the reader to go deeper into the subject if desired.

Acknowledgments

For Wm. E. Hathaway: The personnel of The Special Coagulation Laboratory of the University Hospital and the Coagulation Research Laboratory of the Department of Pediatrics of the University of Colorado School of Medicine, in particular Susan Clarke and Linda Jacobson; and Helen S. Hathaway, M.D. and Wm. G. Hathaway for preparation of manuscripts and graphic art.

For Scott Goodnight: The Hemostasis and Thrombosis Laboratory at the Oregon Health Sciences University (including Diana Nelson, LeAnne Reif, Sandy Reed, Merlinda Heuschkel, and Mia Shepard); my colleagues Dr. Tom DeLoughery and Dr. Rod Johnson; Judy Jensen for superb secretarial help; and most of all to my family—Cecelia, Kate, and Tracy for their patience and unflagging support.

Disorders
of Hemostasis
and Thrombosis
A Clinical Guide

Hemostasis and

Thrombosis—

General

Considerations

Physiology of Hemostasis and Thrombosis

GENERAL CONSIDERATIONS

Hemostasis may be defined as the arrest of blood flow from or within a blood vessel. Clinical hemostasis or the control of bleeding from an injury site involves (1) the interaction of the blood vessel and supporting structures, (2) the circulating platelet and its interaction with the disrupted vessel, (3) the formation of fibrin by the coagulation system, (4) the regulation of the extension of the blood clot by coagulation factor inhibitors and the fibrinolytic system, and (5) the remodeling and repair of the injury site after arrest of bleeding. *Thrombosis* may be defined as the formation and propagation of a blood clot within the vasculature. Clinical thrombosis involves (1) blood flow and the blood vessels, (2) platelet-vessel interactions related to disruption of the endothelium, and (3) the coagulation system, and in particular the natural anticoagulants and the fibrinolytic system. This chapter presents an overview of the physiologic basis for hemostasis and thrombosis to set the stage for more detailed discussions of pathophysiology related to specific disorders.

OVERVIEW

The same basic mechanisms are involved in the generation of a hemostatic plug that arrests bleeding and the formation of an occlusive thrombus leading to obstruction to blood flow and possible tissue infarction. When a blood vessel is damaged and the normal endothelial cell (EC) barrier is disrupted, exposing tissue factor and collagen, platelets are recruited (by adhesion and aggregation mediated by von Willebrand factor and fibrinogen) from the circulating blood to form an occlusive plug and provide surfaces for blood coagulation reactions. In addition, the coagulation system is triggered because factor VII combines with tissue factor leading to a stepwise activation of a series of proenzymes to produce thrombin.

Thrombin activates platelets leading to exposure of negatively charged phospholipids (phosphatidylserine, PS) on their surfaces for clotting factor assembly (from plasma coagulation factors trapped in the plug and released by the platelets) further fostering thrombin formation. Importantly, thrombin clots soluble fibrinogen to insoluble fibrin which is then cross-linked (factor XIII) and anchored into place by the process of clot retraction. Thus, the formation of the platelet-fibrin plug or clot is mediated by adhesive proteins and their receptors (the platelet-vessel interaction) as well as proenzymes and their activators (the coagulation system).

This complex but precise process is regulated by antithrombins (AT III, thrombomodulin) and the protein C-protein S system which inactivate the accelerators of thrombin formation (factor Va and VIIIa). Subsequently, the clot is lysed by plasmin formed through the fibrinolytic system and the repair process continues. Each component of this hemostatic process is discussed separately even though all are dynamically intertwined.

PLATELET-VESSEL INTERACTION

The Vessel

The blood vasculature forms a circuit, free of leaks, which maintains blood in a fluid state. If a vessel is disrupted and blood loss occurs, the platelets and the coagulation system temporarily close the rent until the cells in the vessel wall permanently repair the leak. Blood vessels are composed of ECs and subendothelial basement membrane (intima), layers of smooth muscle cells and their extracellular matrix (media) surrounded by fibroblasts and their extracellular matrix (adventitia). The blood vessel exhibits many properties that contribute to hemostasis or arrest of hemorrhage as well as prevention of thrombosis. The media and adventitia provide mechanical strength and enable blood vessels to constrict or dilate. The subendothelial basement membranes contain several EC-derived adhesive proteins (collagen microfibrils, laminin, thrombospondin, fibronectin, elastin, vitronectin, and von Willebrand factor) which provide binding sites for platelets and leukocytes.

Endothelial cells have multiple mechanisms to help ensure blood flow. They exhibit vasoconstrictive properties by secreting renin, which produces angiotensin, by inactivating bradykinins, and by secreting endothelin, a potent vasoconstrictor peptide. ECs can induce vasodilatation by synthesizing and releasing endothelium-derived relaxing factor (EDRF), which mimics the effect of nitric oxide, and PGI_2 (prostacyclin), a potent vasodilator and inhibitor of platelet function (see below).

Some anticoagulant properties of ECs include the presence of mucopolysaccharides (heparin sulfate, dermatan sulfate), which accelerate the inhibitory effects of AT III and heparin cofactor II on the coagulation mechanism as well as an EC surface protein, thrombomodulin, which binds thrombin and enhances the activation of protein C. The ECs secrete several substances that modulate vascular repair by altering smooth muscle and fibroblast proliferation and function: platelet-derived growth factor (PDGF), vascular permeability factor, and fibroblast growth factor.

The Platelet

The circulating platelet is a small anuclear discoid cell (1.5 to 3 μm) that arises from megakaryocytes with a maturation time of 4 to 5 days and a circulating life span of 9 to 10 days. The bone marrow reserve of platelets is limited and can be rapidly depleted after sudden platelet loss or destruction. Newly formed platelets are larger in size and termed megathrombocytes. The morphology of a nonactivated platelet is shown diagrammatically in Fig. 1-1.

When the EC surface of a blood vessel is injured or disrupted, a platelet and fibrin hemostatic plug is formed, which halts the bleeding and allows repair processes to begin. The events mediated by platelets that are part of the hemostatic plug formation include platelet adhesion, activation and shape change, secretion or release reaction, and support of local coagulation (fibrin formation and clot retraction). These events are listed in Table 1-1, depicted in Fig. 1-2, and discussed below.

Platelet Adhesion

The movement of platelets toward the vessel wall is one of the main factors determining adherence of platelets to the injury site. Platelet adhesion increases with increased shear rate because the smaller platelets are pushed toward the vessel surface. Platelet adhesion is mediated by glycoprotein (GP) receptors, most of which are members of the integrin family (see Table 1-1). At low shear rates, fibronectin is the main adhesive protein, whereas at high shear rates, von Willebrand factor is necessary for optimal platelet adhesion to injured vessels. Other proteins such as laminin, thrombospondin, and vitronectin may also help support adhesion. Glycoprotein Ib (GPIb) is the main receptor for adhesion (for von Willebrand factor) because it is continually expressed on nonactivated platelets. von Willebrand factor can also bind to another surface glycoprotein, GP IIb-IIIa, which must be expressed by activation of platelets. Natural inhibitors of platelet adhesion include prostacyclin and EDRF (released by intact EC).

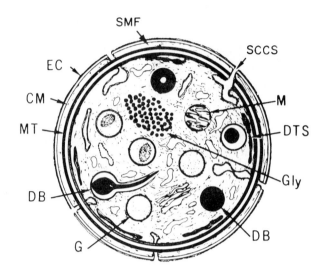

Figure 1-1 Platelet -(equatorial plane) structure as seen by electron microscopy. The surface membrane shows extensive invagination by an open canalicular system (SCCS), which forms an interconnecting network throughout the cell. The canaliculi provide ready access to the interior of the platelet for plasma proteins and facilitate secretion from the cytoplasmic granules during the release reaction. The cytoskeleton of the platelet which is responsible for the disc shape and the alterations in shape induced by activation (spherical with pseudopodia), is comprised of a circumferential band of microtubules (MT), submembrane filaments (SMF), and cytosolic actin and myosin microfilaments. Typical mitochondria (M), Golgi bodies, ribosomes, peroxisomes, and glycogen masses (GLY) are seen within the platelets as well as three types of granules: lysosomes, dense bodies (DB) and α-granules (G). Both dense bodies and α-granules can fuse with the surface connecting system and release their contents to the platelet exterior during contraction. EC, exterior coat, glycocalyx; CM, triaminar unit membrane; SMF, submembrane area; DTS, dense tubular system. (Used with permission from White JG, Gerrard JM: Ultrastructural features of abnormal blood platelets. A review. Am J Path 83:590, 1976.)

Platelet Activation and Secretion

As shown in Fig. 1-2, when platelets are activated by exposure to foreign surfaces, particles, or excitatory agonists (collagen, thrombin, epinephrine, adenosine diphoshate [ADP], thromboxane A_2, calcium ionophores), they rapidly lose their discoid shape, become more spherical and extend short and long pseudopods, a process achieved by altered organization of the cytoskeletal actin filamentous network.

The intracellular processes that are important to platelet activation are the phosphoinositide and the eicosanoid pathways and cyclic adenosine monophosphate (cAMP) levels. The phosphoinositide pathway involves cleaving of PIP_2 (phosphatidylinositol 4,5 biphosphate) by phospholipase C to form IP_3 (inositol 1,4,5-triphosphate) and diacylglycerol, which activates protein kinase C leading to protein phosphorylation, calcium mobilization, granule secretion, and GP IIb-IIIa expression. The eicosanoid pathway is depicted in

TABLE 1-1 Events and Mediators in the Formation of the Hemostatic Platelet-Fibrin Plug

I. Platelet adhesion

Adhesion receptors	Adhesive proteins (ligands)
GP Ib-IX	von Willebrand factor
GP Ic-IIa (static)	fibronectin
GP Ib-IX (flow)	
GP IIb-IIIa (activated)	fibrinogen, von Willebrand factor, fibronectin, vitronectin
GP Ia-IIa	collagen
GP Ic-IIa	laminin
GP IV	thrombospondin

II. Platelet activation and secretion (release reaction)

α-granules
  Fibrinogen
  Fibronectin
  von Willebrand factor
  Thrombospondin
  Vitronectin
  Platelet-derived growth factor
  Platelet factor 4
  β-thromboglobulin
  Immunoglobulin (IgG, IgA)
  Factor V
  C1 esterase inhibitor
  α_2-antiplasmin
  Albumin
  PAI-1
  Protein S
  Factor XI

Lysosomes
  Acid hydrolases
  Glycosidases
  Cathepsins

Cytosol
  Factor XIII
  Platelet-derived endothelial
    cell growth factor

Dense bodies (δ-granules)
  ADP
  ATP
  Serotonin
  Calcium

III. Platelet aggregation

Fibrinogen $\longleftrightarrow$ GP IIb-IIIa
Ca^{++}
(stabilized by thrombospondin)

Agonists	Receptors
ADP	ADP receptor
Epinephrine	α- and β-receptors
Serotonin	5-HT 2

Continued on next page

TABLE 1-1 Events and Mediators in the Formation of the Hemostatic Platelet-Fibrin Plug *(Continued)*

Thromboxane A$_2$	
PGH$_2$	Same receptor
PAF	PAF1
Thrombin	GP Ib
Collagen	GP Ia-IIa

IV. Platelet-associated coagulation

Platelet membrane

HMWK	PF3	PF3
XI	IXa	Xa
IX	VIIIa	Va
	Ca^{++}	II
		Ca^{++}
↓	↓	↓
IXa	X	Thrombin

*ADP, adenosine diphosphate; ATP, adenosine triphosphate; GP, glycoprotein; HMWK, high molecular weight kininogen; 5-HT, 5-hydroxytryptamine; PAF, platelet aggregation factor; PAI, plasminogen activator inhibitor; PF, platelet factor; PGH2, prostaglandin H2

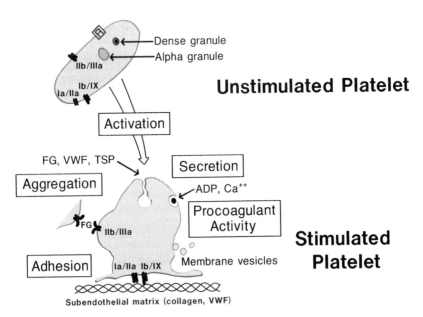

Figure 1-2 Role of platelets in hemostasis. The components of the unstimulated platelet are shown above and described in Table 1-1. R, receptor for agonists. The major responses to platelet activation (adhesion, secretion, aggregation, procoagulant activity) are shown in the stimulated platelet and are detailed in Table 1-1 and the text. (Used with permission from George JN, Shattil SJ: N Engl J Med 324:27, 1991.)

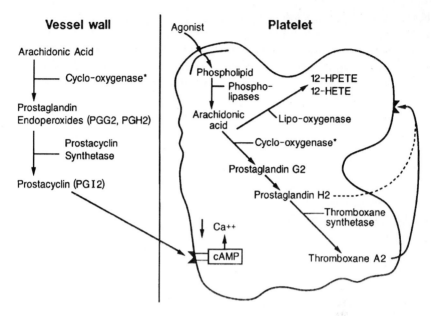

Figure 1-3 Prostaglandin metabolism in vessel wall and platelet. *, site of action of aspirin and sulfinpyrazone; cAMP increases through action of prostacyclin and by inhibition of phosphodiesterase by dipyridamole. Thromboxane A2 causes platelet aggregation and vasoconstriction; prostacyclin inhibits platelet aggregation and causes vasodilatation.

Fig. 1-3 and results in formation of thromboxane A_2, which is a messenger between as well as within platelets. cAMP, formed by adenyl cyclase, is suppressed by most agonists resulting in increased availability of Ca^{++} and platelet contraction; PGI_2 increases cAMP and suppresses platelet responsiveness. In all of these events, the interactions between membrane receptors and the intracellular enzymes are mediated by heterotrimeric, guanosine triphosphate (GTP)-binding proteins ranging in molecular weight from 21 to 28 kDa (G proteins).

Activated platelets release the contents of their granules including the ligands, fibrinogen, von Willebrand factor, ADP, and other substances listed in Table 1-1.

Platelet Aggregation

Glycoprotein IIb-IIIa is the platelet fibrinogen receptor that recognizes fibrinogen and other ligands through exposure of binding sites on platelet activation. Fibrinogen molecules act as bridges (in the presence of Ca^{++}) between receptors on adjacent platelets; their attachment is probably stabilized by thrombospondin. The reaction results in platelet attachment to each other, platelet aggregation. Agonists capable of inducing this reaction in vivo are listed with their receptors, when known, in Table 1-1.

Platelet-Associated Coagulation

Following platelet activation, negatively charged phospholipids (PS, phosphatidylinositol) are translocated to the outer surface of the plasma membrane and phosphatidylcholine moves to the inner half. The exposed phospholipids make up the activity known as platelet factor 3 (PF3) and act as a binding surface for coagulation proteins. Several complexes are formed on the platelet surface (see Table 1-1) resulting in more efficient formation of factors IXa, Xa, and thrombin. The subsequent conversion of fibrinogen to fibrin and further platelet activation by thrombin leads to a platelet-fibrin mass that undergoes clot retraction (interaction of actin and other contractile proteins of the cytoskeleton, fibrin, and GP IIb-IIIa). Platelets also carry protein S which accelerates the conversion of protein C to activated protein C (APC) via the thrombin-thrombomodulin complex and may serve to limit clot growth.

COAGULATION

The Procoagulant System

The procoagulant system of the coagulation process is composed of a series of serine protease enzymes and their cofactors (Table 1-2) which interact usually on a phospholipid surface (platelet membrane or damaged EC) to form a stable fibrin clot. As shown in Fig. 1-4, the system can be divided into an extrinsic pathway (tissue factor-factor VII) and an intrinsic pathway (surface-contact factors). Present evidence suggests that the extrinsic pathway is critical to the initiation of fibrin formation, whereas the intrinsic pathway plays a role in the continued formation of fibrin.

The extrinsic pathway is activated when tissue factor, found in the tissue adventitia or expressed on damaged or stimulated cells, comes in contact with circulating factor VII and forms a complex in the presence of calcium ions. Factor VII is converted to a serine protease by minor proteolysis (possible from trace factor Xa or other protease). The factor VIIa-tissue factor complex then converts factor IX to IXa and factor X to Xa. The newly generated IXa forms a complex with VIIIa (activated by traces of thrombin) in the presence of calcium and phospholipid and subsequently also activates factor X to Xa. Factor Xa binds to Va (again activated by thrombin) which with calcium and the phospholipid is called prothrombinase, the complex that rapidly converts prothrombin to thrombin.

Factor IX may also be activated by factor XIa. Factor XI is converted to XIa by two different mechanisms. In association with a surface (glass, kaolin, dextran sulfate) in vitro or a negatively charged surface or endotoxin in vivo, factor XII may be activated and subsequently cleave prekallikrein to kalli-

TABLE 1-2 The Hemostatic Factors

Name	Description	Concentration in Plasma
I. Procoagulants		
Contact Factors		
XII (Hageman)	Mr 80,000; single-chain serine protease	30 μg/mL (0.04 μM)
HMWK	Mr 110,000; single-chain cofactor: complexed with prekallikrein and XI	70 μg/mL (0.7 μM)
Prekallikrein (Fletcher)	Mr 85,000: single-chain serine protease complexed with HMWK	50 μg/mL (0.6 μM)
XI (plasma thromboplastin antecedent, PTA)	Mr 160,000; two identical sulfide-linked chains; serine protease complexed with HMWK	6μg/mL (0.07 μM)
Vitamin K-dependent		
II (prothrombin)	Mr 72,500; single-chain-serine protease; 10 Gla residues	100 μg/mL (1.5 μM)
VII (proconvertin)	Mr 48,000; single-chain glycoprotein; VIIa activates X and IX	0.5 μg/mL (3 nM)
IX (plasma thromboplastin component, PTC)	Mr 57,100; single-chain glycoprotein; 12 Gla residues	5 μg/mL (140 nM)
X (Stuart-Prower)	Mr 54,800; two-chain glycoprotein serine protease; 11 Gla residues	10 μg/mL (140 nM)
Others		
I (fibrinogen)	Mr 340,000; glycoprotein: Aa_2 Bβ_2 γ_2	300 mg/dL
V (proaccelerin)	Mr 350,000; single-chain nonenzymatic cofactor; activated by thrombin	200 ng/mL
Tissue factor (TF)	Mr 37,000; single-chain glycoprotein complexed to phospholipids	——
VIII (AHF)	Mr 285,000; complexed with von Willebrand factor in plasma	0.1 μg/mL
von Willebrand factor	Mr: multimers of 800.000 to 12 $\times$ 10^6 (subunit 240,000); glycoprotein	10 μg/mL

Continued on next page

TABLE 1-2 The Hemostatic Factors *(Continued)*

Name	Description	Concentration in Plasma
XIII (fibrin-stabilizing factor)	Mr 320,000; zymogen for a transamidating enzyme (A, B subunits)	20 μg/mL
II. Fibrinolytic System		
Plasminogen	Mr 92,000; glycoprotein (Glu, Lys)	1.5–2 μmol/L; 21 mg/dL
Tissue plasminogen activator (tPA)	Mr 68,000 serine protease	4–7 μg/dL
a_2-antiplasmin	Mr 51,000 glycoprotein; specific inhibitor of plasmin (1:1)	1 μM; 7 mg/dL
Plasminogen activator inhibitor-1 (PAI-1)	Mr 52,000; glycoprotein serpin; complexes with tPA, uPA	5 μg/dL
Plasminogen activator inhibitor-2 (PAI-2)	Mr 70,000; glycoprotein serpin; complexes with tPA, uPA	trace
III. Anticoagulants, inhibitors		
Tissue factor pathway inhibitor (TFPI);	Mr 33,000; inhibits VIIa/TF catalytic activity	60–80 ng/mL (2–5 nM)
Protein C	Mr 62,000; two-chain serine protease, vitamin K dependent; 11 Gla residues	2–6 μg/mL
Protein S	Mr 75,000; single-chain cofactor for activated protein C; vitamin K dependent	25 μg/mL
Thrombomodulin	Mr 450 kD; endothelial cell surface receptor for thrombin	——
Antithrombin III (heparin cofactor I)	Mr 58,000; single-chain glycoprotein; forms complexes (1:1) with thrombin, Xa, IXa, XIa, XIIa	3–5 μM; 18–30 mg/dL
Heparin cofactor II	Mr 65,000; forms covalent 1:1 molar complex with thrombin	0.47–1.02 μM; 31–67 μg/mL
C1-esterase inhibitor	Mr 105,000: single-chain 1:1 inhibitor of kallikrein, plasmin, C1, and XIIa	1.7 μM; 18 mg/dL
Protein C inhibitor	Mr 57,000, 1:1 complex with APC; accelerated by heparin	5.3 μg/mL

TABLE 1-2 *(Continued)*

Name	Description	Concentration in Plasma
a_1-Antitrypsin	Mr 60,000; inhibits plasma trypsin, chymotrypsin, XIa and tissue proteases	45 μM; 250 mg/dL
a_2-Macroglobulin	Mr 725,000; dimeric protein; inhibits plasmin, kallikrein, thrombin	3.5 μM; 250 mg/dL
Fibronectin	Mr 440,000; adhesive matrix glycoprotein; mediator of tissue repair	150–700 μg/mL
Vitronectin	Mr 65,000; adhesive glycoprotein; unfolded vitronectin binds heparin; binds PAI-1 and increases T1/2	0.25–0.45 ng/mL
Thrombospondin	Mr 420,000; adhesive glycoprotein in many cells including a-granules of platelets; T 1/2 = 9 h; acute phase reactant	0–3 ng/mL
Platelet activating factor (PAF)	Acetyl glyceryl ether phosphorylcholine; made in many cells; activates platelets and polymorphonuclear cells; causes increased vascular permeability and hypotension	intracellular
β-thromboglobulin	Mr 8,800; synthesized by cleavage of low affinity platelet factor 4; T 1/2 = 100 min	10–40 ng/mL
Platelet factor 4	Mr 30,000; cationic protein; neutralizes heparin; inhibits collagenase; T 1/2 = 20 min	1.5–16 ng/mL

krein and factor XI to XIa. Kallikrein accelerates the process by increasing the rate of factor XII activation (positive feedback). High molecular weight kininogen (HMWK) bound to prekallikrein and factor XI in the plasma functions as a cofactor in the factor XII-dependent surface-mediated reac-

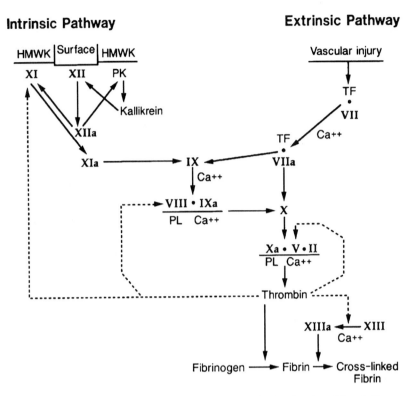

Figure 1-4 The procoagulant system and formation of a fibrin clot. The dotted lines indicate thrombin effects in addition to clotting of fibrinogen.

tions. Recently the activation of factor XI by thrombin in the presence of a negatively charged surface has been demonstrated. Thus, factor XI can be activated independent of the remainder of the contact pathway, which provides a possible explanation for the absence of bleeding manifestations seen in individuals lacking factors XII, prekallikrein, and HMWK.

In addition to its role as the structural framework of a thrombus and a site for cell attachment during the repair process, fibrin has several other cofactor and regulatory activities (see Chap. 19). Examples include modulating thrombin activity, regulating cross-linking activity by factor XIII, and enhancing fibrinolysis by binding a_2-antiplasmin (a_2-AP), tissue plasminogen activator (t-PA), and plasminogen.

The hemostatic effect of the extrinsic pathway is short-lived due to the presence of a Kunitz-type inhibitor, or tissue factor pathway inhibitor (TFPI) which inactivates the factor VIIa-tissue factor complex by binding both VIIa and Xa. The effectiveness of TFPI is less in the presence of factors IX and VIII and therefore is greater in their absence (hemophilia A and B). This observation is offered as one explanation for why hemophiliacs bleed despite normal levels of VII, X, and tissue factor at the site of injury.

The Inhibitor System

The natural anticoagulant mechanism limits and localizes the formation of the hemostatic plug or thrombus at the site of injury to blood vessels. The majority of the coagulation factor inhibitors or natural anticoagulants are directed against the formation or action of thrombin and include anti-thrombins and the protein C–protein S system (Fig. 1-5). Antithrombin III (AT III) inactivates thrombin and other serine proteases (XIIa, XIa, Xa, IXa) by binding irreversibly through an arginine residue to the active serine site of the protease (serine protease inhibitor or serpin). In the absence of heparin, the rate of inactivation is relatively slow, but when heparin or vessel wall heparan sulfate binds to a lysine residue on the AT III molecule, a confirmational change occurs in the AT III, resulting in almost instanta-

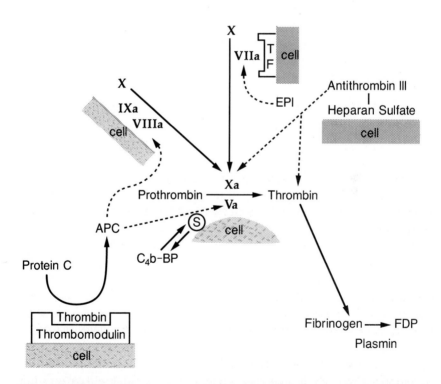

Figure 1-5 The physiologic anticoagulant system. Dotted lines indicate anticoagulant (inhibitor) actions. TF, tissue factor; EPI, extrinsic pathway inhibitor or tissue factor pathway inhibitor; APC, activated protein C; C4b-BP, C4b-binding protein. (Adapted from Bauer KA and Rosenberg RD: Semin Haematol 28:10–18, 1991.)

neous inactivation of thrombin. AT III is therefore called heparin cofactor I. Heparin cofactor II, a second inhibitor, can also be activated by heparin (although larger amounts are needed) or another vessel wall glycosaminoglycan, dermatan sulfate, to inactive thrombin. Thrombin may also be bound to the endothelial or platelet surface by the thrombomodulin receptor and removed from the circulation. Other serpins such as a_1-antitrypsin and a_2-macroglobulin can inactivate thrombin but are physiologically less important.

Thrombin also activates the protein C system which limits the rate of thrombin formation by inactivating the cofactors Va and VIIIa. The major site of protein C activation is the EC surface where thrombin binds to a constitutively expressed cellular membrane protein, thrombomodulin, and ceases to function as procoagulant. The thrombomodulin-thrombin complex activates protein C to APC, which as a serine protease cleaves the activated cofactors Va and VIIIa, thus decreasing thrombin formation by downregulating the coagulation cascade. APC functions most efficiently in the presence of its cofactor protein S (which exists in plasma as free protein and in a bimolecular complex with the complement component, C4b-binding protein) at the cell surface. APC also has inhibiting activity against the major inhibitor of plasminogen activation, PAI-1. APC is inactivated by a third heparin cofactor called APC inhibitor. For further details of the protein C–protein S system, see Chapters 40 and 41.

The Fibrinolytic System

The general overall scheme for fibrinolysis is shown in Fig. 1-6. Plasminogen, which circulates partly (50 percent) in a reversible complex with histidine-rich glycoprotein (HRG), a competitive inhibitor, is converted to the two-chain active plasmin molecule by cleavage of a single peptide bond. Native plasminogen has Glu 1 as the NH_2 terminal amino acid (Glu-plasminogen) but due to catalytic degradation the terminal 76 residues are cleaved resulting in the more active (in vitro) Lys 77 form (Lys-plasminogen). In physiologic circumstances, the activation of plasminogen is mainly by t-PA synthesized and released from vascular endothelial cells. The activity of t-PA is enhanced when it is bound to the surface of fibrin, facilitating the conversion of clot bound plasminogen to plasmin. Another activator, urokinase (u-PA), is produced in the kidney and is found mostly in the urine. However, trace amounts of plasma prourokinase or single-chain u-PA (scuPA) can be converted to active form through the contact system by kallikrein. After stimulation of t-PA release by exercise, stasis, or desmopressin (DDAVP), its half-life in the circulation is very short (about 5 min) due to inhibition by PAI-1 and clearance in the liver.

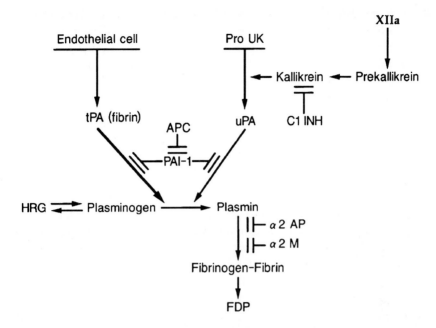

Figure 1-6 The Fibrinolytic System. Activation is shown by arrows; inhibition is shown by double bars; $\rightleftharpoons$, reversible complex. HRG, histidine-rich glycoprotein; t-PA, tissue plasminogen activator; uPA, urokinase; Pro UK, prourokinase; C1 INH, C1 esterase inhibitor; a_2AP, a_2-antiplasmin; a_2M, a_2-macroglobulin; FDP, fibrinogen-fibrin degradation products; PAI-1, plasminogen activator inhibitor-1; APC, activated protein C. The relatively greater activation of plasminogen by t-PA in association with fibrin is shown by the heavy arrow.

The fibrinolytic process is regulated at each enzymatic step by specific protease inhibitors. The plasminogen activators are rapidly inhibited by PAI-1 (sources are platelets, ECs, plasma) and PAI-2 produced in the placenta and neutrophils. PAI-1 is an acute phase reactant that may result in high levels following stress. PAI-1 is quickly inactivated by physiologic conditions (neutral pH and 37°C) resulting in a half-life of about 2 h; the molecule is stable at pH 5.5 and 0°C. PAI-2 is found in the plasma usually only during pregnancy.

Plasmin is rapidly inhibited by a_2-AP, backed up by a_2-macroglobulin. These inhibitors protect the normal constituents in plasma (fibrinogen, factor VIII, factor V) from proteolysis by unopposed plasmin. However a_2-AP is not an efficient inhibitor of plasmin at or near the fibrin surface of a clot (fibrin-bound plasmin covers the lysine sites and slows the reaction with a_2-AP), thus allowing fibrinolytic activity where it is most useful. Even though APC has been shown to inactivate PAI-1 in vitro, there is little evidence that this reaction significantly alters fibrinolysis.

Plasmin has fibrinogen and fibrin as its major substrates leading to the production of specific fragments collectively called fibrinogen-fibrin degradation products (FDP). Cleavage of fibrinogen first produces X fragments (237 to 246 Kd) which are clottable and are often measured as fibrinogen in standard assays. The transiently produced X fragment continues to degrade into smaller D and E fragments or a transient Y fragment composed of a D-E core. Plasmin cleavage of intact fibrinogen also produces $B\beta$ peptide 1-42 which has been used as a clinical marker for primary fibrinolysis.

Fibrin lysis by plasmin leads to a different pattern of fragments because of the cross-linking of the molecule by factor XIII after clotting by thrombin (even though the plasmin cleavage sites are generally the same). These unique fragments such as DD (D-dimer), DY, and YY are characteristic of fibrin breakdown. In addition, non–cross-linked fibrin (fibrin I or early polymers) may complex with fibrinogen and early proteolytic products (X, Y) to produce large macromolecular complexes. Under physiologic conditions fibrinogen is spared plasmin action more than fibrin because of the circulating plasmin inhibitors; however, during pathologic proteolysis (disseminated intravascular coagulation, liver disease, and thrombolytic therapy) significant fibrinogenolysis may occur. Accumulation of FDP in the circulation is associated with inhibition of fibrin formation as reflected in prolongation of screening tests (activated partial thromboplastin time [APTT], prothrombin time [PT], thrombin time) and with decreased platelet function.

Details of FDP production and their application to detection of disease states are discussed in Chap. 25.

RELATION OF HEMOSTATIC SYSTEM TO OTHER BIOLOGIC SYSTEMS

The hemostatic system (blood vessels, platelets, coagulation schemes) is related to several other biologic systems important in host defense in humans and are mentioned briefly.

1. *Vascular Growth Factors and Angiogenesis.* Many cells such as platelets, endothelium, smooth muscle cells, fibroblasts, and monocyte-macrophages are involved in the development of vascular lesions (atherosclerosis, neovascularization of ophthalmic lesions, hemangiomas, arteriovenous malformations, abnormal tissue healing of skin, connective tissue, bone and solid tumors). The abnormal proliferation of the vascular tissue is controlled by well-characterized small molecular weight mediators found in platelets and ECs such as PDGF, fibroblast growth factor, angiogenic and transforming growth factors, a and β. Certain of these factors such PDGF are operative in the normal repair process.

2. *Neutrophil-platelet Interaction.* In addition to the well-known role of leukocyte procoagulants in fibrin function in inflammatory disorders, neu-

trophils also inhibit platelet reactivity by multiple mechanisms. Neutrophil-derived EDRF inhibits platelet aggregation. Cell-free releasates from neutrophils inhibit both platelet activation and recruitment. Neutrophil elastase acting on platelet membrane glycoproteins downregulates platelet activation; these roles in thromboregulation suggest that the neutrophil may be more than an innocent bystander in the thrombus. Other cooperative ventures include the platelet stimulator, platelet aggregation factor, which is produced in the neutrophil and the cell collaboration that occurs in the biosynthesis of leukotrienes.

3. *Inflammatory Response.* Four principal systems in blood that interact with the coagulation system are almost always involved in development of inflammation in the tissues:

a. The complement system: factor XIIa fragments activate C1 to C1 esterase; kallikrein destroys C1 components and activates the alternative pathway; plasmin and thrombin can convert C3 to C3a; C4b-binding protein indirectly controls free protein S levels.

b. The contact system: kallikrein cleaves HMWK and LMWK, releasing bradykinin, which cause vasodilatation, increased permeability, smooth muscle contraction, and cellular glucose uptake; kininogens inhibit cysteine proteases.

c. The acute phase reaction: several factors increase in response to interleukins and secondary cytokines: fibrinogen, factor V, factor VIII, von Willebrand factor, t-PA, PAI, a_1-antitrypsin; others (thrombomodulin and protein C system) are downregulated.

d. The inflammatory cellular response: monocyte-macrophages, lymphocytes, neutrophils, eosinophils, basophils, mast cells, and platelets interact with plasma components, release cytokines, or their inhibitors (examples are thrombospondin, fibronectin).

BIBLIOGRAPHY

Bauer KA, Rosenberg RD: Role of antithrombin III as a regulator of in vitro coagulation. *Semin Hematol* 28:10, 1991.

Davie EW et al: The coagulation cascade: Initiation, maintenance, and regulation. *Biochemistry* 30:10363, 1991.

De Groot PG, Sixma JJ: Platelet adhesion. *Br J Haematol* 75:308, 1990.

Esmon CT: The roles of protein C and thrombomodulin in the regulation of blood coagulation. *J Biol Chem* 164:4743, 1989.

Folkman J: Angiogenesis. In: Verstraete M, Vermylen J, Lijnen R, Arnout J (eds): *Thrombosis and Haemostasis*, Leuven, Belgium, Leuven University Press, 1987, pp 583–596.

Gentry PA: The mammalian blood platelet: Its role in haemostasis, inflammation, and tissue repair. *J Comp Path* 107:243, 1992.

Henkin J et al: The plasminogen-plasmin system. *Prog Cardiovasc Dis* 34:135, 1991.

Jaffe EA: Endothelial cell structure and function. In: Hoffman R, Benz EJ Jr, Shattil SJ, Furie B, Cohen HJ (eds): *Hematology, Basic Principles and Practice*, New York, Churchill-Livingstone, 1991, pp 1198–1213.

Kaplan AP, Silverberg N: The coagulation-kinin pathway of human plasma. *Blood* 70:1, 1987.

Kunick TJ, Newman PJ: The molecular immunology of human platelet proteins. *Blood* 80:1386, 1992.

Naito K, Fujikawa K: Activation of human blood coagulation factor XI independent of factor XII. *J Biol Chem* 266:7353, 1991.

Nemerson Y: The tissue factor pathway of blood coagulation. *Semin Hematol* 29:170, 1992.

Rapaport SI: The extrinsic pathway inhibitor: A regulator of tissue factor dependent blood coagulation. *Thromb Haemost* 66:6, 1991.

Tuffin DP: The platelet surface membrane: Ultrastructure, receptor binding and function. In: Page CP (ed): *The Platelet in Health and Disease*, London, Blackwell Scientific Publications, 1991, pp 10–60.

Wiman B, Hamsten A: The fibrinolytic enzyme system and its role in the etiology of thromboembolic disease. *Semin Thromb Hemost* 16:207, 1990.

Laboratory
Measurements
of Hemostasis
and Thrombosis

The accurate and efficient diagnosis and monitoring of disorders of hemostasis and thrombosis depend on a high quality hematology laboratory. This laboratory, often designated for "special coagulation," is essential for optimal diagnosis and management of hemorrhagic and thrombotic disorders, and the measurement of hemostatic variables in solving basic and applied research problems. Tests derived for each of these purposes frequently overlap in their use. These tests are discussed below and in subsequent chapters.

PLATELET-VESSEL INTERACTION

Several measurements can be made of platelets and their interaction with key components of the vessel wall (endothelial cell and plasma components), as it occurs in physiologic platelet plug formation. Platelets may be enumerated and their morphology observed on peripheral blood smear or electron microscopy. Platelet aggregation to standard agonists can be measured in photo-optical instruments recorded over time (platelet aggregation tests, see Fig. 10-1). More specific measures of platelet adhesive receptors and their ligands include glycoprotein Ib (GPIb)-von Willebrand factor and GPIIb-IIIa–fibrinogen, each component of which may be quantitated by specific assay. The bleeding time test, an in vivo measurement of platelet plug formation reflecting platelet number and function, is commonly used in clinical practice.

SCREENING TESTS, CONTROLS, STANDARDS, AND PREDICTIVE VALUE

Screening or global tests of hemostasis are usually performed on citrated plasma samples and are designed to measure a portion of the coagulation scheme (both procoagulant and acquired inhibitory activities). These simple, one-stage clotting tests (APTT, PT, thrombin clotting time [TCT], etc.) are discussed in detail in Chap. 4. The results of these tests are usually expressed as a clotting time in seconds and are compared to the range as calculated from the mean ± 2 or 3 standard deviations (SD) of test values in a group of normal adults (at least 25 subjects). The test result and the "normal range" (usually ± 2 SD) are supplied to the clinician. In addition a "normal control" that ensures the reproducibility of the test system is performed on standard normal or reference plasma, which has been frozen or from lyophilized normal pooled plasma. Other abnormal "controls" besides the normal control are often used to indicate the ability of the test system to detect mild abnormalities.

The *predictive value* (ability of a test to detect an abnormality) is the interaction of test sensitivity and test specificity. *Sensitivity* refers to the percentage of positive results in patients with a known defect. A sensitivity of 95 percent means that 95 percent of patients with the defect will be detected by the test (true positives, TP) and 5 percent of patients with the defect will have false negative (FN) results:

$$\text{Sensitivity} = \frac{\text{TP}}{\text{TP} + \text{FN}} \times 100$$

Specificity refers to the percentage of negative test results in persons without the defect. A specificity of 95 percent means that 95 percent of persons without the defect will test negative (true negatives, TN) and 5 percent of patients without the defect will have false positive results (FP):

$$\text{Specificity} = \frac{\text{TN}}{\text{TN} + \text{FP}} \times 100$$

The predictive value of a laboratory measurement depends on sensitivity, specificity, and the *prevalence* (the frequency of patients with a certain disease in the group being tested). For example, these parameters can be used to compute receiver operating characteristic curves (ROC) for a measurement like the bleeding time (see Channing Rodgers and Levin reference). The ROC method assumes that values above a predetermined precision level (cutoff point) are considered abnormal (e.g., a prolonged bleeding time) and those below it are normal. The sensitivity of the bleeding time is the fraction of abnormal (diseased) subjects that have an abnormal test result and the specificity is the fraction of nondiseased subjects classified by the test as normal. Combined with prevalence information these measurements allow estimation of the positive and negative predictive power of the test. Sensitivity and specificity summarize the performance of the test when prior knowledge of the state of the test subjects is available, whereas positive and negative predictive values provide information about a "patient" given prior experience with the test.

WHOLE BLOOD CLOT FORMATION

Whole blood (native or without anticoagulation) or anticoagulated whole blood may be studied for time of clot formation with (activated clotting time) or without (whole blood clotting time) particulate activators as well as for dynamics of fibrin formation and lysis by instruments such as the thromboelastograph (TEG) or sonoclot. Platelet-rich plasma or platelet-poor plasma prepared by appropriate centrifugation of anticoagulated whole blood is used in procedures as the thrombin generation test, or platelet-rich plasma clotting time to detect the influence of platelets on fibrin formation. When native blood is allowed to clot, the centrifuged supernatant or serum can be used in tests such as the prothrombin consumption (tests platelet factor 3, factor VIII, and IX contribution to prothrombinase) and the thromboplastin generation test, which is sometimes used as procedure for factor VIII assays (see Chap. 14).

Tests using whole blood have an advantage over plasma clotting tests because they measure platelet, leukocyte, and erythrocyte contributions to coagulability. However, they frequently lack sensitivity in detection of mild to moderate abnormalities of the coagulation system, that is, the whole blood clotting time is not sensitive to levels of factor VIII above 2 percent. At present, the most frequent use of whole blood clotting tests are in detecting heparinization during renal dialysis and cardiovascular surgery and detection of severe hypocoagulability and fibrin lysis during liver transplantation (TEG).

QUALITATIVE OR FUNCTIONAL ASSAYS OF SPECIFIC COAGULATION FACTOR ASSAYS

Qualitative coagulation factor activity assays are of two major types: clotting assays and chromogenic substrate assays. Clotting time assays use a reagent system depleted of the factor activity to be measured by using a specific congenitally deficient plasma or artificially factor-depleted plasma. The length of the time for final clot formation is indirectly proportional to the concentration of the coagulation factor in question (see Fig. 2-1). Chromogenic (amidolytic) assays take advantage of the principle that clotting proteases or enzymes generally act specifically toward their natural substrates.

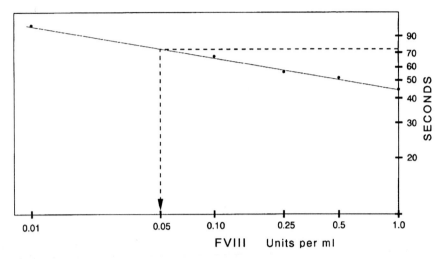

Figure 2-1 The standard normal curve used to determine factor VIII activity from clotting times of mixtures of diluted "pooled normal plasma" or "unknown plasma" in the assay system. When the unknown or patient plasma was assayed at a dilution equal to 1.0 U/mL of standard, the clotting time was 75 s or (as the dashed line indicates) 0.05 U/mL.

Chromogenic substrates are synthetic short peptide chains that mimic the natural substrate and are attached to color markers such as *p*-nitroaniline. Fluorogenic, luminogenic, and radioactive markers are also feasible. The rate of color generated on release of the chromophore is proportional to the enzyme activity. Commonly used chromogenic substrates are S-2222 (thrombin), S-2302 (kallikrein), S-2251 (plasmin), and S-2336 (activated protein C).

Both the clotting activity assay and the chromogenic assay must be standardized and related to a calibration curve of normal enzyme (see Fig. 2-1.). The reference plasma used to develop the standard curve is a critical determinant of the overall accuracy of the assay. Pooled (at least 25 donors) normal adult plasma preferably measured against a known standard (WHO or CAP) is assigned a 100 percent value.

The clotting time and chromogenic assays may be automated using instruments such as the Fibrometer (electromechanical detection of fibrin strands formed during clotting), the Coag-A-Mate (interruption of light path to detect a clot), the Multistat centrifugal analyzer, MLA (photometric detection of increased turbidity), and the Automated Coagulation Laboratory, ACL (centrifugal analysis with nephelometric detection of increased turbidity) as well as kinetic spectrophotometry is used for chromogenic assays. These qualitative assays measure enzyme function available under test conditions regardless of the amount of protein present. That is, nonfunctional proteins may have normal amounts of protein (antigen) as measured by a quantitative assay, but reduced or nondetectable amounts of enzyme (activity) as measured by the qualitative tests.

QUANTITATIVE ASSAYS OF SPECIFIC COAGULATION FACTORS

The measurement of the total amount of a clotting protein (procoagulant, anticoagulant, fibrinolytic component, or activation peptide or complex) is frequently accomplished with immunologic techniques using heterologous, monoclonal, or naturally occurring antibodies. The major techniques used are agglutination of antibody-coated beads, immunoelectrophoresis, radio-immunoassay, and most popularly, enzyme-linked immunosorbent assay (ELISA). These quantitative tests (also called antigen tests) do not measure function of the protein.

ACTIVATION PEPTIDES, FRAGMENTS, AND COMPLEXES

With the exception of diagnosis and management of hereditary defects, specific clotting factor assay levels, whether quantitative or qualitative, may be less helpful to the clinician than measurements of fragments or peptides released during the clotting process (activation peptides, enzyme-inhibitor complexes, clot lysis products) or abnormally formed during synthesis (non-carboxylated proteins). Examples of these products include prothrombin fragment 1·2, thrombin-antithrombin III, fibrinopeptide A, D-dimer and other fibrin degradation products, and noncarboxylated prothrombin (see Chap. 25). Most of these circulating protein fragments are detected by immunoassays (often ELISA).

COAGULATION TESTS ARE NO BETTER THAN THE TEST SPECIMEN

A major axiom of clinical hemostasis is that the results of a coagulation test or assay is only as good as the sample collection. Details of sample collection and processing must be adhered to if the results are to be meaningful. Unusual or spurious results are often related to problems with blood procurement. Artifacts to avoid are discussed below.

Correction for the Hematocrit

Several investigators have stressed the necessity of proportionately decreasing the anticoagulant used when the subject's hematocrit is elevated above the normal adult values, as it frequently is in the term infant (preterm infants have hematocrit levels comparable to those of normal adults) and polycythemic adult (see Hellum reference). The anticoagulant is decreased to avoid excess citrate which binds calcium and prolongs the clotting time. A nomogram based on hematocrit and amount of anticoagulant to use is available and representative values to maintain a constant ratio of anticoagulant to plasma volume are given in Table 2-1. Anemia (unless extremely severe) does not significantly influence the clotting tests.

Anticoagulation and Plasma Preparation

To maintain the pH of the blood near physiologic values and to bind calcium, a buffered citrate (three parts, 0.1 mol/L of sodium citrate to two parts, 0.1 mol/L of citric acid) anticoagulant or its equivalent is used. The collection tube is plastic or silicone coated and is kept covered at 4°C during processing to platelet-poor plasma by centrifugation at 1400g (minimum) to remove platelets. Various inhibitors may be added to the basic citrate anticoagulant to prevent proteolytic changes during transport and storage of sample (EDTA, adenosine, heparin, aprotinin).

Tissue "Juice" Contamination

Whenever possible, a two-syringe venipuncture technique or free-flowing (without squeezing) puncture technique should be used to avoid contamination of the specimen by procoagulant materials (tissue factor or thrombin). Traumatic and repeated punctures as well as slow flow of blood may produce this artifact, which characteristically shortens the APTT and elevates fibrin monomer or even produces fibrin clots in the specimen.

Heparin Contamination of Specimens

Heparin contamination of specimens obtained from indwelling arterial and venous catheters is a common problem. Others have studied this problem and have concluded that at least 4 to 6 mL blood (or five to six times the

TABLE 2-1 Values to Maintain a Constant Ratio of Anticoagulant in Blood of 1:10

Hematocrit	Anticoagulant (mL)	Final volume (mL)
70	0.3	5
60	0.37	5
50	0.45	5
40	0.5	5
70	0.12	2
60	0.15	2
50	0.18	2
40	0.2	2

volume of the catheter dead space) must be withdrawn through a catheter to prevent heparin contamination of the specimen. After the sample arrives in the laboratory, neutralization of heparin by protamine, polybrene, or anion exchange resins is difficult and may give unreliable results. Recognition of heparin contamination can also be difficult in the infant; characteristically, heparin prolongs the partial thromboplastin time (PTT) and TCT with only minor effect of the PT. In vitro mixtures of cord blood plasma with heparin gave the results listed in Table 2-2. The reptilase time (not affected by heparin) can be helpful in determining whether a prolonged TCT is due to heparin.

In vitro Fibrinolysis

Specimens of plasma or serum to be tested for presence of degradation products of fibrinogen or fibrin should be collected in tubes containing a fibrinolytic inhibitor such as ε-aminocaproic acid, soybean trypsin inhibitor, tranexamic acid, or aprotinin to prevent in vitro fibrinolysis, which is particularly apt to occur in cord or newborn blood samples.

Cord Blood Collection

Two techniques have proven adequate for collection of cord blood to be used for coagulation assays. As soon as the infant is delivered, the cord is clamped with two clamps and is cut between the clamps; the infant is removed from

TABLE 2-2 Effect of Heparin on Screening Tests (in vitro Mixtures). Cord Studies Performed with Kaolin PTT (NA = 37–50 seconds)

Heparin Concentration (U/mL)	APTT (s)	PT (s)	TCT(s)
Adult plasma			
2.0	>150	15	>55
1.0	>150	12	>55
0.5	105	11	>55
0.3	67	11	>55
0.1	33	10	20
0.05	29	10	13.5
0	28	10	12
Cord Plasma			
0.5	>300	22	>120
0.25	165	18.5	>120
0.10	96	17	90
0.05	78	16.5	19
0	70	15	13

the field, and immediately before separation of the placenta, the umbilical vein is punctured and the sample is withdrawn. Alternatively, as soon as the infant is delivered, a segment of cord is double-clamped with four clamps (Fig. 2-2) and is cut between the clamps, freeing a long cord segment, which is given to another member of the team to procure the specimen. Both techniques are done with a two-syringe technique with the anticoagulant in the second syringe. Five to 10 mL blood can be obtained in this manner. The amount of anticoagulant necessary for a hematocrit of 55 percent is used in term deliveries. The first procedure is faster but requires that aseptic technique be observed by the blood procurer; the second procedure is a few seconds slower but allows the cord segment to be handed to the blood procurer, who may work in an adjacent area.

Micromethods

The need to evaluate hemostatic problems in small infants has led to many attempts to establish "micromethodology." The components of these efforts are efficient and safe sample procurement, and the ability to perform multiple tests on a small sample. Our own experience has caused us to use methods that require very small amounts of plasma from blood obtained by venipuncture, indwelling catheters, or occasionally arterial punctures (rather than "capillary" samples). Four to six clotting factor assays can be done on 100 μL of plasma when appropriately diluted. When screening tests like the PT, TCT, APTT, or fibrinogen are done, undiluted plasma samples must be used, and the minimal amount of plasma is 500 μL, which requires a whole blood sample up to 2 mL depending on the infant's hematocrit. In special situations blood can be obtained by heel stick (warmed heel, B-D microlance) directly

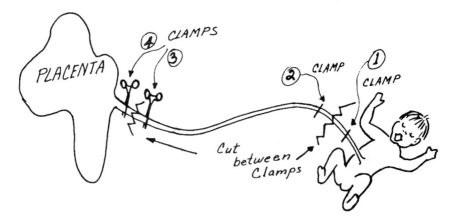

Figure 2-2. Cord blood collection. Clamps are placed immediately after delivery of infant in order shown (1 through 4) and cord is cut as illustrated to free segment for blood procurement.

into plastic collection tubes (B-D microcontainer containing the anticoagu-lant). As discussed in the Hathaway and Bonnar reference, the successful use of micromethods is directly proportional to the energy and effort input of the personnel responsible for the procedures.

BIBLIOGRAPHY

Castillo JB et al: Prothrombin times and clottable fibrinogen determination on an automated coagulation laboratory (ACL-810). *Thromb Res* 55:213, 1989.

Channing Rodgers RP, Levin J: A critical reappraisal of the bleeding time. *Semin Thromb Hemost* 16:1, 1990.

Cumming AM et al: In vitro neutralization of heparin in plasma prior to the activated partial thromboplastin time test: An assessment of four heparin antagonists and two anion exchange resins. *Thromb Res* 41:43, 1986.

Friberger P: Synthetic peptide substrate assays in coagulation and fibrinolysis and their application on automates. *Semin Thromb Hemost* 9:281, 1983.

Hathaway WE, Bonnar J: *Hemostatic Disorders of the Pregnant Woman and Newborn Infant.* New York, Elsevier, 1987, Chap. 1.

Hellum AJ: The assay of platelet adhesiveness. *Scand J Clin Lab Invest* 12 (suppl 51):18, 1960.

Johnston J, Zipursky A: Microtechnology for the study of the blood coagulation system in newborn infants. In: Lusher JM, Barnhart MI (eds): *Acquired Bleeding Disorders in Children,* New York, Masson, 1981, pp 133–148.

Koepke JA, Koepke JF: *Guide to Clinical Laboratory Diagnosis,* 3rd ed. Norwalk, Los Altos, Appleton and Lange, 1987, Chap. 1.

Molyneaux RD Jr et al: Coagulation studies and the indwelling heparinized catheter. *Heart Lung* 16:20, 1987.

Peters M et al: Rapid microanalysis of coagulation parameters by automated chromo-genic substrated methods—Application in neonatal patients. *Thromb Res* 28:773, 1982.

Peterson P, Gottfried EL: The effects of inaccurate blood sample volume on pro-thrombin time (PT) and activated partial thromboplastin time (aPTT). *Thromb Hemost* 47:101, 1982.

Triplett DA: *Laboratory evaluation of coagulation.* Chicago, American Society of Clinical Pathology Press, 1982.

White JG, Gerrard JM: Ultrastructural features of abnormal blood platelets. *Am J Pathol* 83:590, 1976.

Normal Values for
the Hemostatic System

Normal values for measurements of the hemostatic system can be tabulated according to age and other physiologic alterations such as development, pregnancy, stress, or exercise. Values (taken from the recent literature) for each of the biologic subsets are displayed in Table 3-1. Comparisons were made with adult pooled plasma obtained from young males and females aged 20 to 40 years (normal adult). In most reports, the range was calculated from ± 2 or 3 standard deviations (SD) from the mean. In Table 3-1, the lower limit of normal is ± 2 SD and therefore will exclude 2.5 percent of the values (mean ± 2 SD includes 95 percent of values). However, this lower limit provides practical help in deciding what is abnormal and deserving of further evaluation. Whenever possible the values used are based on functional or activity tests that in most instances are equal to quantitative or immunologic values. Examples of discrepancies between activity and antigen for the clotting protein are occasionally seen in the fetus and newborn (fetal proteins as noted below), during pregnancy (factor VII), and during exercise (activation of factors VIII and VII). Certain generalizations may be made from study of Table 3-1 and are discussed below.

FETUS AND NEWBORN

A recent review of the available data for the newborn infant was accomplished by the subcommittee on Perinatal Hemostasis of the International Committee of Thrombosis and Hemostasis (see Hathaway reference). This report included guidelines for obtaining normal data in the newborn infant and stressed the need for selection of gestational-age matched subgroups of well infants in whom careful attention was paid to specimen procurement. Of interest, only a few clotting factors display unique characteristics that suggest structural and functional differences from the mature "adult" protein. Examples of such "fetal" proteins and the described differences include: (1) fibrinogen (represents a postsynthetic modification of the fibrinogen molecule re-

TABLE 3-1 Physiologic Alterations in Measurements of the Hemostatic System

				Subjects				
Measurement	Normal adults	Fetus (20 wk)	Preterm (25–32 wk)	Term Infant	Infant (6 mo)	Pregnancy (term)	Exercise (acute)†	Aging (70–80 y)†
A. Platelets								
Count								
μL × 10³	250	107–297	293	332	—	260	↑18–40%	225
Size (fl)	9.0	8.9	8.5	9.06	—	9.6	↑	—
Aggregation								
ADP	N	+	↓	↓	—	↑	N	—
Collagen	N	↓	↓	↓	—	N	N	—
Ristocetin	N	—	↑	↑	—	—	—	—
BT (min)	2–9	—	3.6±2	3.4±1.8	—	2.8 (or↑)	—	5.6
B. Procoagulant System								
PTT*	1.0	2.2	1.4–2.4	1.3	1.1	1.09	↓15%	↓
PT*	1.0	1.3	1.3	1.1	1.0	0.95	N	—
TCT*	1.0	—	1.3	1.1	1.0	0.92	N	—
Fibrinogen mg/dL	278 ±0.61	96 (40)	250 (100)	240 (150)	251 (160)	450 ±100	↑10%	↑15%
II, U/mL	1.0 (0.7)	0.16 (0.10)	0.32 (0.18)	0.52 (0.25)	0.88 (0.6)	1.15 (0.68–1.9)	—	N
V, U/mL	1.0 (0.6)	0.70 (0.40)	0.80 (0.43)	1.00 (0.54)	0.91 (0.55)	0.85 (0.40–1.9)	—	N
VII, U/mL	1.0 (0.6)	0.21 (0.12)	0.37 (0.24)	0.57 (0.35)	0.87 (0.50)	1.71 (0.87–3.3)	↑200%	↑25%

Continued on next page

TABLE 3-1 Physiologic Alterations in Measurements of the Hemostatic System (Continued)

	Subjects							
Measurement	Normal adults	Fetus (20 wk)	Preterm (25–32 wk)	Term Infant	Infant (6 mo)	Pregnancy (term)	Exercise (acute)†	Aging (70–80 y)†
VIII, U/mL	1.0 (0.6)	0.50 (0.23)	0.75 (0.40)	1.50 (0.55)	0.90 (0.50)	2.12 (0.8–6.0)	↑200%	↓27%
vWf, U/mL	1.0 (0.6)	0.65 (0.40)	1.50 (0.90)	1.60 (0.84)	1.07 (0.60)	1.70	↑75–200%	↑
IX, U/mL	1.0 (0.5)	0.10 (0.05)	0.22 (0.17)	0.35 (0.15)	0.86 (0.36)	0.81–2.15	↑25%	—
X, U/mL	1.0 (0.6)	0.19 (0.15)	0.38 (0.20)	0.45 (0.3)	0.78 (0.38)	1.30 (1.6–6.0)	—	↑16%
XI, U/mL	1.0 (0.6)	—	0.20 (0.12)	0.42 (0.20)	0.86 (0.38)	0.7	—	—
XII, U/mL	1.0 (0.6)	—	0.22 (0.09)	0.44 (0.16)	0.77 (0.39)	1.3±0.24	—	↑16%
XIII, U/mL	1.04 (0.55)	0.30	0.1–0.4	0.61 (0.36)	1.04 (0.50)	0.96	—	—
PreK, U/mL	1.12 (0.6)	—	0.26 (0.14)	0.35 (0.16)	0.86 (0.56)	1.18±.25	—	↑27%
HMWK, U/mL	0.92 (0.48)	—	0.28 (0.20)	0.64 (0.50)	0.82 (0.36)	1.6	—	↑32%
C. Anticoagulant System								
AT III, U/mL	1.0 (0.8)	0.23 (0.12)	0.35 (0.20)	0.56 (0.32)	1.04 (0.84)	1.02 ±0.11	↑14%	↓10%

PC, U/mL	1.0 (0.7)	0.10 (0.06)	0.29 (0.20)	0.50 (0.30)	0.59 (0.37)	1.07 (0.9–1.2)	N	↑16%
PS, total, U/mL	1.0 (0.6)	—	—	0.24 (0.1)	0.87 (0.55)	0.61	—	—
PS, free, U/mL	1.0 (0.5)	0.37	0.48	0.42	—	0.63	—	—
Heparin cofactor II, U/mL	1.01 (0.73)	0.30	0.25 (0.10)	0.49 (0.36)	0.97 (0.59)	—	—	↓10%
D. Fibrinolytic System								
Plasminogen U/mL	1.0	0.20	0.35 (0.20)	0.37 (0.18)	0.9	1.39 (±0.20)	↓10%	N
t-PA, ng/mL	3.5 (3.0)	—	—	2.3 (0.4)	—	—	↑300%	—
α_2-AP U/mL	1.0	1.0	0.74 (0.5)	0.83 (0.65)	1.11 (0.83)	0.95	N	N
PAI-1, U/mL	1.0	—	—	1.0	1.07	4.0–8.0	—	—
Histidine rich glycoprotein, μg/mL	86 (45)	—	—	16 (7)	40 (27)	—	—	—
Overall fibrinolysis	N	↑	↓	↓	—	↓	↑100% (or ↓)	—

Except as otherwise indicated values are mean ±2 SD or values in ( ) are lower limits (−2SD or lower range): +, positive or present; ↓, decreased; ↑, increased; N, normal adult or no change; * values as ratio or subject/mean of reference range; †, value as %↓ or ↑; BT, bleeding time; TCT, thrombin clotting time; PreK, prekallikrein; HMWK, high molecular weight kininogen; PC, protein C; PS, protein S; t-PA, tissue plasminogen activator; PAI, plasminogen activator inhibitor; overall fibrinolysis as measured by euglobulin lysis; vWf, von Willebrand factor; AT III, antithrombin III; ADP, adenosine diphosphate; α_2-AP, α_2-antiplasmin.

sulting in increased phosphorous and sialic acid content associated with a prolonged reptilase and thrombin time); (2) plasminogen (adult amino acid sequence but increased mannose and sialic acid content producing decreased activation kinetics); (3) von Willebrand factor (altered multimeric structure with increased high molecular weight forms producing increased reactivity with ristocetin); and (4) protein C (altered migration in agarose gel).

In the fetus and newborn infant, the procoagulant system shows decreased levels of the contact and vitamin K-dependent factors inversely related to gestational age, that is, the younger the fetus, the lower the factor. However, cofactors such as factor VIII and V, as well as fibrinogen, are within the normal adult range even in the small preterm infant. Most of the naturally occurring anticoagulants (antithrombin III [AT III], proteins C and S) are decreased in activity; an exception is a modest elevation of a_2 macroglobulin. Native whole blood clots faster than the blood of adults even though the plasma screening tests (especially the APTT) are prolonged. Plasminogen, tissue plasminogen activator (t-PA) activity, and antigen are decreased; plasminogen activator inhibitor (PAI-1) and a_2-antiplasmin (a_2-AP) are normal to increased; and overall plasmin generation is slow, suggesting impaired fibrinolysis. The platelet count is normal and despite reduced platelet aggregation the bleeding time of the infant is shorter than that of adults (possibly due to the increased hematocrit and altered von Willebrand factor of the newborn). Despite these paradoxical changes, the normal infant is not a "bleeder" and shows no undue thrombotic tendency. However, the balance of the coagulation system appears to be weighted toward hypercoagulability and potential thrombosis in the sick infant.

The decreased hemostatic factors (note that von Willebrand factor is elevated and associated with a slight increase in factor VIII in the term infant) of the newborn infant gradually reach normal adult levels during the first 3 to 6 months of life. A notable exception is protein C, which does not reach the adult range until puberty. Indeed, low normal means for protein C activity (0.83 and 0.95 U/mL) are recorded in 15- and 30-year-old normal males. A recent study (Andrew reference) indicates that the range of normal is slightly lower for general factors (V, II, VII, IX, X, XI, XII) throughout childhood. The upper limit of the bleeding time is slightly longer in children (11 min; see Chap. 4).

PREGNANCY

During pregnancy, major changes occur in the coagulation system and to a lesser extent in platelets and their interaction with blood vessels. Levels of most procoagulants (factors VII, VIII, IX, XII, and fibrinogen) rise during pregnancy and are associated with laboratory evidence of enhanced thrombin generation. Pregnant women, oral contraceptive users, and some normal women show a cold-promoted activation of factor VII related to activation of factor XII and prekallikrein. The anticoagulants AT III and protein C remain at normal levels while the protein S level falls. Apparently to secure hemostasis at the uteroplacental level, systemic fibrinolysis is deficient during pregnancy (prolonged euglobulin lysis time [ELT], normal t-PA, and plasminogen with increased levels of PAI of both endothelial cell type [PAI-1] and placental-derived type [PAI-2]). At delivery, the coagulation system is activated and overall fibrinolytic activity is increased. Coagulation changes similar to those seen during pregnancy (except that fibrinolysis is normal and AT III is decreased) are observed after the use of oral contraceptive agents. These changes are dose dependent with ethinyl estradiol and mestranol.

STRESS OR INFLAMMATION

Stimuli such as cell injury, inflammation, and pregnancy promote the production of increased levels of a heterogeneous group of proteins called acute phase reactants. In addition to C-reactive protein and complement components including C4b-binding protein and ceruloplasmin, several coagulation proteins also behave as acute phase reactants: fibrinogen, von Willebrand factor, factor VIII, factor V, a_1-antitrypsin, PAI-1, t-PA, a_2-macroglobulin, plasminogen, and possibly factor VII. The acute phase response of fibrinogen involves monocyte production of interleukin-6, which regulates transcription of mRNA for the a-, β-, and γ-chains of fibrinogen; the increase of fibrinogen level is observed by 12 to 96 h after stimulus. Stress, whether in the form of strenuous acute exercise, high altitude, or mental stress, is associated with an increase in some acute phase reactants (fibrinogen, factor VIII, von Willebrand factor, and factor VII) and enhanced coagulability with an activation of the fibrinolytic system (increased t-PA, decreased plasminogen and a_2-AP, increased fibrinogen degradation products). Platelet number may increase and the bleeding time is shortened.

Diurnal variations in hemostasis include decreased fibrinolytic activity in the morning which is probably due to the circadian variations in the t-PA (lowest in morning and highest in afternoon) and PAI-1 activity (peaks in early morning and shows a trough in the afternoon). Platelet reactivity also can be increased in the early morning.

THE ELDERLY

Studies of hemostasis in the elderly have shown shortening of the bleeding time and APTT, an increase in factors II, VIII, X, high molecular weight kininogen, and prekallikrein, as well as a decrease in AT III (see Table 3-1). Fibrinogen is increased and fibrinolysis may be decreased. These alterations associated with advancing age may create a potential for hypercoagulability.

Evaluation of patients with hemorrhagic or thrombotic tendencies should be accomplished in the resting state whenever possible, and the results should be interpreted in light of age-related normal values. The resting state for both patients and normal controls refers to a consistent time of day (preferably morning) prior to eating, following a night's rest without early morning exercise. The effects of oral contraceptive agents and pregnancy must also be considered.

BIBLIOGRAPHY

Andrew M et al: Development of the human coagulation system in the full term infant. *Blood* 70:165, 1987.

Andrew M et al: Development of the human coagulation system in the healthy premature infant. *Blood* 72:1651, 1988.

Andrew M et al: Maturation of the hemostatic system during childhood. *Blood* 80:1998, 1992.

Bahakim H et al: Coagulation parameters in maternal and cord blood at delivery. *Ann Saudi Med* 10:149, 1990.

Bremme K et al: Enhanced thrombin generation and fibrinolytic activity in normal pregnancy and the puerperium. *Obstet Gynecol* 80:132, 1992.

Bourey RE, Santoro SA: Interactions of exercise, coagulation, platelets, and fibrinolysis—a brief review. *Med Sci Sports Exerc* 20:439, 1988.

Corrigan JJ Jr et al: Newborn's fibrinolytic mechanism: components and plasmin generation. *Am J Hematol* 32:273, 1989.

Corrigan JJ Jr et al: Histidine-rich glycoprotein levels in children: The effect of age. *Thromb Res* 59:681, 1990.

Edelberg JM et al: Neonatal plasminogen displays altered cell surface binding and activation kinetics, correlation with increased glycosylation of the protein. *J Clin Invest* 86:107, 1990.

Forestier F et al: Hematological values of 163 normal fetuses between 18 and 30 weeks of gestation. *Pediatr Res* 20:342, 1986.

Greffe BS et al: Neonatal protein C: Molecular composition and distribution in normal term infants. *Thromb Res* 56:91, 1989.

Hager K et al: Blood coagulation factors in the elderly. *Arch Gerontol Geriatr* 9:277, 1989.

Hathaway W, Corrigan J: Report of Scientific and Standardization Subcommittee on Neonatal Hemostasis. Normal coagulation data for fetuses and newborn infants. *Thromb Haemost* 65:323, 1991.

Jern C et al: Changes of plasma coagulation and fibrinolysis in response to mental stress. *Thromb Haemost* 62:767, 1989.

LaCroix KA et al: The effects of acute exercise and increased atmospheric pressure on the hemostatic mechanism and plasma catecholamine levels. *Thromb Res* 57:717, 1990.

Macpherson CR, Jacobs P: Bleeding time decreases with age. *Arch Pathol Lab Med* 111:328, 1987.

Melissari E et al: Protein S and C4b-binding protein in fetal and neonatal blood. *Br J Haematol* 70:199, 1988.

Rocker L et al: Effect of prolonged physical exercise on the fibrinolytic system. *Eur J Appl Physiol* 60:478, 1990.

Stratton JR et al: Effects of physical conditioning on fibrinolytic variables and fibrinogen in young and old healthy adults. *Circulation* 83:1692, 1991.

Toulon P et al: Antithrombin III (ATIII) and heparin cofactor II (HCII) in normal human fetuses (21st-27th week). *Thromb Haemost* 56:237, 1986.

Tygart SG et al: Longitudinal study of platelet indices during normal pregnancy. *Am J Obstet Gynecol* 154:883, 1986.

Hemorrhagic

Disorders

Screening Tests
of Hemostasis

When historical or physical examination assessment indicates that a bleeding tendency should be evaluated, appropriate laboratory tests are performed. These tests, called hemostatic screening tests, are designed to detect both severe and mild defects and should lead to a definitive diagnosis (which may require further procedures and assays). The initial screening tests are selected and performed as a group depending on the age and clinical condition of the patient. The use of the screening tests will be discussed further for the bleeding infant (see Chap. 7), ambulatory patients with history of bleeding (see Chap. 5), and ill inpatients who are bleeding (see Chap. 6).

PLATELET COUNT AND SIZE

At all ages the normal platelet count ranges from 150,000 to 450,000/μL. Any instances of thrombocytopenia (platelet count <150,000/μL) should be confirmed by an estimation of platelets from a stained peripheral blood smear. Examination of the blood smear is particularly important because most laboratories use an electronic counter that counts particles by size and that may over- or underestimate the true platelet count. For example, an observed platelet count higher than actual may be caused by microspherocytes, fragmented red blood cells, leukocyte fragments, Pappenheimer bodies, and bacteria. Conversely, pseudothrombocytopenia (due to platelet clumping) may be caused by poor collection techniques (blood clotting in the specimen), EDTA-dependent platelet agglutination (EDTA anticoagulant plus a plasma factor such as an IgG or IgM platelet antibody), platelet cold agglutinins, or platelet satellitism (platelet adherence to neutrophils or monocytes). In these instances, an accurate platelet count can usually be obtained by performing a phase contrast count on a freshly obtained finger stick blood sample.

Measurement of the mean platelet volume (MPV) or average platelet size is additional information provided by the electronic particle counter (Coulter counter). When confirmed by the blood smear, the MPV is usually >10 fL in hereditary giant platelet syndromes, recurrent myocardial infarction, and immune thrombocytopenias. A MPV <6 fL is suggestive of the Wiskott-Aldrich syndrome.

BLEEDING TIME

In 1910 Duke described a bleeding time method in which a small cut was made in the lobe of the ear (normal bleeding time, 1 to 3 min) and related bleeding time prolongation to thrombocytopenia. The sensitivity was improved by Ivy who used a puncture wound of the forearm while a blood pressure cuff was applied. The Ivy bleeding time was further "standardized" by use of a 9 × 1 mm template (Mielke) guided cut (normal, up to 10 min). Currently, modifications of the template bleeding time are widely used (Simplate, Surgicut); the upper limit of normal is approximately 9 min. Prolongation of the bleeding time indicates an abnormality in hemostatic plug formation.

Physiologic Variables Influencing the Bleeding Time

The bleeding time is shorter in newborn infants than in adults, tends to be longer in females, and decreases with aging. Dietary habits, such as the ingestion of fish oil, can prolong it. The bleeding time is inversely related to platelet count (begins to increase at levels <100,000/μL), platelet mass, and hematocrit (in general, anemia prolongs and erythrocytosis decreases the bleeding time). Recent reports indicate that the bleeding time (Simplate) may be slightly longer in children (ages 1 to 12) with the upper limits of normal being 10 to 13 min. Otherwise our experience indicates that the bleeding time is a useful test in children.

Relation of the Bleeding Time to Platelet-Vessel Interaction

Extensive literature on the bleeding time indicates that a prolonged bleeding time is found in many patients with excessive bleeding. A long bleeding time can usually be related to defects in specific components of the platelet-vessel interaction and platelet-fibrin plug formation. For example: (1) abnormal vessel components (connective tissue disorders such as Ehlers-Danlos syndrome); (2) abnormal platelet adhesion to subendothelial vascular components (von Willebrand's disease); (3) specific platelet function disorders (intrinsic platelet defects as in platelet storage pool disease and defects in platelet and adhesive proteins); (4) acquired platelet function defects due to drugs (ASA, antibiotics); (5) defects in fibrin formation in the platelet plug—coagulopathies, both hereditary (hemophilia, fibrinogen deficiencies) and acquired (disseminated intravascular coagulation [DIC], abnormal proteins, and antibodies). In many disorders the bleeding time may be prolonged and platelet-vessel interaction altered by as yet undetermined mechanisms including congenital heart disease, hypothyroidism, leukemias, renal diseases, hepatic disorders, and anemia.

Relationship of Bleeding Time to Platelet Count

Because the bleeding time is determined by platelet mass and function, a variable relation to number of platelets is observed (Fig. 4-1). Nevertheless, the bleeding time is usually prolonged in thrombocytopenic disorders when the platelet count is <50,000 to 100,000/μL. The bleeding time test is most helpful when prolonged despite a normal platelet count, that is, indicating platelet dysfunction.

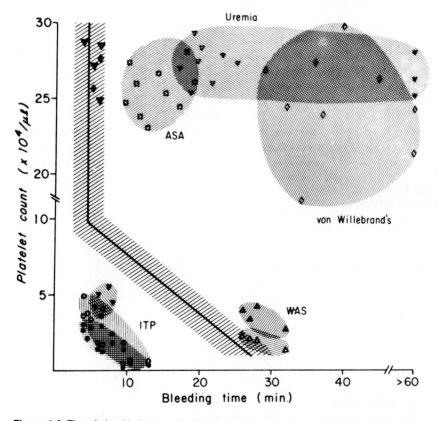

Figure 4-1 The relationship between the bleeding time and the platelet count in various patient groups. Note the disparate bleeding times in Wiscott-Aldrich syndrome (WAS) with small, poorly functioning platelets as compared to ITP patients (ITP) with larger, better functioning platelets. (Used with permission from Harker LA, Slichter SJ: The bleeding time as a screening test for evaluation of platelet function. N Engl J Med 287:155, 1972.)

Evaluation of the Prolonged Bleeding Time

The bleeding time is frequently used in two clinical situations: (1) as part of the diagnostic screening tests and (2) to determine a bleeding tendency in a patient prior to an invasive procedure. Little literature exists to aid the determination of risk for bleeding in different disease states. The degree of prolongation, history of previous bleeding, current drug therapy, associated hemostatic defects, and response to trials of DDAVP should be considered in evaluation of the prolonged bleeding time. Currently there is no evidence that the bleeding time alone is predictive of a bleeding tendency at surgery or other invasive procedures. A prolonged bleeding time is most helpful in evaluating an unknown bleeding disorder (see Chap. 5).

ACTIVATED PARTIAL THROMBOPLASTIN TIME

The PTT time has been used as a screening test for coagulation factor deficiencies since the early 1950s. The modern test, a recalcification clotting time of citrated plasma with added surface contact activation (kaolin, celite, ellagic acid) and a source of phospholipid (the "partial" thromboplastin), is especially sensitive to coagulation abnormalities of the "intrinsic" pathway (factors XII, XI, IX, and VIII) and less sensitive to deficiencies of prothrombin and fibrinogen. The test is usually designated as APTT (activated PTT). The range of APTT values for normal subjects and the sensitivity of the test in detecting factor deficiencies or inhibitors varies considerably depending on the reagents (activator, phospholipid) used and should be determined for each clinical laboratory especially when reagents or equipment are changed.

Prolongation of the APTT indicates a deficiency of one or more coagulation factors (prekallikrein; high molecular weight kininogen; factors XII, XI, IX, VIII, X, V, II; or fibrinogen) or inhibition of the coagulation process by heparin, the lupus anticoagulant, fibrin-fibrinogen degradation products, or specific factor inhibitors. When a prolonged APTT plasma is mixed with normal plasma in the proportion of equal parts (1:1) and the resultant APTT is within the normal range, a factor deficiency is suggested; if "correction" is not complete, then an inhibitor is suspected. This 1:1 mixing is often the first step in the investigation of a prolonged APTT of unknown cause.

Factor Deficiencies

The APTT is commonly used to screen for disorders of the "intrinsic pathway," that is, contact factor deficiencies and hemophilia A (factor VIII deficiency), hemophilia B (factor IX deficiency), and hemophilia C (factor XI deficiency). Several studies (Fig. 4-2) have demonstrated that the APTT

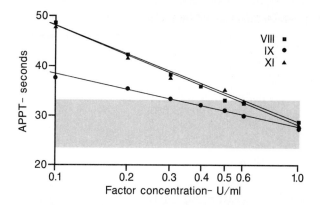

Figure 4-2 APTT sensitivity curves. Each curve represents the APTT (s) for the various in vitro mixtures of normal plasma in factor XI, IX, or VIII-deficient plasma. The shaded area indicates the normal range for the APTT.

is abnormal with factor deficiencies of <0.3 to 0.4 U/mL. Since the minimal hemostatic level of factors VIII, IX, and XI is approximately 30 percent, the APTT is particularly useful as a hemostatic screening test. However, some APTT procedures have failed to detect mild hemophilia at levels of 25 to 30 percent of normal. Therefore, specific factor assays should be performed when there is strong suspicion of mild hemophilia even when the APTT is normal. The degree of prolongation of the APTT reflects the level of factor VIII in most patients with hemophilia A (the rare exception may be certain hereditary variants, see Chap. 14). The correlation of factor level and APTT prolongation is less precise in patients with factor IX- and XI-deficient hemophilia and von Willebrand's disease (Table 4-1).

Inhibitors

The APTT is a good screening test for inhibitors such as the lupus anticoagulant when a sensitive reagent is used. The inhibitory effects of fibrin degradation products (FDP) in DIC may prolong the APTT. In addition, depending on the reagent system used, heparin effect (therapeutic or sample contamination) can be detected in amounts as low as 0.05 U/mL (see Chap. 61). Specific factor inhibitors such as factor VIII antibodies may prolong the APTT by reducing the level of the clotting factor. In these instances, the 1:1 mixture may "correct" immediately but is prolonged after incubation for 1 to 2 h at 37°C.

Artifacts

A spuriously prolonged APTT may be observed in several clinical situations: (1) a polycythemic adult or infant when the citrate/plasma ratio has not been

TABLE 4-1 Representative APTTs in Various Conditions

Condition	APTT (s)
Normal adult (range)	23.5–33.0
Term infant	30.0–54.0
Factor VIII deficient hemophilia	
Severe (VIII = <0.01 U/mL)	82.5
Moderate (VIII = 0.03 U/mL)	57.5
Mild (VIII = 0.18 U/mL)	35.0
Acquired factor VIII Inhibitor (VIII =<0.01 U/mL)	64.0
von Willebrand's disease (VIII = 0.02 U/mL)	55.0
von Willebrand's disease (VIII = 0.25 U/mL)	36.0
Factor IX-deficient hemophilia	
Severe (IX = <0.01 U/mL)	55.6
Mild (IX = 0.20 U/mL)	34.0
Factor XI-deficient hemophilia	
Severe (XI = <0.01 U/mL)	86.0
Mild (XI = 0.50 U/mL)	40.0
Factor XII deficiency	
Severe (XII = <0.01 U/ml)	200.0
Mild (XII = 0.32 U/mL)	37.0
Lupus anticoagulant	72.0
Heparin therapy	
0.1 U/mL	34.0
0.3 U/mL	66.0

*APTT performed with micronized silica in a photo-optical detecting instrument.

corrected during blood procurement, (2) partially filled blood collection tubes (excess citrate), (3) other pretesting variables such as prolonged storage or warming of samples before processing, (4) a clotted sample, and (5) heparin contamination. An incompletely characterized deficiency state with a prolonged APTT has been reported in some bleeding patients (Passovoy deficiency); however, a recent report indicates the commercially available deficient plasma used in evaluation is defective (see Foster reference).

PROTHROMBIN TIME

The PT, first introduced by Quick in 1935, is performed by adding brain tissue thromboplastin and calcium to citrated plasma and recording the clotting time. The PT is a measure of the "extrinsic" system and reflects the procoagulant activity of factors VII, X, V, and II. The test is usually not prolonged by low fibrinogen unless the level is <100 mg/dL.

The PT is particularly useful in monitoring the effect of coumarin-type agents (dicumarol, warfarin) during anticoagulant therapy or in screening for vitamin K deficiency from other causes. The PT is less sensitive to nonspecific inhibition by FDP and heparin than the PTT or thrombin time. The PT is abnormally prolonged when the level of one or more factors (VII, X, V, or II) is below 0.4 to 0.5 U/mL. A major cause of an isolated prolongation (2 to 3 s) of the PT is heterozygous factor VII deficiency.

THROMBIN CLOTTING TIME

The TCT, performed by adding thrombin (usually of bovine or human origin) to citrated plasma (with or without added calcium), measures the amount and quality of fibrinogen and the rate of conversion of fibrinogen to fibrin. Thus, a prolonged TCT may indicate a deficiency of normal fibrinogen (usually 100 mg/dL) as seen in congenital hypofibrinogenemia or afibrinogenemia. The TCT may rarely be prolonged in conditions with abnormally high levels of fibrinogen (inflammation) or more commonly, qualitatively abnormal fibrinogen (hereditary dysfibrinogenemia, cirrhosis, hepatocellular carcinoma, newborn infants). Substances interfering with the thrombin-induced fibrinogen conversion to fibrin are associated with a prolonged TCT (heparin, antithrombin antibodies), proteolytic products of fibrin and fibrinogen (FDP), procainamide-induced anticoagulant, systemic amyloidosis, abnormal serum proteins). Combinations of these mechanisms producing an increased TCT are seen in renal diseases and DIC. A TCT reported as an infinite clotting time usually means heparin effect. The snake venom Bathrop's atrox (Reptilase) clots fibrinogen in the presence of heparin and therefore can be used to identify heparin as the cause of a prolonged TCT.

FIBRINOGEN

Fibrinogen, the clotting factor present in highest concentration in plasma, is significantly reduced in both acquired (DIC, liver dysfunction, fibrinolytic states) and hereditary (afibrinogenemia, dysfibrinogenemia, and hypofibrinogenemia) coagulopathies. Although the normal adult level ranges from 175 to 400 mg/dL, the commonly used screening tests (APTT, PT, thrombin time) usually are not prolonged until the fibrinogen level falls to <100 mg/dL. Therefore a specific assay for fibrinogen, most frequently done by a functional assay, must be included in the basic screening tests. A fibrinogen level that is low by a functional method (thrombin clotting) but near normal by an immunologic or heat precipitation method is suggestive of a dysfibrinogenemia. The minimal level for normal hemostasis is approximately 75 to 100 mg/dL.

EUGLOBULIN LYSIS TIME

The euglobulin lysis time (ELT) is a screening test for accelerated fibrinolytic activity of blood. The euglobulin fraction of citrated plasma (prepared by acidification of dilute plasma) is clotted and the time for spontaneous lysis of the clot at 37°C is recorded (normal range is 60 to 300 min). A shortened lysis time may be detected after severe stress or DDAVP infusion in normal individuals and during hyperfibrinolytic states (liver disease, a_2-anti-plasminogen deficiency, plasminogen activator inhibitor-1 [PAI-1] deficiency, postplasminogen activator infusions) or systemic fibrinolysis. Only rarely is the test abnormally decreased in DIC or secondary fibrinolysis. Prolonged lysis times have been observed in venous thrombosis (in association with increased PAI-1 levels) and renal disease.

FIBRINOGEN-FIBRIN DEGRADATION PRODUCTS

Commonly used screening tests for detection of FDP include the Thrombo-Wellco test (performed on serum, detects D and E fragments) and the Dimertest (performed on citrated plasma, detects D-dimer). These tests are frequently used to screen for or confirm the diagnosis of DIC in a sick patient. Their use is further discussed in Chap. 25.

USE OF THE SCREENING TESTS IN COMBINATION

When determining the etiology of a bleeding diathesis, the use of the screening tests as a group or "battery" is recommended, even though the tests included in each battery will vary according to the clinical situation. In outpatients with a history of bleeding or potential bleeding, the following tests are routinely performed: platelet count, bleeding time, APTT, PT, TCT, and fibrinogen. Inpatients who are ill and bleeding usually have the same tests plus a determination for FDP and consideration of the ELT; the bleeding time is less often done. Bleeding newborn infants have the platelet count, PT, fibrinogen, and FDP performed; the bleeding time and APTT are seldom indicated. The rationale and strategy of using these groups of tests will be discussed in the following three chapters.

Another advantage of using the tests together is the diagnostic help provided when only one or two tests are abnormal with the other tests in the group being normal. For example, if only the APTT is abnormal, consider factors XII, XI, IX, or VIII deficiency; if only the PT is abnormal, consider factor VII deficiency; if both PT and APTT are abnormal, consider early liver disease or vitamin K deficiency; if only the bleeding time is abnormal, platelet function defects should be considered.

BIBLIOGRAPHY

Berkman N et al: EDTA-dependent thrombocytopenia: A clinical study of 18 patients and a review of the literature. *Am J Hematol* 36:195, 1991.

Bessman JD et al: Mean platelet volume. The inverse relation of platelet size and count in normal subjects, and an artifact of other particles. *Am J Clin Pathol* 76:289, 1981.

Carr ME Jr, Gabriel DA: Hyperfibrinogenemia as a cause of prolonged thrombin clotting time. *South Med J* 79:563, 1986.

Duke WW: The relationship of blood platelets to hemorrhagic disease. Description of a method for determining the bleeding time and coagulation time and report of three cases of hemorrhagic disease relieved by transfusion. *JAMA* 55:1185, 1910.

Foster et al: Multiple coagulation factor abnormalities in commercially available Passovoy-deficient plasma. *Blood* 80:3260, 1992.

Galanakis DK et al: Circulating thrombin time anticoagulant in a procainamide-induced syndrome. *JAMA* 239:1873, 1978.

Gastineau DA et al: Inhibitor of the thrombin time in systemic amyloidosis: A common coagulation abnormality. *Blood* 77:2637, 1991.

Hathaway WE et al: Activated partial thromboplastin time and minor coagulopathies. *Am J Clin Pathol* 71:22, 1979.

Koepke JA: Partial thromboplastin time test—proposed performance guidelines. ICSH panel on the PTT. *Thromb Haemost* 55:143, 1986.

Lind SE: The bleeding time does not predict surgical bleeding. *Blood* 77:2547, 1991.

Martin JF et al: Influence of platelet size on outcome after myocardial infarction. *Lancet* 338:1409, 1991.

Mielke CH Jr et al: The standardized normal Ivy bleeding time and its prolongation by aspirin. *Blood* 34:204, 1969.

Peterson P, Gottfried EL: The effects of inaccurate blood sample volume on pro-thrombin time (PT) and activated partial thromboplastin time (aPTT). *Thromb Haemost* 47:101, 1982.

Quick AJ et al: A study of the coagulation defect in hemophilia and in jaundice. *Am J Med Sci* 190:501, 1935.

Rapaport SI et al: Clinical significance of antibodies to bovine and human thrombin and factor V after surgical use of bovine thrombin. *Am J Clin Pathol* 97:84, 1992.

Rodgers RP, Levin J: A critical reappraisal of the bleeding time. *Semin Thromb Hemost* 16:1, 1990.

Evaluation of Bleeding Tendency in Outpatient Child and Adult

The clinician is frequently asked to evaluate the cause of acute or chronic bleeding or to determine the potential for excess bleeding prior to invasive diagnostic or surgical procedures. The patient evaluation includes assessment of historical information (Table 5-1), physical examination, and performance of basic hemostatic screening tests.

HISTORY

Obtaining a meaningful history of excessive hemorrhage can be more difficult than it sounds. Many individuals are convinced that they or their children are "bleeders" or have a bleeding tendency even though no real defect can be determined. Others consider significant episodes of bleeding as "normal." A carefully taken history covering the areas listed in Table 5-1 should be interpreted to answer the following questions: Does the patient display excessive, prolonged, recurrent, or delayed bleeding? Has the patient ever had the opportunity to bleed excessively (physical trauma, skin lacerations, surgery)? Is there a family history of significant bleeding?

PHYSICAL EXAMINATION

Bleeding manifestations can be the presenting symptoms and signs of an underlying disorder which may be suggested by certain physical findings. Consider, for example, petechiae in thrombocytopenia, palpable purpura in anaphylactoid purpura, enlarged spleen and lymph nodes in chronic infections or malignancies, signs of liver decompensation, telangiectasias in Osler-

TABLE 5-1 The Hemostatic History Questionnaire: Historical Information to be Obtained From Patient or Parent

1. Abnormal bruising (ecchymoses or petechiae). Are bruises extensive (larger than quarter, indurated), located where trauma is unlikely or unexplained by minor injury? Are petechiae ever seen? Gum bleeding?
2. Prolonged bleeding after laceration or surgery. Has there been prolonged (hours) or recurrent bleeding after lacerations (cuts, oral injury), surgery (circumcision, skin biopsy, tonsillectomy) tooth extractions or childbirth? Poor wound healing? List all operations and significant trauma.
3. Epistaxis or menorrhagia. Has there been prolonged and heavy menstrual bleeding or severe or recurrent epistaxis? If so, was anemia present or need for iron therapy or transfusion?
4. Soft tissue or joint hemorrhage. Is there a history of unusual hematomas or unexplained "arthritis" or joint swelling?
5. Has there been hematemesis, melena, hematuria, hemoptysis without obvious cause?
6. Family history. Has any blood relative had a problem with excessive bleeding as noted in questions 1–4?
7. General health. Is there evidence for a disorder known to be associated with a bleeding tendency (chronic liver or renal disease, connective tissue disorder, malabsorption syndrome, systemic lupus erythematosus, myeloproliferative disorder, leukemia, amyloidosis)? Is there evidence for abuse or self-inflicted injury?
8. Drugs or medications. Has aspirin, an antibiotic, or warfarin been taken in last 10–14 days? Has vitamin K been used? History of transfusion?

Weber-Rendu disease, albinism in Hermansky-Pudlak syndrome, mitral valve prolapse and von Willebrand's disease, hyperextensible joints and paper-thin scars in Ehlers-Danlos syndrome, Noonan's syndrome and factor XI-platelet function defects, skin plaques and scalloped tongue in amyloidosis, and musculoskeletal defects in the hemophilias.

HEMOSTATIC SCREENING TESTS

The basic screening tests are performed as a group and include:

- Platelet count and blood smear
- Bleeding time
- Activated partial thromboplastin time
- Prothrombin time
- Thrombin clotting time
- Fibrinogen

Each of these tests may be the single abnormal test in bleeding disorders present in an outpatient (Table 5-2).

TABLE 5-2 Abnormal Screening Tests in Various Hemorrhagic Disorders

Disorder	Screening tests					
	Platelet count	Bleeding time	APTT	PT	TCT	Fibrinogen
Thrombocytopenia	X					
Platelet dysfunction		X				
Hemophilia			X			
Factor VII deficiency				X		
Dysfibrinogenemia (mild)					X	
Hypofibrinogenemia						X

*X, abnormal tests. Note that only one test is abnormal in each disorder. This observation emphasizes the need to perform the tests as a group since omission of one test may miss a disorder.

STRATEGY FOR EVALUATION OF BLEEDING TENDENCY

Fig. 5-1 outlines the strategy used for the diagnosis of the potential bleeder. With the information obtained through the history and physical examination, the patient is classified as (1) definite bleeding disorder; (2) questionable bleeding disorder; (3) negative findings but patient has not had sufficient stress to cause bleeding (too young, no trauma or surgery) and/or prior to high-risk procedure (these procedures are associated with considerable bleeding in "normal" persons: tonsillectomy, complicated cardiovascular surgery, scoliosis corrective surgery, CNS surgery, prostatectomy, closed needle biopsies of liver and kidney); or (4) negative findings including history of hemostatic challenge (i.e., surgery, tooth extractions).

All patients receive the basic screening battery except those in category 4. If the basic screening tests are normal, no further tests are done except for patients in category 1. These patients with a definite history of bleeding and a negative hemostatic screening battery should have further diagnostic evaluation to consider mild hemophilia, von Willebrand's disease, factor XIII deficiency, α_2-antiplasmin, or plasminogen activator inhibitor-1 deficiencies, and vascular defects. The questionably positive patients (category 2) with a negative basic screen are occasionally candidates for further testing, particularly if high risk surgery is planned. If the patient has a history suggestive of mild von Willebrand's disease or platelet function disorder and the bleeding time is normal, tests for von Willebrand's disease or platelet aggregation tests are indicated. Sometimes repeated von Willebrand factor testing is necessary to establish the diagnosis in mild cases. Rarely a mild hemophilic patient has a normal APTT (especially if factor IX deficient) and specific factor assays are indicated if the history is suspicious.

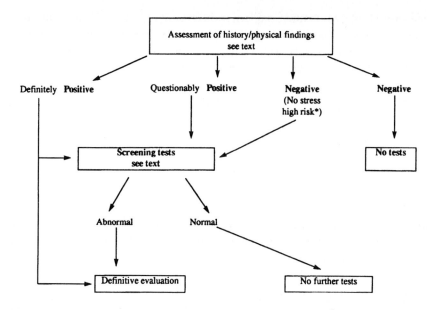

Figure 5-1 Outline of diagnostic evaluation of potential bleeding diathesis. *High-risk patients are those who will have procedures frequently associated with excess bleeding in "normal" persons (tonsillectomy in child; complicated cardiovascular surgery; scoliosis corrective surgery; CNS surgery; prostatectomy) or closed (needle) liver and renal biopsies.

Preoperative Hemostatic Evaluation

The routine preoperative performance of bleeding screening tests such as the APTT and bleeding time has not been demonstrated to be significantly predictive of hemorrhagic complications or cost effective. As indicated in Fig. 5-1, basic screening laboratory tests are reserved for those patients with a positive assessment or who are at higher risk of bleeding because of special circumstances. For example, the basic screening tests are indicated in all children prior to tonsillectomy and adenoidectomy because the procedure has a significant incidence of postoperative bleeding, and a personal history of bleeding may not be available in the young child (no previous stress).

Easy Bruising

Complaints or signs of easy bruising are common in children and many elderly people. Small bruises (smaller than the size of a quarter) are frequently seen on the lower extremities of active youngsters; up to 30 percent of children report bruises as often as weekly. However, it is rare for children < age 1 year to show bruising. Trauma (accidental, nonaccidental, or self-inflicted) should be considered as a cause of multiple or unusual bruises at any age. Nonaccidental trauma is a major differential point in the evaluation of easy bruising or unusually large hematomas. A positive family history for hemorrhagic tendencies or the suspicion of nonaccidental trauma is an indication for basic screening tests in patients with easy bruising. Large (> 2 inches in diameter) or indurated purpuric lesions of the skin evoke the differential diagnosis of skin purpura (see Chap. 22).

Chronic Epistaxis

Chronic or habitual epistaxis may be the only indication of a mild bleeding disorder. Recurrent brief nosebleeds are frequently seen in children; nose bleeds that occur every 1 to 2 months, last longer than 10 min, involve both nares, and require medical attention or transfusion are suspicious of a bleeding defect. As many as 25 percent of these patients may have an underlying hemostatic defect, particularly of the platelet-vessel interaction type (platelet dysfunction, von Willebrand's disease).

MILD BLEEDING DISORDERS

The evaluation of a bleeding tendency in an ambulatory setting is often the differential diagnosis of the mild bleeding disorder. Older children and young adults who are otherwise healthy will present with a history of easy bruising, epistaxis, excessive postoperative or postpartum bleeding, menorrhagia, gingival bleeding, excessive bleeding after a tooth extraction, or the concern of a positive family history for excess bleeding. The diagnoses most frequently confirmed in the patient with a mild bleeding disorder (incidence ranging from 3 to 50/100,000) are von Willebrand's disease, mild hemophilia A or B, platelet function disorder, or factor XI deficiency. Frequently these patients delay seeking medical attention and may only be diagnosed after persistent postoperative or postdental extraction bleeding. A carefully taken history is usually suggestive and leads to the screening tests which starts the diagnostic evaluation. A precise diagnosis of the mild defect is difficult and sometimes requires repeated testing using the most sensitive tests and assays available. Often the most cost-effective method is referral to a reference or consulting laboratory if the initial screening battery is inconclusive.

ISOLATED PROLONGATION OF THE ACTIVATED PARTIAL THROMBOPLASTIN TIME

A challenging clinical problem is the investigation of prolonged APTT in a person who does not have an obvious bleeding diathesis but in whom a

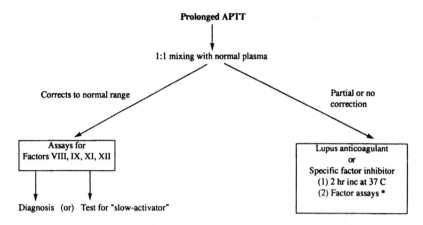

Figure 5-2 Evaluation of APTT when other screening tests are normal and heparin effect has been eliminated.* Do complete standard curves and look for inhibitor effect.

surgical procedure is contemplated. Complete hemostatic screening tests (PT, TCT, platelet count, bleeding time, fibrinogen level) are normal except for a slight or moderately prolonged APTT. The approach to this problem is outlined in Fig. 5-2. An investigation of 41 patients with the presenting complaint of a "prolonged APTT" prior to a surgical procedure indicated that most of these patients had a defect in the contact system (i.e., either a deficiency of factor XII or a "slow activator" [see Chap. 17]). Many of the patients subsequently had surgery without excessive bleeding. Possible causes of an isolated prolonged APTT in an outpatient also include the conditions listed in Table 5-3.

ISOLATED PROLONGATION OF THE BLEEDING TIME

Occasionally only the bleeding time will be prolonged in patients with normal hemostatic screening tests. The platelet count is normal and examination of

TABLE 5-3 Causes of an Isolated Prolonged APTT in an Ambulatory Patient

I. No bleeding

Factor XII deficiency
(probable heterozygote)
Lupus anticoagulant
"Slow-activator" (see Chap. 17)

II. Potential bleeding

Mild hemophilia (factors VIII, IX, XI deficiency)
Mild von Willebrand's disease

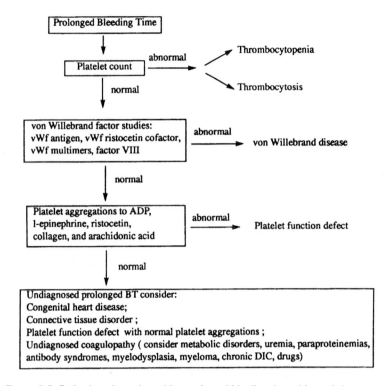

Figure 5-3 Evaluation of a patient with a prolonged bleeding time without obvious cause.

the blood smear reveals no abnormal platelet size or staining. The diagnostic possibilities include hereditary and acquired disorders of platelet-vessel interaction. Since the most common abnormalities will be von Willebrand's disease or platelet function defects on a hereditary basis, the approach is presented in Fig. 5-3. If prolongation of the bleeding time persists, repeat von Willebrand's disease studies may be indicated because of variation in these studies over time in patients with mild disease.

BIBLIOGRAPHY

Bachmann F: Diagnostic approach to mild bleeding disorders. In: Miescher PA, Jaffe EF (eds): *Seminars in Hematology: Mild Bleeding Disorders*, New York, Grune and Stratton, 1980, pp 292–305.

Barber A et al: The bleeding time as a preoperative screening test. *Am J Med* 78:761, 1985.

Beran M et al: Haemostatic disorders in habitual nose-bleeders. *J Laryngol Otol* 101:1020, 1987.

Katsanis E et al: Prevalence and significance of mild bleeding disorders in children with recurrent epistaxis. *J Pediatr* 113:73, 1988.

Kiley V et al: Coagulation studies in children with isolated recurrent epistaxis. *J Pediatr* 100:579, 1982.

Kitchens CS: Occult hemophilia. *Johns Hopkins Med J* 146:255, 1980.

Kitchens CS: Prolonged activated partial thromboplastin time of unknown etiology: A prospective study of 100 consecutive cases referred for consultation. *Am J Hematol* 27:38, 1988.

Manning SC et al: An assessment of preoperative coagulation screening for tonsillectomy and adenoidectomy. *Int J Pediatr Otorhinolaryn* 13:237, 1987.

Nosek-Cenkowska B et al: Bleeding/bruising symptomatology in children with and without bleeding disorders. *Thromb Haemost* 65:237, 1991.

Suchman AL, Mushlin AI: How well does the activated partial thromboplastin time predict postoperative hemorrhage? *JAMA* 256:750, 1986.

Werner EJ et al: Relative value of diagnostic studies for von Willebrand disease. *J Pediatr* 121:34, 1992.

Evaluation of

Bleeding in the

Hospitalized Patient

GENERAL APPROACH

Excessive bleeding in hospitalized patients is a common and challenging clinical problem. Most of the time, the bleeding is surgical and quickly controlled with a few well-placed sutures (factor XIV). All too frequently, however, the bleeding is accentuated by generalized hemostatic defects that require prompt identification and therapy. A correct diagnosis can usually be rapidly made using data gathered from the patient's history, the physical examination, and the laboratory. A general approach to these patients is outlined in Tables 6-1 and 6-2. Note that the laboratory studies should be obtained early, so that results are available by the time the rest of the evaluation is complete.

HISTORY AND MEDICAL RECORD

Data must be collected from several sources, including the patient, family, nurses, the medical record, and the laboratory information system. If there is extensive data from a long or complex hospital course, a simple flow sheet should be constructed to include key test results, major clinical events (e.g., surgery, episodes of bleeding), changes in medications, and blood product administration. While the new laboratory studies are pending, the information gathered from these sources should be reviewed to determine:

TABLE 6-1 An Approach to the Actively Bleeding Hospitalized Patient

See the patient; make an initial assessment
↓
Draw screening tests of hemostasis
↓
Collect historical data:
history
medical record
laboratory information system
construct a flow sheet (if needed)
↓
Do the physical exam
↓
Analyze the data
Make a presumptive diagnosis
Construct a plan of action
↓
Write orders for therapy and/or further diagnostic tests

Has the bleeding been prolonged, delayed, or recurrent; or is it simply more rapid than normal?

In general, brisk bleeding from a site of obvious trauma suggests a local vascular defect. In contrast, bleeding that is prolonged, delayed, or recurrent is characteristic of a generalized hemostatic disorder. Sudden resumption of bleeding from a previously injured site raises the possibility of systemic fibrinolysis.

Is the bleeding from a single site or from several different locations?

Bleeding from multiple sites strongly suggests a generalized hemostatic disorder, whereas hemorrhage from a single location is more likely due to a local defect.

TABLE 6-2 Key Questions

- Is the bleeding serious or trivial?
- Is the bleeding due to a generalized disorder of hemostasis or to a local vascular defect?
- Is the disorder hereditary or acquired?
- What is the relationship of the bleeding to medical or surgical management?
- What is the urgency of the situation?

Is the bleeding appropriate for the injury?

Although rather subjective, extensive bleeding from small injuries (e.g., venipuncture sites, nasogastric tubes) suggests a hemostatic disorder.

Is there a past history of bleeding?

Bleeding symptoms could be lifelong (suggesting a hereditary defect) or associated with an illness (more likely an acquired disorder).

What medications have been given?

Particular attention should be directed toward antiplatelet agents (aspirin, nonsteroidal anti-inflammatory drugs), anticoagulants, and antibiotics.

Are diseases present that are associated with known hemorrhagic syndromes?

Examples include the combinations of acute promyelocytic leukemia and disseminated intravascular coagulation (DIC); liver disease and systemic fibrinolysis; antibiotic therapy and vitamin K deficiency; or trauma and a dilutional coagulopathy.

Is there a family history of bleeding?

Although most hemostatic defects in hospitalized patients are acquired, underlying hereditary disorders may become manifest in the hospital setting. For example, von Willebrand's disease might be discovered because of hemorrhage after a surgical procedure.

PHYSICAL EXAMINATION

The objective of the physical examination is to determine whether bleeding seems appropriate for the injury and whether single or multiple sites are involved. A careful examination may also uncover diseases associated with hemostatic defects (e.g., splenomegaly in myeloproliferative disease, lymphadenopathy in malignancy, hepatomegaly in liver disease). Areas to examine with particular care are wounds, intravenous or other catheter sites, fluid collection bags (urine, gastric, wound drainage, pleural fluid), and the patient's clothing and bedding. The skin should be examined in detail looking for oozing or bleeding from previous finger or heel sticks, and injection or bleeding time sites. Petechiae, particularly in dependent locations, and ecchymoses should be sought. The patient should be turned to one side to seek evidence of bruising over the flank (suggesting retroperitoneal hemorrhage). Ultrasound scans can be useful for the identification of deep-seated hematomas.

LABORATORY STUDIES

After an initial assessment of the clinical situation, laboratory tests of hemostasis should be obtained as soon as possible in patients who are actively bleeding, without waiting for the completion of the history, medical record review, and physical examination. Platelet function, coagulation, DIC, and systemic fibrinolysis must be assessed (Table 6-3). The tests should be ordered as a battery to save time and to obtain an overview of all facets of hemostasis. Often, the bleeding time is not routinely obtained in children and is reserved for adult patients suspected of a platelet function defect after initial screening. The euglobulin lysis time (ELT) could also be limited to patients with known liver disease or those suspected of complex coagulopathies. Based on the results of these tests, more definitive assays should be ordered as necessary.

Care must be taken in obtaining, labeling, and processing the blood samples. Generally, in adults one or two citrate (blue top) tubes are needed for coagulation tests, with an EDTA (lavender top) tube for the complete blood and platelet counts. Smaller volumes are collected from pediatric patients. Ideally, the blood samples should be obtained from a separate clean venipuncture with efforts made to avoid contamination with heparin or dilution by intravenous fluids, and then transported promptly to the laboratory for analysis.

Some comments about the use and interpretation of the laboratory screening tests are listed below.

■ Isolated prolongation of the PT by 2 to 3 s is seen frequently in adults who have undergone major surgery or trauma or who are seriously ill. Although probably related to a fall in factor VII, the mechanisms are unknown. Considerations include early liver insufficiency or vitamin K deficiency. In adults, excessive bleeding is unusual when the sole laboratory abnormality is a mild prolongation of the PT. In children, a prolonged PT more often reflects a propensity for hemorrhage, especially when associated with a long APTT.

TABLE 6-3 Screening Tests of Hemostasis for Hospitalized Patients

Coagulation disorders	PT, APTT, TCT, fibrinogen
Platelet function defects	Platelet count, bleeding time
Disseminated intravascular coagulation	Fibrin degradation products (e.g., D-dimer)
Systemic fibrinolysis	Euglobulin lysis time

- If both the PT and APTT are prolonged, and the disorder is acquired, then the cause is more likely to involve multiple clotting factor deficiencies than an abnormality of a single factor in the common pathway (i.e., factors X, V, or prothrombin).

- The TCT is mildly prolonged in both renal and liver disease, but when it is greatly prolonged (e.g., > 100 s), severe hypofibrinogenemia or heparin effect should be considered.

- A separate measurement of fibrinogen is always warranted because the PT and APTT are not sensitive to moderate hypofibrinogenemia. The fibrinogen concentration is an excellent reflection of the severity of DIC, systemic fibrinolysis, or liver disease.

- In acutely ill hospitalized patients, the bleeding time is of less diagnostic value if the platelet count is < 50,000/μL. In general, if the bleeding time is normal (and the patient does not have von Willebrand's disease), bleeding is unlikely to be due to a platelet function defect. However, a prolonged bleeding time does not always predict future hemorrhage.

- Bleeding times are infrequently performed in sick children except when specifically indicated to rule out inherited von Willebrand's disease, platelet function defects, or when the use of DDAVP is being considered.

- Modern tests for fibrin degradation products (FDP; e.g., D-dimer) make the older paracoagulation tests for fibrin monomer (protamine or ethanol gel tests) less valuable in patients suspected of DIC.

- A shortened ELT is a sensitive measure of systemic fibrinolysis but is not always predictive of fibrinolytic bleeding. Because systemic fibrinolysis is so rare in a pediatric population, the ELT is usually not ordered in infants or children.

Once results of the initial battery of laboratory tests have been obtained, then consideration should be given to follow-up testing to guide therapy in an actively bleeding patient. Serial hematocrits will be needed as well as the PT, APTT, fibrinogen, and platelet count. The bleeding time, D-dimer test, and ELT are usually not repeated unless they are abnormal. Intervals between tests may be as short as hourly in a severely injured trauma patient with massive hemorrhage or as infrequently as daily in patients with less severe but chronic bleeding.

ANALYSIS OF THE DATA

A limited number of hemorrhagic defects account for most of the bleeding in hospitalized patients. These disorders are usually acquired rather than hereditary and involve multiple rather than single hemostatic defects (Table 6-4). In children, with a less informative past history, bleeding after surgery or other trauma suggests a hereditary disorder (see Chap. 5).

Vitamin K Deficiency

Seriously ill patients can easily become deficient in vitamin K due to poor nutrition or long-term antibiotic therapy. Because vitamin K deficiency reduces the activity of clotting factors II, VII, IX, and X, the PT and APTT are both prolonged, but the fibrinogen concentration and TCT are normal. The PT lengthens before the APTT because of the short half-life of factor VII (5 hr).

Liver Disease

Because the liver is the site of synthesis of most of the clotting factors, the PT and APTT are often prolonged in advanced liver disease. As in vitamin K deficiency, the PT is first to increase. The TCT is often mildly prolonged, which is most likely a result of hepatic synthesis of a dysfunctional fibrinogen or inhibition of fibrin polymerization by circulating FDP. As liver failure becomes more profound, the concentration of fibrinogen begins to fall. The platelet count can be low due to hypersplenism. The bleeding time is often mildly or moderately prolonged although the mechanism is unclear. The ELT is shortened in up to 40 percent of patients with advanced liver disease due to circulating fibrinolytic enzymes that are not cleared by the liver or are ineffectively neutralized by a_2-antiplasmin.

Disseminated Intravascular Coagulation

The classic pattern of laboratory abnormalities in acute severe DIC includes low concentrations of fibrinogen (< 100 mg/dL), high levels of FDP (D-dimer > 2 μg/mL), prolonged PT and APTT, thrombocytopenia, and a prolonged bleeding time. The ELT will be normal in most patients with DIC. In mild DIC, fibrinogen concentrations are often normal since synthesis is increased due to acute phase reactions, but this is balanced by accelerated consumption of fibrinogen. The APTT can be short, presumably due to circulating activated clotting factors. Concentrations of FDP are almost always elevated (see Chap. 25).

Systemic Fibrinolysis

Bleeding due to circulating fibrinolytic enzymes occurs with some regularity in two clinical situations: (1) as a complication of therapeutic thrombolysis

TABLE 6-4 Representative Test Results for Common Bleeding Disorders in Hospitalized Patients

	PT	APTT	TCT	Fibrinogen	Platelet Count	D-Dimer	ELT
Normal Range	11–13.5 s	25–35 s	<30 s	150–450 mg/dL	150–350K/μL	<0.5 μg/mL	<60 min
Vitamin K deficiency							
Early	18	32	21	225	250	<0.5	>60
Late	26	58	21	225	250	<0.5	>60
Liver disease							
Early	16	32	23	225	185	<0.5	>60
Late	22	63	45	75	60	1.0	30
Disseminated Intravascular Coagulation							
Mild	12.5	22	36	190	250	1.5	>60
Severe	24	86	45	65	40	4-8	>60

Systemic fibrinolysis							
Mild	12.5	32	35	225	250	<0.5	15
Severe	22	72	60	55	250	<0.5	<15
Dilutional coagulopathy							
Mild	16	38	21	150	125	<0.5	>60
Severe	28	90	21	55	25	1.0	>60
Heparin							
Small	12.5	36	>100	225	250	<0.5	>60
Large	18	>100	>100	225	250	<0.5	>60

and (2) in patients with advanced liver disease, particularly in conjunction with trauma or surgery. In both of these settings, the ELT is short. If fibrinolysis is severe, fibrinogen concentrations are low, and the PT, APTT, and TCT are mildly to moderately prolonged. Concentrations of D-dimer are usually normal, but have been reported to be elevated in some patients with severe systemic fibrinolysis due to plasmin digestion of circulating soluble fibrin.

Dilutional Coagulopathy

In patients with extensive trauma or surgery, blood loss is often temporarily replaced with large volumes of intravenous fluids, which produce substantial dilution of clotting factors and platelets. This "washout" syndrome may be enhanced by consumption of clotting factors and platelets at sites of massive tissue injury. Almost all screening tests of hemostasis are abnormal due to depletion of clotting factors and platelets. D-dimer is usually normal or only slightly elevated except in cases of DIC in patients with brain injury or prolonged hypotension. The ELT is normal except in some patients with advanced liver disease.

Heparin Excess

The presence of heparin in plasma commonly causes confusion in the interpretation of coagulation tests. The blood sample may be contaminated by residual heparin in central venous or arterial lines, which produces abnormal laboratory tests, but not bleeding. Rarely, heparin may be inadvertently administered to patients producing both bleeding and abnormal laboratory studies. Heparin in the plasma may be strongly suspected if the TCT and APTT are greatly prolonged, particularly if the fibrinogen concentration is > 100 mg/dL. In case of doubt, the most practical approach is to redraw the sample using a peripheral venipuncture site. Alternatively, the plasma can be passed through a heparin-retaining filter, or the heparin neutralized with polybrene or protamine prior to repeating the coagulation screening tests (see Chap. 2).

The conditions described above represent a large proportion of the serious hemostatic defects in hospitalized patients. Other disorders necessitate more specific laboratory assays. For example, a patient with a spontaneous inhibitor to factor VIII will require mixing studies and quantification of the circulating anticoagulant. In children, specific assays for hereditary disorders of hemostasis may be necessary. However, in the great majority of patients, simple screening tests are usually sufficient for a presumptive diagnosis and can serve as guides for clotting factor and platelet replacement therapy to treat the bleeding.

BIBLIOGRAPHY

Bowie EJW, Owen CA: Hemostatic failure in clinical medicine. *Semin Hematol* 14:341, 1977.

Bowie EJW, Owen CA: The significance of abnormal preoperative hemostatic tests. *Prog Hemost Thromb* 5:179, 1980.

Channing Rodgers RP, Levin J: A critical reappraisal of the bleeding time. *Semin Thromb Hemost* 16:1, 1990.

Coller BS, Schneiderman P: Clinical evaluation of hemorrhagic disorders: The bleeding history and differential diagnosis of purpura. In: Hoffman R, Benz EJ Jr, Shattil SJ, Furie B, Cohen HJ (eds): *Hematology. Basic Principles and Practice*, New York, Churchill Livingstone, 1991, pp 1252–1266.

Feinstein DI: Diagnosis and management of disseminated intravascular coagulation: The role of heparin therapy. *Blood* 60:284, 1982.

Harker LA, Slichter SJ: The bleeding time as a screening test for evaluation of platelet function. *N Engl J Med* 287:155, 1972.

Rapaport SI: Preoperative hemostatic evaluation: Which test if any? *Blood* 61:229, 1983.

Suchman AL, Griner PF: Diagnostic uses of the activated partial thromboplastin time and prothrombin time. *Ann Intern Med* 104:810, 1986.

White GC et al: Approach to the bleeding patient. In: Colman RW, Hirsh J, Marder VJ, Salzman EW (eds): *Hemostasis and Thrombosis. Basic Principles and Clinical Practice,* 2d ed., Philadelphia, Lippincott, 1987, pp 1048–1060.

CHAPTER
7

Evaluation of Bleeding
in the Newborn

Physiologic alterations of the hemostatic system in the fetus and newborn plus consideration of hemorrhagic disorders unique to the perinatal period demand that a different approach than that for children and adults be taken for the evaluation of a bleeding tendency in the newborn infant. Information available before the delivery of the infant is frequently helpful in planning the evaluation. A family history of a bleeding disorder which could be inherited in a dominant (von Willebrand disease, dysfibrinogenemia) or X-linked (hemophilia A and B) manner requires planning prior to delivery so that a cord blood sample (see Chap. 2) will be obtained. Such planning prevents the need for subsequent vessel puncture which may lead to excessive bleeding if the infant is affected. If the mother has immune thrombocytopenic purpura (ITP), a fetal scalp sample for a platelet count may be indicated; or if a previous infant was thrombocytopenic, platelet alloimmunization should be considered. Prenatal and obstetric complications which should alert the physician to potential bleeding in the infant include maternal medications (anticonvulsants and warfarin), intrauterine hypoxia, abruptio placenta, and dead twin fetus (disseminated intravascular coagulation, DIC).

Routine screening tests used in the newborn include the platelet count, PT, APTT, and TCT or fibrinogen. Because physiologic alterations in the contact factors result in a significant prolongation of the APTT (especially in preterm infants), the test is usually not helpful but may be included to detect heparin; the TCT is also used to detect heparin effect. If hemophilia is suspected, factor assays should be performed rather than using the APTT as a screening test. The bleeding time is rarely used as a screening test in the newborn for two reasons: (1) the normal range is shorter and slight abnormalities are difficult to interpret; and (2) follow-up evaluation of a prolonged bleeding time requires von Willebrand disease studies and platelet aggregation tests which are also difficult to interpret in the newborn because of

TABLE 7-1 Mean Values for Newborn Screening Tests

	Adult	Term Infant	Preterm Infant (33-week gestation)
Platelet count (per μL)	250,000	330,000	290,000
Bleeding time (Simplate, min)	5.5	3.5	3.5
APTT, s	28	36	45
PT, s	10.5	11.5	13.5
TCT, s	11	12	14
Fibrinogen (mg/dL)	270	250	240

physiologic alterations (see Chap. 3). The precise role of the bleeding time as a neonatal screening test remains to be established. Unless there are urgent reasons (i.e., specific therapy), it is more practical to defer the bleeding time and associated studies until 6 months of age or later in suspected cases of von Willebrand disease and platelet function disorder. Determinations of fibrin degradation products (FDP) are usually done routinely in sick infants. Table 7-1 summarizes the results of screening tests in the newborn infant. The values shown demonstrate the relative differences for these tests in the neonate as compared to the adult.

DIFFERENTIAL DIAGNOSIS OF THE BLEEDING INFANT

Fig. 7-1 presents an outline of the differential diagnosis of the bleeding infant. The assessment is based on the history and physical findings which allows classification into "well" and "sick." The "well"-appearing infant is usually of term gestation and presents with bleeding from one or more orifices (oral or rectal bleeding, hematuria), skin purpura or petechiae, cephalohematoma, or persistent oozing after the trauma of skin punctures or minor surgery (circumcision). One or more of these manifestations may occur in an otherwise well-appearing infant (vital signs are normal).

The basic screening tests (platelet count, APTT, PT) will indicate the following:

1. Decreased platelet count as the only abnormality in an infant with petechiae suggests the differential diagnosis of thrombocytopenia
2. Prolongation of both the PT (slight) and APTT (marked) with failure of correction of 1:1 mixing suggests heparin effect (iatrogenic overdose or contamination of catheters); or if corrected in 1:1 mixing, vitamin K deficiency (breast-fed infant, no vitamin K at birth)

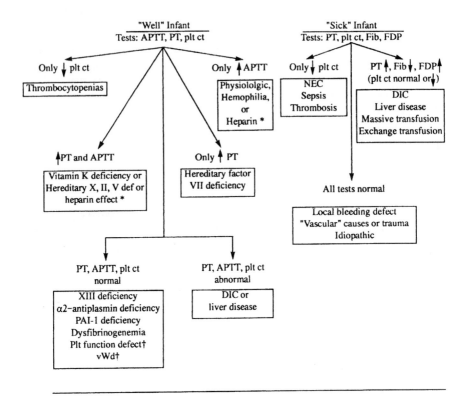

Figure 7-1 Differential diagnosis of the bleeding infant.

3. Prolongation of the APTT alone suggests hemophilia A or B (or physiologic contact factor deficiency [perform factor assays])

4. Isolated prolongation of the PT suggests hereditary factor VII deficiency

5. If all tests are normal, consider factor XIII, a_2-antiplasmin (a_2-AP) or plasminogen activator inhibitor-1 deficiency (especially if delayed or persistent umbilical cord stump bleeding, do factor assays) or consider a platelet function defect or von Willebrand's disease (plan subsequent bleeding time and other studies).

6. If all screening studies are abnormal, reevaluate the infant for liver disease or "missed" DIC.

In summary, the history, type of bleeding, and results of these tests allow a diagnosis to be made which can be confirmed at a later date when the neonatal physiologic alterations in clotting tests are no longer present.

The "sick"-appearing infant who displays evidence of a bleeding tendency may be either a preterm infant (usually with respiratory distress, hypoxia, unstable vital signs) or a term infant with evidence of CNS bleeding or sepsis (viral or bacterial). The only sign of bleeding may be shock and pallor (hematoma of liver, adrenal, or kidney, or severe intracranial hemorrhage). Tracheal bleeding in an intubated infant may be due to trauma aggravated by a bleeding tendency. The screening tests (PT, platelet count, fibrinogen, FDP) are usually slightly or markedly abnormal. If the most abnormal test is the platelet count, consider sepsis, bowel necrosis (necrotizing enterocolitis), or major vessel thrombosis. Abnormalities in the fibrinogen level and PT with increased FDP confirm the diagnosis of DIC, or less commonly, severe liver disease. Rarely the bleeding and sick infant will have normal screening studies; this combination is particularly seen in intraventricular hemorrhage (IVH) in the premature infant or postoperatively (congenital cardiac lesions) where the bleeding is due to a local lesion or an ill-defined platelet function defect (see below).

GASTROINTESTINAL BLEEDING

Infants with signs of gastrointestinal bleeding (melena or hematemesis) particularly in the first few hours of life may have swallowed maternal blood during delivery. A gastric aspirate, vomitus, or stool containing gross blood should be tested for adult hemoglobin by the Apt test. The addition of 1% sodium hydroxide to a pink solution containing adult blood will result in a color change from pink to yellow-brown. When the pink color remains, the solution contains mostly fetal hemoglobin and a neonatal origin for the blood is confirmed (a hemolyzed sample of the infant's blood is a good control for the test).

INTRACRANIAL HEMORRHAGE

Neonatal intracranial bleeding may result from many etiologies including birth trauma, hereditary bleeding diatheses, hemorrhagic cerebral necrosis due to infection, vascular malformations, and acquired bleeding disorders. The hemorrhagic syndrome of IVH has been studied extensively in the past few years and remains one of the challenging problems in perinatal medicine. Recent evidence yielded by many new techniques including ultrasonography, positron emission tomography, and cerebral blood flow studies has led to a reappraisal of the potential etiologies of IVH. The associated parenchymal hemorrhage and the delayed onset of IVH extension of the early subependymal hemorrhage may represent a hemorrhagic component of an initial ischemic lesion. Thus, alterations of the coagulation system may have a more direct etiologic role; that is, an initial ischemic lesion may be due to "microthrombosis" or "infarct," and the hemorrhagic extension may be secondary to a concomitant hemostatic impairment.

From a diagnostic viewpoint, it is recommended that all term infants with intracranial hemorrhage (not otherwise explained) have a hemostatic screening battery to include factor XIII and a_2-AP levels; preterm infants (usually < 33 weeks' gestation) should have the basic screening tests (PT, fibrinogen, platelet count) to determine whether correctable deficiencies are present.

BIBLIOGRAPHY

Feusner JH et al: Acquired haemostatic defects in the ill newborn. *Br J Haematol* 53:73, 1983.

Gordon EM et al: Studies on some coagulation factors (Hageman factor, plasma prekallikrein, and high molecular weight kininogen) in the normal newborn. *Am J Pediatr Hematol Oncol* 2:213, 1980.

Hathaway WE, Bonnar J: *Hemostatic Disorders of the Pregnant Woman and Newborn Infant*, New York, Elsevier, 1987.

Kisker CT: Pathophysiology of bleeding disorders in newborn. In: Polin RA, Fox WW (eds): *Fetal and Neonatal Physiology*, Philadelphia, Saunders, 1992, pp 1381–1394.

McDonald MM et al: Role of coagulopathy in newborn intracranial hemorrhage. *Pediatrics* 74:26, 1984.

Montgomery RR et al: Newborn haemostasis. *Clin Haematol* 14:443, 1985.

Pramanik AK: Bleeding disorders in neonates. *Pediatr Rev* 13:163, 1992.

Susuki S, Hathaway WE, Bonnar J, Sutor AH (eds): *Perinatal Thrombosis and Hemostasis*, Tokyo, Springer-Verlag, 1991.

Thrombocytopenias

Thrombocytopenia is defined as a platelet count $< 150,000/\mu L$ for all ages (from the small premature infant to the elderly adult). However, the most common etiologic events and associations vary with age and development. The newborn infant is particularly susceptible to decreased platelets. As many as 20 percent of sick infants have thrombocytopenia which is usually based on increased destruction. Pregnancy is associated with several unique causes of thrombocytopenia including preeclampsia and pregnancy-induced thrombocytopenia. Thrombocytopenias based on decreased production are prominent in adults (bone marrow depression caused by chemotherapeutic agents).

CAUSES OF THROMBOCYTOPENIA IN THE NEWBORN INFANT

Although the causes of newborn thrombocytopenia are many, the approach to determination of etiology is simplified by looking for the most common causes in the particular clinical setting. In the sick preterm infant, consider sepsis, disseminated intravascular coagulation (DIC), large vessel thrombosis, necrotizing enterocolitis, or pulmonary syndromes (infant respiratory disease syndrome [IRDS], meconium and amniotic fluid aspiration, pulmonary hypertension). In the full-term infant who appears to be well, the most likely diagnosis is antibody-mediated (maternal immune thrombocytopenia [ITP] or systemic lupus erythematosis [SLE] or alloimmune, see Chap. 9), viral syndrome, hyperviscosity syndrome, or occult large vessel thrombosis. Infection and DIC are the most common causes of decreased platelets in both term and preterm infants. Bacterial sepsis frequently (up to 60 percent of cases) is associated with acute thrombocytopenia which often takes 6 to 10 days to resolve. Congenital viral infections may produce severe thrombocytopenia by several mechanisms including megakaryocytic injury, splenic removal, hepatic disease, and platelet-endothelial cell injury.

An unusual mechanism for thrombocytopenia in the newborn is decreased platelet production due to marrow involvement in the disorders displayed in Table 8-1. Other causes of neonatal thrombocytopenia include infants small for gestational age, postexchange transfusion ("wash-out"), neonatal thyrotoxicosis, metabolic disorders (hyperglycinemia, mucolipidosis, propionic

TABLE 8-1 Bone Marrow Abnormality Associated with Neonatal Thrombocytopenia

Congenital megakaryocytic hypoplasia
Absent radii (TAR) syndrome (leukemoid reaction, absent radius, digits present)
Phocomelia syndrome
Aplastic anemia
Trisomy syndromes (myeloproliferative syndrome)
Osteopetrosis (myeloproliferative syndrome)
Congenital leukemia
Fanconi's pancytopenia (deformed or absent radius and thumb, onset is later in life)

acidemia), maternal hypertension, erythroblastosis fetalis, giant heman-gioma, placental chorioangioma, and maternal (tolbutamide, hydantoin, azathioprine) and infant (intralipid, tolazoline) drugs. Hereditary thrombo-cytopenias (see below) may present in the neonatal period.

CAUSES OF THROMBOCYTOPENIA IN THE CHILD AND ADULT

Thrombocytopenia in the child and adult may be classified as to increased destruction or sequestration or decreased production; these disorders are listed in Table 8-2. The antibody-mediated syndromes are discussed in Chap. 9. Nonimmune causes of increased platelet destruction include the DIC syn-dromes, Kasabach-Merritt syndrome, hemolytic uremic syndrome/throm-bocytic thrombocytopenic purpura (HUS-TTP) and hypersplenism. Throm-bocytopenias due to decreased platelet production have a greater role in older children and adults as do the mixed or miscellaneous causes shown in Table 8-2.

DIAGNOSIS OF THROMBOCYTOPENIAS

The clinical context of the occurrence of thrombocytopenia frequently indicates the etiology or mechanism involved. For example, bacterial sepsis, a frequent complication of the ill hospitalized patient, can produce a profound decrease in the platelet count which will rise gradually to normal levels over the ensuing 7 to 10 days under successful treatment. The HUS/TTP syndrome is an easily recognized cause of reduced platelet count (see Chap. 29). The characteristic infection in postinfectious ITP (rubella, varicella, mumps, Epstein-Barr virus, HIV-1) provide a distinctive cause. However, the finding of a bleeding tendency in a patient who has been well and who shows few other symptoms raises a diagnostic problem addressed by the algorithm displayed in Fig. 8-1.

The diagnosis of "isolated thrombocytopenia" is usually made by follow-

TABLE 8-2   Causes of Thrombocytopenia in Children and Adults

Increased platelet destruction and/or sequestration
  Immune thrombocytopenias
    Primary
      ITP, posttransfusion purpura
    Secondary
      Infections: Viral, bacterial, protozoan
      Autoimmune disorders (SLE, Evan's syndrome)
      Lymphoma
      Hodgkin's disease
      Carcinomatosis
      Drugs: Heparin   Cimetidine
          Gold   Digoxin
          Quinidine   Valproic acid
          Quinine α-interferon
          Penicillins
  Nonimmune
    DIC syndromes
    Kasabach-Merritt syndrome
    Hemolytic uremic syndrome
    Thrombotic thrombocytopenic purpura
    Chronic hemolytic anemia and thrombocytopenia
    Congenital or acquired heart disease
    Hypersplenism
    Catheters, protheses, cardiopulmonary bypass
    Familial hemophagocytic reticulosis
Decreased platelet production
  Aplastic anemia, Fanconi's pancytopenia
  Marrow infiltrative processes
    Leukemias
    Metastatic carcinoma
    Myelofibrosis
    Multiple myeloma
    Histiocytoses
    Osteopetrosis
    Infections
  Megakaryocytic thrombocytopenia
    Ethanol abuse
    HIV-1
    Parvovirus infections
    Myelodysplastic syndrome
    Antibody and T-cell suppression
  Nutritional deficiencies
    Iron
    Folate
    B_{12}
  Drug or radiation induced
    Ethanol

TABLE 8-2 *(Continued)*

Phenylbutazone
Chloramphenicol
Chemotherapeutic agents
Paroxysmal nocturnal hemoglobinuria
Cyclic thrombocytopenia (Garcia's disease)
Hereditary thrombocytopenias (see Table 8-4)
Miscellaneous
   Liver disease
   Uremia, renal diseases, renal transplant rejection
   Exchange transfusion, massive transfusions, extracorporeal circulation
   Heat or cold injury
   Thyroid diseases (hyper-, hypo-)
   Fat embolism
   Allogeneic bone marrow transplantation
   Graft-versus-host disease

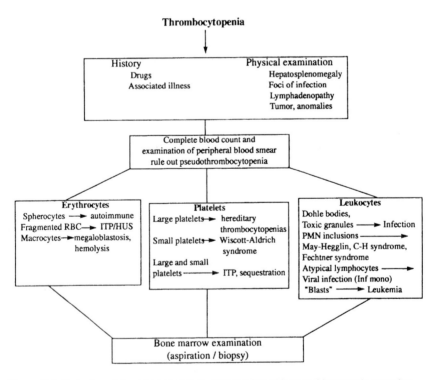

Figure 8-1 Evaluation of thrombocytopenia in child or adult with normal hemostatic screening tests and who is not acutely ill. C-H, Chediak Higashi.

ing a systematic approach using (1) the history (associated illnesses, pharmacologic agents, specific symptoms) and (2) physical examination (anomalies, hepatosplenomegaly, foci of infection, tumor, lymphadenopathy) for overall direction followed by (3) careful interpretation of the complete blood count and examination of the peripheral blood smear for clues to the diagnosis. The complete blood count and blood smear confirm the degree of thrombocytopenia, rule out spuriously decreased platelets, provide clues to associated hematologic disorders and offer an estimation of platelet size (confirmed by Coulter counter mean platelet volume). If the diagnosis is not secure at that point, and frequently it is not, (4) a bone marrow examination including both needle aspiration and biopsy is indicated. Even in children, the marrow biopsy as well as aspiration should be done to accurately estimate cellularity and look for infiltrative disease (tumor cells). In some instances of suspected childhood ITP, the bone marrow examination is deferred or omitted if (1) the history is typical (preceding viral infection in otherwise well child); (2) normal physical examination except bleeding signs; (3) normal blood count and blood smear except low platelets; and most importantly (4) a decision not to treat (particularly with corticosteroids). Watchful waiting without treatment will confirm the diagnosis after recovery in a few weeks. However, if any aspect of the case appears atypical or if specific treatment is planned, a marrow examination should be performed in order not to confound the diagnosis of leukemia or early aplasia.

The use of the bone marrow examination as a guide to the diagnosis is shown in Table 8-3. Although the presence of normal or increased numbers of megakaryocytes may exclude the possibility of decreased platelet production, that conclusion may not be correct when megakaryocyte maturation is impaired.

Fig. 8-1 and Table 8-2 suggest that other tests may be required to confirm a specific diagnosis or mechanism for the thrombocytopenia in addition to the morphology of blood and bone marrow cells. More commonly used adjunctive tests are quantitative immunoglobulins, platelet-associated immunoglobulins (PAIgG), antinuclear antibody (ANA), direct antiglobulin test, monospot test, HIV serology, and lupus anticoagulant (LA) test as well as specific organ-related function tests (renal, hepatic, thyroid). Less commonly, bone marrow chromosome analysis is helpful in the diagnosis of older patients who present with isolated thrombocytopenia (refractory thrombocytopenia, myelodysplastic syndrome).

HEREDITARY THROMBOCYTOPENIAS

The familial occurrence of thrombocytopenia has been reported with increasing frequency. The diagnosis is suspected when the history reveals

TABLE 8-3 Bone Marrow Examination as a Guide to the Etiology of Thrombocytopenia

Decreased Megakarycotes in Normal Marrow	Decreased Megakaryocytes in Abnormal Marrow	Increased or Normal Megakaryocytes in Normal Marrow
Thrombocytopenia with absent radius (TAR)	Aplastic anemia	ITP/SLE
Early Fanconi's syndrome or aplastic anemia	Leukemia, myeloma, tumor	Hypersplenism
Idiopathic megakaryocytic hypoplasia	Myelofibrosis, osteopetrosis Myelodysplasia	Infection (AIDS)
Immune mediated (SLE, AIDS)	Preleukemia	Hereditary thrombocytopenia
	Megaloblastosis	Vascular neoplasms Congenital heart disease

family members with low platelets, the onset of undiagnosed thrombocytopenia in infancy, the detection of giant or tiny platelets on the blood smear, the observation of mild thrombocytopenia with significant bleeding, or during the differential diagnosis of ITP. A classification of hereditary thrombocytopenia is shown in Table 8-4 and is limited to those reported disorders which have characteristic findings allowing differentiation from the others. Platelet size is estimated by both morphologic appearance on blood smears and mean platelet volume by Coulter counter since platelet shape-change defects may produce giant platelets during preparation of the smear (see Milton reference). For example, the diameter of platelets with severe hereditary giant platelet syndromes (Bernard-Soulier syndrome, Montreal platelet syndrome) is considerably larger on blood smears than on phase contrast microscopy of freshly fixed platelets. Overlap between the disorders in Table 8-4 and the hereditary platelet function diseases can be observed (see Chap. 10).

Most of the hereditary thrombocytopenias are characterized by platelet counts of 50,000 to 100,000/μL and are relatively mild or asymptomatic. Exceptions include the following syndromes with severe bleeding manifestations: Wiscott-Aldrich syndrome (see Table 8-4); thrombocytopenia with absent radii (TAR; leukemoid reaction with severe thrombocytopenia in the newborn, tendency for spontaneous remissions), Chediak-Higashi syndrome (storage pool defect in platelets, abnormal leukocyte function, albinism, increased infections), and Bernard-Soulier syndrome.

TABLE 8-4   Hereditary Thrombocytopenias

Disorder	Inheritance	Platelet Function Tests	Other Findings
I. Macrothrombocytes			
Bernard-Soulier syndrome	AR	↓agg to ristocetin BT markedly increased	Decreased membrane GP Ib-IX (V)
Montreal platelet syndrome	AD	↓agg to thrombin; normal agg to ristocetin, ADP, collagen	Normal to reduced GP Ib
May-Hegglin anomaly	AD	Normal	Dohle bodies in leukocytes
Epstein's syndrome Alport's syndrome	AD	Abnormal agg to ADP, collagen	Renal disease, nerve deafness
(Fechtner variant)		Normal	Leukocyte inclusions
(Sebastian variant)		Normal	Leukocyte inclusions; no associated defect
Gray platelet syndrome	Autosomal	Abnormal agg to ADP, collagen thrombin	↓alpha granules; pale-staining platelets and agranular megakaryocytes
Genetic thrombo- cytopenia (Najean- Lecompte)	AD	Normal	Normal microscopy and platelet survival
II. Normothrombocyte			
Thrombocytopenia with absent radius (TAR)	AR	↓agg to L-epi and collagen	↓megakaryocytes; absent radii, normal thumbs; presenta- tion at birth
Chediak-Higashi syndrome	AR	↓agg to L-epi and collagen	Oculocutaneous albinism, recurrent infections, large abnormal granules in leukocytes, macrophages
Hereditary intrinsic platelet defect (Murphy)	AD	Normal	↓platelet survival

TABLE 8-4 *(Continued)*

Disorder	Inheritance	Platelet Function Tests	Other Findings
Familial platelet disorder (Dowton)	AD	Abnormal agg to L-epi and collagen	Hematologic neoplasms; normal GPs
Pseudo-von Willebrand disease	AD	↑agg to ristocetin	↑plt binding of vWf; plt agg with normal plasma; abnormality of GP Ib
III. Microthrombocytes			
Wiskott-Aldrich syndrome	X-linked	Abnormal agg to ADP, collagen thrombin	↓plt survival; eczema, recurrent infections, immune deficiency due to failure of lymphocytes maturation (decreased CD43)

*Classification based on platelet size; bone marrow examination is normal unless noted otherwise. AR, autosomal recessive; AD, autosomal dominant; epi, epinephrine; agg, aggregation; plt, platelet; BT, bleeding time; ADP, adenosine diphosphate; GP, glycoprotein; ↓, decrease; ↑, increase.

RELATIONSHIP OF BLEEDING MANIFESTATIONS TO PLATELET COUNT

The usual manifestations of thrombocytopenic bleeding are petechiae and small ecchymoses, mucous membrane bleeding (epistaxis, gastrointestinal, and menorrhagia), cerebral hemorrhage, and immediate-type bleeding after surgery or trauma. These manifestations are rarely seen if the platelet count is at least 50,000/μL. The level of platelet count that is associated with risk of bleeding in thrombocytopenia is often related to the mechanism of the thrombocytopenia; that is, patients with randomly aged or "old" platelets circulating in conditions such as leukemia or marrow failure (production deficits) or in diseases with a platelet function defect (hereditary or acquired) will display bleeding at a higher platelet count than patients with disorders such as ITP who have a population of rapidly turning over young platelets. This concept was presented by Harker and Slichter in 1972 using the standardized bleeding time (see Fig. 4-1) as an index of bleeding. In many thrombocytopenic conditions, factors other than the level of the platelet count may influence the bleeding tendency. Such factors include platelet function-altering drugs (ASA, antibiotics), intravascular coagulation syndromes, platelet activation or "exhausted platelets" (congenital heart lesions, prosthetic valves), and the coexistence of other hemostatic defects in liver disease and uremia.

MANAGEMENT

Guidelines for management of the immune thrombocytopenias are discussed in Chap. 9. In general, the management for the other thrombocytopenic disorders is treatment or elimination of the underlying cause plus management of the ongoing bleeding manifestations.

The thrombocytopenia of hypersplenism is primarily due to increased platelet pooling in an enlarged spleen of any etiology. A massively enlarged spleen can hold up to 90 percent of the total platelet mass (part of the exchangeable pool). The thrombocytopenia is rarely severe and most patients are asymptomatic. When thrombocytopenic bleeding is of clinical significance and therapy by medical means (antibiotics, chemotherapy, immunosuppression) has been used optimally or the cause of the splenomegaly is unknown, splenectomy should be considered. These conditions include Gaucher's disease, chronic hemolytic disorders, hairy cell leukemia, and rarely lymphoproliferative and myeloproliferative disorders. Partial splenectomy or splenic embolism may be an alternative in children. Splenectomy is also effective in raising the platelet count in Wiscott-Aldrich syndrome but increases the risk of severe infections in these immunocompromised patients.

Specific treatment in acquired pure megakaryocytic thrombocytopenic purpura include management of underlying disorder (ethanol abuse, HIV-1, or parvovirus infection) or immunosuppression (prednisone, intravenous immunoglobulin, cyclophosphamide, cyclosporine, antithymocyte globulin) in the antibody or T cell-mediated disorders. Infants with the TAR syndrome can show spontaneous remission after several months so that comprehensive platelet transfusion support should be planned for that interval.

The management of acute bleeding episodes in nonimmune-mediated thrombocytopenic patients involves the use of platelet concentrate transfusions or intravenous infusions of DDAVP. For therapy of the immune disorders see Chap. 9. Patients with at least $50,000/\mu L$ platelets and who are displaying a bleeding tendency (indicating a platelet function disorder) can be treated with DDAVP except for those hereditary syndromes which have been shown not to respond, for example, Glanzmann's thrombasthenia and Scott syndrome. Other bleeding thrombopenic patients (with counts usually $< 20,000/\mu L$) will require platelet concentrate transfusions. All patients at risk for bleeding should be advised to avoid platelet function inhibiting drugs (ASA, nonsteroidal anti-inflammatory agents, and synthetic penicillins). Patients requiring long-term treatment should be given leukocyte-poor platelet concentrates from limited numbers of donors (apheresis) to decrease alloimmunization (see Chap. 53).

BIBLIOGRAPHY

Bryckaert MC et al: Abnormality of glycoprotein Ib in two cases of "pseudo"-von Willebrand's disease. *J Lab Clin Med* 106:393, 1985.

Castle V et al: Frequency and mechanism of neonatal thrombocytopenia. *J Pediatr* 108:749, 1986.

Dowton SB et al: Studies of a familial platelet disorder. *Blood* 65:557, 1985.

Epstein CJ et al: Hereditary macrothrombocytopathia, nephritis and deafness. *Am J Med* 52:299, 1972.

Greinacher A et al: Sebastian platelet syndrome: A new variant of hereditary macrothrombocytopenia with leukocyte inclusions. *Blut* 61:282, 1990.

Hamilton RW et al: Platelet function, ultrastructure, and survival in the May-Hegglin anomaly. *Am J Clin Pathol* 74:663, 1980.

Hedberg VA, Lipton JM: Thrombocytopenia with absent radii. *Am J Pediatr Hematol Oncol* 10:51, 1988.

Hoffman R: Acquired pure amegakaryocytic thrombocytopenic purpura. *Semin Hematol* 28:303, 1991.

Menke DM et al: Refractory thrombocytopenia. A myelodysplastic syndrome that may mimic ITP. *Am J Clin Pathol* 98:502, 1992.

Milton JG et al: Platelet size and shape in hereditary giant platelet syndromes on blood smear and in suspension: Evidence for two types of abnormalities. *J Lab Clin Med* 106:326, 1985.

Miura M et al: Efficacy of several plasma components in a young boy with chronic thrombocytopenia and hemolytic anemia who responds repeatedly to normal plasma infusions. *Am J Hematol* 17:307, 1984.

Murphy S et al: Hereditary thrombocytopenia with an intrinsic platelet defect. *N Engl J Med* 281:857, 1969.

Najean Y, Lecompte T: Genetic thrombocytopenia with autosomal dominant transmission: A review of 54 cases. *Br J Haematol* 74:203, 1990.

Rodgers RPC, Levin J: A critical reappraisal of the bleeding time. *Semin Thromb Hemost* 16:1, 1990.

Stuart MJ, Kelton JG: The platelet: Quantitative and qualitative abnormalities. In: Nathan DG, Oski FA (eds): *Hematology of Infancy and Childhood*, Philadelphia, Saunders, 1987, chap. 47.

Tomer A et al: Autologous platelet kinetics in patients with severe thrombocytopenia: Discrimination between disorders of production and destruction. *J Lab Clin Med* 118:546, 1991.

Weiss HJ et al: Pseudo-von Willebrand's disease. An intrinsic platelet defect with aggregation by unmodified human factor VIII/von Willebrand factor and enhanced adsorption of its high-molecular-weight multimers. *N Engl J Med* 306:326, 1982.

Immune
Thrombocytopenia

The fact that thrombocytopenia could have a humoral or immunologic basis was established in the 1950s by Harrington and others. At present it is known that IgG and IgM antibodies interact with platelet surface antigens and mediate, with the help of complement activation, macrophage Fc receptor expression, and the reticuloendothelial system (liver, spleen) clearance of platelets. The process produces increased platelet destruction and compensatory increased production usually with variable thrombocytopenia. Immune thrombocytopenia (ITP) includes autoimmune thrombocytopenia with both primary (ITP, adult and childhood) and secondary (systemic lupus erythematosis [SLE], rheumatoid arthritis, thyroid disease, lymphoproliferative diseases, infections, drugs) types, alloimmune thrombocytopenias (post-transfusion purpura and neonatal alloimmune thrombocytopenia, [NAIT]), and platelet transfusion refractoriness.

PLATELET ANTIGENS AND ANTIBODIES

The platelet membrane components that may serve as targets for auto- and alloantibodies include glycoproteins (GP), alloantigens, blood group, and HLA. Autoantibodies (ITP, SLE) are commonly specific for GP IIb-IIIa and other GPs and glycolipids. Alloantibodies associated with NAIT and post-transfusion purpura are specific for platelet alloantigens while refractoriness to platelet transfusions may be associated with both HLA and specific alloantigens found on platelets.

Measurement of Platelet Antibodies

For measurements of platelet antibodies to be clinically useful, several facts must be kept in mind: (1) > 90 percent of platelet IgG is located within the a-granule (acquired by endocytosis of plasma proteins) and is unlikely to be platelet antibody; (2) < 1 percent of total platelet IgG is located on the cell surface and can be platelet antibody. Normal subjects have 5 femtograms or 20,000 molecules of *total* IgG per platelet and only 0.05 femtograms or 200 molecules of platelet *surface* IgG. Measurements of platelet-associated IgG (PAIgG) should give useful estimates of only surface IgG and not be contaminated by total IgG. For this reason, techniques using intact platelets and fluorescent-labeled heterologous or monoclonal anti-immunoglobulin antibodies are the most precise. Specificity is increased even further when antibodies to specific platelet proteins are measured (i.e., anti-GP IIb-IIIa in ITP and anti platelet antibody [PLA-1] in NAIT).

Measurements of total PAIgG are consistently increased in ITP as compared to normal subjects, but total PAIgG is also increased in many nonimmune causes of thrombocytopenia due to platelet destruction. The increase is associated with increased platelet volume (increased platelet turnover) and a greater platelet IgG content. In some infections (HIV-1, for example) patient's platelets may also have elevated levels of complement, IgM, and immune complexes in addition to PAIgG.

IMMUNOLOGIC (AUTOIMMUNE) THROMBOCYTOPENIA

As noted above, the occurrence of platelet autoantibodies causes thrombocytopenia in both secondary (malignancies, infections, SLE, rheumatoid disorders, lymphoproliferative diseases, drugs) and primary (ITP) disorders. ITP is a mild to severe bleeding disorder that can occur at any age (after 3 to 6 months) and is characterized by petechiae, skin and mucous membrane bleeding, menorrhagia, gastrointestinal hemorrhage, and rarely, intracranial bleeding (about 1 percent). Two forms of the disorder are recognized: childhood or acute and adult or chronic (Table 9-1 lists distinguishing characteristics). The childhood type commonly follows viral infections and runs a self-limited course with spontaneous remission in 90 percent of cases within 3 months. The other 10 percent represents the chronic or adult type; this type occurs in adults and children over the age of 8 years and may persist for years.

The diagnosis of ITP is confirmed by exclusion of secondary causes and hereditary thrombocytopenias (see Chap. 8) and confirmation of a normal physical examination without splenomegaly and a normal bone marrow examination. Although not necessary for the diagnosis, demonstration of platelet autoantibodies (anti-GP IIb-IIIa, Ib-IX) may be seen in 75 percent or more of patients (both children and adults) with the chronic type. Activation of the complement system and more severe thrombocytopenia is seen in chronic ITP with GP Ib autoantibodies. PAIgG levels are also elevated but are less helpful in confirmation of diagnosis or prognosis. Greatly elevated

TABLE 9-1 Distinguishing Features of Childhood and Adult-Type Immune Thrombocytopenic Purpura.

	Acute (Childhood)	Chronic (Adult)
Duration of thrombocytopenia	< 6 months (usually several weeks)	> 6 months (often many years)
Onset	Sudden	Insidious
Antecedent or concomitant viral infection	Common	Infrequent
Age incidence	2–8 years (may occur at any age)	All ages (most common in teenages and young adults)
Sex incidence	Males = females	Females > males
Level of PAIgG	Extremely increased	Increased
Associated immunologic abnormalities	Rare	Common (20–30% of patients have positive Coombs' test, positive antinuclear antibody, reduced serum immunoglobulins)
Associated disorders	None	Uncommon (SLE, AIDS)

*Adapted from Buchanan, GR: The nontreatment of childhood idiopathic thrombocytopenic purpura. *Eur J Pediatr* 146:107, 1987.

levels of PAIgG (immune complexes) are seen in immune thrombocytopenia associated with viral infections (childhood type and HIV infection).

Immune Thrombocytopenia in Pregnancy

Pregnant women who have ITP or who have a history of chronic ITP are at risk for delivering an infant with passively acquired thrombocytopenia (platelet count < 50,000 in 10 to 30 percent of cases). IgG platelet antibodies readily cross the placenta and cause immune destruction of fetal platelets. The absence of circulating maternal platelet antibody reduces the risk of fetal thrombocytopenia. Although the correlation between maternal and fetal platelet counts is poor, about half the infants will show a low platelet count especially if the maternal count is < 100,000/μL. However, a normal maternal platelet count can be associated with severe neonatal thrombocytopenia, in particular when the mother has had a previous splenectomy. Interestingly, about 4 to 8 percent of normal women will develop mild thrombocytopenia during uncomplicated pregnancy (pregnancy-associated [PAT] or gestational thrombocytopenia) without a history or other evidence of chronic ITP except for increased mean platelet size and elevated PAIgG. The offspring of women with PAT rarely show thrombocytopenia and no special management considerations are indicated.

Management

Children

No specific treatment is necessary unless the platelet count is < 20,000/μL or the patient displays bleeding manifestations such as severe epistaxis or oral mucosal bleeding ("wet" purpura). Depending on the urgency of the situation, either oral prednisone (2 to 4 mg/kg daily, divided three times a day), intravenous methylprednisolone (30 mg/kg), or intravenous immunoglobulin (IVIG) are given. Maintenance therapy with oral prednisone or repeated doses of IVIG may be used if the platelet count remains < 20,000/μL. Usually no further treatment is indicated after 2 to 3 weeks since the platelet count will begin to rise and in most cases a complete recovery will be seen in 3 to 6 months. If oral prednisone is used, the dose is tapered and stopped after 3 to 4 weeks regardless of the platelet count. Impending or established intracranial hemorrhage may be treated by IVIG plus intravenous methylprednisolone or emergency splenectomy. Platelet concentrate transfusions are usually not indicated except in a seriously bleeding patient until other treatment is effective. The child should avoid platelet function-inhibiting drugs like ASA (antihistamines, glyceryl guaiacolate, acetaminophen are safe to use) and should avoid contact sports or similar activity.

Chronic ITP in children (persistence after 6 to 12 months) is managed essentially the same as in adults with consideration of splenectomy followed by other methods of therapy if needed to control bleeding symptoms. Because of the increased risk of postsplenectomy sepsis, the operation is usually postponed until after the age of 5 years and pneumococcal, H flu B vaccines, and prophylactic antibiotics are employed.

Adult

The goal of therapy of ITP in adults is to induce a long-term (i.e., unmaintained by therapy) remission that results in an adequate but not necessarily normal platelet count. A platelet count of 25,000/μL or higher is not usually associated with bleeding. Corticosteroid therapy is usually the first treatment which consists of oral prednisone, 1 mg/kg per day. Although 40 to 75 percent of patients will respond to steroids initially, only about 15 percent will have a complete remission. The magnitude of response to prednisone correlates with long-term prognosis and if successful will show a rise of platelets within 3 weeks. IVIG may produce good responses initially, but relapses are common and a refractoriness to repeated infusions often occurs.

Splenectomy is the treatment of choice in patients who fail to respond to steroids or to maintain adequate platelet levels after tapering steroids; over 80 percent of patients will have a long-term remission after splenectomy. Responding patients frequently show a good initial response to steroids with a brisk rise in platelets. Only a few patients (< 10 percent in most series) fail to show a satisfactory level of platelets after treatment with steroids, splenectomy, and a period of waiting for spontaneous improvement.

Refractory patients who are having bleeding symptoms with a low platelet count or who are at risk for bleeding (platelet count consistently < 20,000/μL) are candidates for other therapy. The attenuated androgen, danazol (400 to 800 mg/day orally), may produce remissions in refractory cases. For patients failing danazol, cyclophosphamide (3 to 4 mg/kg per day orally for 6 months; slow response), vincristine (2 mg intravenously weekly for weeks; brisk response); colchicine (1.2 to 2.4 mg/day; only 30 percent response), and azathioprine (3 to 6 mg/kg/day orally; slow response, needs maintenance) may be tried. Lasting unmaintained remissions of up to 5 years have been observed in patients treated successfully for a year. Most of these drugs have undesirable side effects and patients should be carefully selected for treatment. In many instances, if the platelet count is at least 10,000/μL and no bleeding is present, it may be best to "watch and wait." IVIG can be used for temporary effect (as in children) for acute bleeding episodes. Relapses may be related to splenic regrowth and can be confirmed by ultrasound excommunications or splenic scan.

Pregnancy

A woman with ITP during pregnancy should be treated with oral prednisone therapy if the platelet count falls below 25,000/μL or a bleeding tendency occurs. Prednisone at a dosage of 1 mg/kg per day in two divided doses is given for 2 weeks, then tapered to the lowest dose to maintain a platelet count of at least 50,000/μL. About 70 percent of patients will show a complete or partial remission. Nonresponders may be given IVIG 400 mg/kg per day times 5 days. Maintenance therapy using a single day's dose can be used at monthly intervals. Splenectomy should be used only as a last resort and done during the second trimester, if necessary, to control severe bleeding.

If the infant's platelet count is determined to be < 50,000/μL by intrauterine cord blood or scalp sampling at time of labor, the most atraumatic form of delivery possible should be used based on degree of risk for fetal thrombocytopenia. A recent review has indicated that of 475 infants born of mothers with ITP, 10 percent were born with moderate thrombocytopenia and 15 percent with severe thrombocytopenia; intracranial hemorrhage occurred in 3 percent and was not affected by mode of delivery. Other studies have shown considerably less neonatal thrombocytopenia and intracranial hemorrhage. Severe maternal bleeding at time of delivery (which rarely occurs) is treated with platelet transfusions, IVIG, and possibly splenectomy.

Platelet count in the infant at time of delivery (cord) and repeated daily (platelet count usually decreases) will indicate how severely the infant is affected. Bleeding manifestations are usually only in those infants with counts < 50,000 or even 20,000/μL. The thrombopenic infants should have ultrasonography or CT scan to determine CNS bleeding. The count will rise slowly to normal levels over 1 to 2 months. If the infant is bleeding, treatment may include one or all of the following: corticosteroids, IVIG, or exchange transfusion followed by random donor platelet transfusion.

Association with Autoimmune Disorders

Autoimmune hemolytic anemia and ITP may occur together (Evan's syndrome) or with neutropenia with or without manifestations of an underlying disease, usually SLE, rheumatoid arthritis, or thyroid disease. Older children and adults with ITP should be considered as candidates for a genetic predisposition to immunoregulatory abnormalities. Basic evaluation should include a careful family history for autoimmune disorders and appropriate screening tests to include Coombs' test, possibly antiplatelet antibodies, and antinuclear antibody test.

Association with HIV Infection

Individuals at risk for AIDS may have an immunologic thrombocytopenia that is clinically indistinguishable from classic ITP. Of interest is the observation that HIV seropositive hemophiliacs show an inverse relationship between platelet count and platelet-bound IgG, presence of antiplatelet 7S IgG in the serum, and platelet eluates containing antiplatelet IgG. These findings are like those in classic ITP while other HIV-positive patients (narcotic addicts, homosexuals) with thrombocytopenia usually have immune complex deposition on platelets. Significant thrombocytopenia in HIV-ITP patients is probably best treated with IVIG for bleeding episodes and zidovudine (AZT) or splenectomy for chronic symptomatic thrombocytopenia (especially in HIV-positive hemophiliacs) while avoiding prednisone in most cases.

DRUG-INDUCED IMMUNE THROMBOCYTOPENIA

A clinical syndrome resembling ITP can occur in susceptible individuals after ingestion of certain drugs. The offending drug (quinidine, quinine, sulfonamides, valproic acid, chlorothiazide) binds to antidrug IgG on the platelet surface resulting in platelet activation and aggregation (Fig. 9-1). One of the

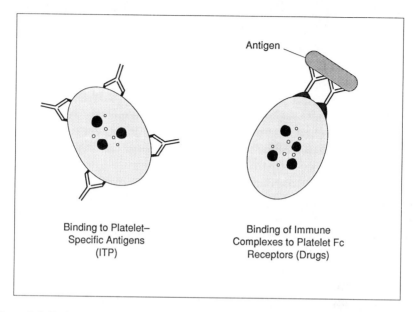

Antigen

Binding to Platelet–
Specific Antigens
(ITP)

Binding of Immune
Complexes to Platelet Fc
Receptors (Drugs)

Figure 9-1 Mechanisms for immune thrombocytopenia in ITP and by drugs. IgG molecules are depicted binding to platelet-specific antigens (GP IIb-IIIa, GP Ib-IX) through the Fab segment in ITP. Also depicted are binding of immune complexes (drugs + antibody; viruses + antibody) to platelet Fc receptors through the IgG Fc segment. Both mechanisms lead to clearance of the platelet by the reticuloendothelial system. (Used with permission from Kelton JG: Hosp Pract June:95, 1985.)

most common drugs to cause thrombocytopenia is heparin, which forms a heparin-antibody immune complex binding to and activating the platelet through the Fc receptors (see Chap. 46).

ALLOIMMUNE THROMBOCYTOPENIA

Neonatal Alloimmune Thrombocytopenia

Neonatal alloimmune thrombocytopenia is the platelet equivalent of Rh hemolytic disease of the newborn. Alloantibodies are produced by the mother to specific fetal platelet antigens (lacking in the mother, present in the fetus and father). The most commonly involved antigen is PLA-1 (Zwa) in 75 percent of cases. Although HLA antigens are involved in platelet sensitization after transfusions, they are probably not a cause of NAIT even though HLA type DR3 (DR$_w$52) is associated with a greater risk of antiplatelet antibody production. The incidence of NAIT is about 1/5000 deliveries.

The neonatal diagnosis of NAIT can be suspected by detection of alloantibodies in (1) a pregnant or previously pregnant woman who has had an affected infant; or (2) is directly related to such a woman; or (3) who is known to be negative for a specific platelet antigen. Optimal serologic evaluation should include determination of platelet alloantigen phenotype of parents and measurement of platelet antibody in the mother. If maternal serum antiplatelet antibody is detected, it should be determined whether it is specific for the platelet antigen involved. Because these assays are difficult, this evaluation is best performed in an experienced reference laboratory. Prenatal detection of thrombocytopenia in the infant has been done by cordocentesis after 20 weeks of gestation. Platelet phenotype of the fetus can be done on nucleated cells from routine amniocentesis with fetal DNA by polymerase chain reaction for Pla or Bak.

In many instances the diagnosis of NAIT is first suspected in a newborn infant (usually term, often firstborn child, and without other obvious causes of thrombocytopenia) who shows evidence of multiple petechiae, skin bleeding or, in up to 20 percent of cases, intracranial hemorrhage (which can occur in utero). A tentative diagnosis of NAIT can be confirmed by later serologic evaluation. An adjunct to clinical diagnosis is the response to platelet transfusions if given. As in autoimmune thrombocytopenia, random donor platelets are short lived (< 12 to 24 h); however, a normal life span of washed maternal platelets is supportive of the diagnosis of NAIT. The differential diagnosis of NAIT versus an infant of a mother with ITP is detailed in Table 9-2. The coincidental association of NAIT with maternal thrombocytopenia (ITP or PAT) has been reported.

Management

Because intracranial hemorrhage may occur antenatally in a high percentage of cases, considerations for intrauterine diagnosis in pregnant women at high risk (especially those with a previously severely affected child and a homozygous father) will often require fetal blood sampling for platelet count and typing. The risk of intrauterine bleeding in seriously thrombocytopenic infants suggests consideration of early intervention, that is, maternal IVIG, in utero platelet transfusion near term, elective cesarean-section at 34 to 36 weeks, or a combination of these strategies.

Treatment of the newborn infant who has a platelet count $< 25,000/\mu L$ or shows any evidence of CNS bleeding by ultrasonography includes IVIG or washed maternal platelet transfusion (or specific platelet antigen negative platelets).

Posttransfusion Purpura

Another platelet alloimmunization syndrome is the rare disorder called posttransfusion purpura which often presents as severe thrombocytopenic

TABLE 9-2 Differential Diagnosis of Antibody-Induced Thrombocytopenia in the Newborn Infant

| Category | Antibodies | Platelets Decreased in Mother | Maternal Platelet-Associated IgG | | Survival of Transfused Platelets in Infant | |
			Serum	Platelets	Random Donor	Maternal Donor
Passive transfer of maternal platelet antibodies to baby (ITP, SLE)	Auto-antibodies to GP-IIb-IIIa Ib-IX, etc.	Usually (can have normal platelet count)	Increased	Increased	Decreased	Decreased
Active formation of allo-antibodies in mother with transfer to baby	Antibodies to PLA[-1] or Zw[a], Br, Bak, Ko, Duzo, etc.	No	Increased	Normal	Decreased	Normal

bleeding about 1 week after exposure to a blood product. The patient, frequently a woman with a history of pregnancy, has been sensitized previously to a platelet alloantigen (usually PLA-1) which is lacking on her platelets. A proposed mechanism is that the transfused antigen (PLA-1) may interact with the antiplatelet antibody (anti-PLA-1) to form an immune complex which binds to the autologous platelets (FcR receptor) which lack PLA-1 thus producing thrombocytopenia. Predisposing factors include HLA-DR3 positivity and increased amounts of PAIgG on the patient's platelets. The thrombocytopenic bleeding may be exceedingly serious and even life-threatening (CNS hemorrhage) and can persist for several days. The recommended treatment is IVIG and corticosteroids or plasmapheresis. Platelet concentrate transfusions are contraindicated.

Platelet Refractoriness

The most common alloimmunization syndrome is the failure to achieve adequate platelet increments in multiply transfused thrombocytopenic patients. These patients may have increased levels of detectable HLA or platelet alloantibodies. Platelet refractoriness due to alloimmunization after random donor platelet transfusions is most often due to incompatibilities in the HLA system; however, 20 to 35 percent of alloimmunized patients do not respond even to fully HLA-matched platelets. To identify platelet alloimmunization, antiplatelet or lymphocytotoxic antibodies must be demonstrated.

Some measures to prevent platelet refractoriness are based on following strict indications for platelet transfusions, limiting the number of transfusions, limiting the number of donors (single donor, apheresis), using leukocyte-poor blood products (to decrease class II HLA antigen), and using UV-irradiated donor platelets (to limit antigen presenting cell function; see Chap. 53).

BIBLIOGRAPHY

Brannan DP, Guthrie TH: Idiopathic thrombocytopenic purpura in adults. *South Med J* 81:75, 1988.

Burrows RF, Kelton JG: Incidentally detected thrombocytopenia in healthy mothers and their infants. *N Engl J* Med 319:142, 1988.

Bussel J, Kaplan C, McFarland J, and the working party on neonatal immune thrombocytopenia of the Neonatal Hemostasis Subcommittee of the Scientific and Standardization Committee of the ISTH: Recommendations for the evaluation and treatment of neonatal autoimmune and alloimmune thrombocytopenia. *Thromb Haemost* 65:631, 1991.

Cook RL et al: Immune thrombocytopenic purpura in pregnancy: A reappraisal of management. *Obstet Gynecol* 78:578, 1991.

Donner M et al: Platelet surface-bound IgG and platelet-specific IgG in plasma in childhood thrombocytopenia. *Acta Paediatr Scand* 79:328, 1990.

Eden OB et al: Guidelines for management of idiopathic thrombocytopenic purpura. *Arch Dis Childh* 67:1056, 1992.

George JN: Platelet IgG: Measurement, interpretation, and clinical significance. *Prog Hemost Thromb* 10:97, 1991.

Imbach P et al: Different forms of chronic childhood thrombocytopenic purpura defined by antiplatelet autoantibodies. *J Pediatr* 118:535, 1991.

Karpartkin S: HIV-1 related thrombocytopenia. *Hematol Oncol Clin North Am* 4:193, 1990.

Lippman SM et al: Genetic factors predisposing to autoimmune diseases. Autoimmune hemolytic anemia, chronic thrombocytopenic purpura, and systemic lupus erythematosus. *Am J Med* 73:827, 1982.

McCrae KR et al: Pregnancy associated thrombocytopenia: Pathogenesis and management. *Blood* 80:2697, 1992.

McMillan R et al: Platelet-associated and plasma anti-glycoprotein autoantibodies in chronic ITP. *Blood* 70:1040, 1987.

Nugent DJ: Alloimmunization to platelet antigens. *Semin Hematol* 29:83, 1991.

Pietz J et al: High-dose intravenous gamma globulin for neonatal alloimmune thrombocytopenia in twins. *Acta Pediatr Scand* 80:129, 1991.

Schreiber AD et al: Effect of danazol in immune thrombocytopenic purpura. *N Engl J Med* 316:503, 1987.

Wang WC: Evans syndrome in childhood: Pathophysiology, clinical course, and treatment. *Am J Pediatr Hematol Oncol* 10:330, 1988.

Hereditary Platelet
Function Defects

As one reviews the structure-function relationships of platelet-vessel inter-action (Fig. 1.2), it is apparent that there are many opportunities for defects to occur, resulting in abnormal platelet plug formation and prolonged bleed-ing. A few of these genetic defects have been characterized and are associated with specific disorders of platelet function (Table 10-1). For example, a deficiency (protein amount or function) of platelet membrane glycoprotein (GP) Ib-IX results in an adhesion disorder called Bernard-Soulier syndrome (BSS); a deficiency of membrane GP IIb-IIIa causes an aggregation abnor-mality, Glanzmann's thrombasthenia; defects in specific platelet agonist receptors such as the collagen receptor may produce platelets which cannot be optimally activated and a bleeding disorder; platelet secretion disorders include signal-processing defects and storage pool deficiency syndromes due to decreased or absent dense bodies, a-granules, or both; functional defects in secretion or release are also due to specific abnormalities in the prosta-glandin pathway (cyclooxygenase deficiency, thromboxane synthetase defi-ciency); syndromes with specific deficiencies in the platelet contribution to prothrombinase activity occur. Specific deficiencies in plasma adhesive pro-teins such as fibrinogen and von Willebrand factor, are also causes of defec-tive platelet plug formation.

CLINICAL MANIFESTATIONS

Patients with hereditary platelet function defects (PFDs) display hemor-rhagic patterns much like thrombocytopenic bleeding, that is, skin and mu-cous membrane bleeding (petechiae, ecchymoses), recurrent epistaxis, gas-trointestinal hemorrhage, menorrhagia, and immediate-type bleeding after trauma and surgical procedures. Intracranial bleeding is rare; neonatal pur-pura may occur; joint and muscle bleeding is distinctly uncommon. Bleeding manifestations may be severe or mild depending on the defect. Although

TABLE 10-1 Hereditary Platelet Function Disorders

Disorder	Heredity	Platelet Morphology	Platelet aggregation				
			L-epi	ADP	Collagen	Ristocetin	AA
Glanzmann's thrombasthenia	AR	Normal	−	−	−	+	−
Bernard-Soulier syndrome	AR	Giant platelets thrombocytopenia	+	+	+	−	+
Pseudo von Willebrand disease	AD	Normal (thrombocytopenia)	+	+	+	Increased	?
Storage pool defects:							
Dense body deficiency	AR	Decreased, absent dense bodies	−	+/−	−	+/−	+/−
α-granule deficiency (gray platelet syndrome)	AR	Large platelets Decreased α-granules	+	+/−	+/−	+	+
Mixed-α + dense body deficiency	AD	Decreased α- and dense granules	+/−	+/−	−	+/−	+/−
Secretion defects (failure to release)	Variable	Normal	−	+/−	−	+/−	−
Scott syndrome (PF3 deficiency)	AR	Normal	+	+	+	+	+

(Continued on next page)

TABLE 10-1 Hereditary Platelet Function Disorders (*Continued*)

Disorder	Heredity	Platelet Morphology	Platelet aggregation				
			L-epi	ADP	Collagen	Ristocetin	AA
Platelet factor V deficiency (Factor V Quebec)	AD	Normal thrombocytopenia			"Normal"		
Familial α_2-adrenergic receptor defect	AD	Normal	−	+	+	+	+
Isolated collagen aggregation defect	?	Normal	+	+	−	+	+

Disorder	Specific defects
Glanzmann's thrombasthenia	Variable deficiency of GP IIb-IIa; platelet fibrinogen
Bernard-Soulier syndrome	GP Ib-IX complex deficiency
Pseudo von Willebrand disease	Intrinsic GP Ib defect; increased binding of von Willebrand factor
Storage pool defects:	
(a) Dense body deficiency	Decreased thrombin release of ADP and serotonin; Decreased dense bodies
(b) α-granule deficiency (Gray platelet syndrome)	Decreased α-granules and contents
(c) Mixed α-granule-dense body deficiency	Decreased α-granules and dense bodies

Secretion defects (failure to release)

Cyclooxygenase deficiency
Thromboxane synthetase deficiency
Impaired release of AA
Defects in phosphotidylinositol metabolism
Defects in calcium mobilization

Scott syndrome

Impaired response to thromboxane A_2
Decreased platelet prothrombinase and tenase activity; impaired membrane microvesicle formation

Platelet factor V deficiency (Factor V Quebec)

Qualitative platelet factor V deficiency; decreased platelet prothrombinase activity

Familal a_2-adrenergic receptor defect
Isolated collagen aggregation defect

a_2-Receptor deficiency
GP Ia-IIa deficiency

*L-epi, L-epinephrine; AA, arachidonic acid; −, absent or decreased; +, present, normal; +/−, variable, slight increase; AR, autosomal recessive; AD, autosomal dominant; ADP, adenosine diphosphate; PF, platelet factor; GP, glycoprotein.

exceptions are known, the more severe the specific defect, the worse the bleeding tendency; that is, severe bleeders with thrombasthenia (type I) have < 10 percent platelet GP IIb-IIIa, whereas type II patients (about 30 percent GP) are less severe. A similar pattern is observed in BSS. A moderately severe bleeding tendency is observed in the Hermansky-Pudlak syndrome (oculocutaneous albinism in association with dense body deficiency in the platelets). In our experience the majority of patients with inherited platelet function defects fall into the secretion defect category (storage pool defects and failure-to-release disorders) and have mild bleeding tendencies.

LABORATORY MANIFESTATIONS

The major laboratory indicator of a PFD is a prolonged bleeding time despite a normal platelet count (a few disorders are associated with decreased platelets) in patients in whom von Willebrand disease has been eliminated. Mild to moderate thrombocytopenia is common in BSS and in the other hereditary thrombocytopenias which may also have associated PFDs (see Chap. 8). Bleeding time may be normal or slightly prolonged in some mild bleeders but usually becomes greatly prolonged after aspirin. Since the mid 1960s, platelet aggregation testing has been the mainstay of the procedures used to diagnose and classify the hereditary PFDs. With careful attention to technical details, the aggregation curves produced by various agonists (L-epinephrine, adenosine diphosphate [ADP], collagen, ristocetin, arachidonic acid) when added to platelet-rich plasma, provides sensitive detection of most disorders. The pattern of the abnormalities in the aggregation curves can be used to tentatively classify the PFD (see Fig. 10-1). More detailed or confirmatory procedures are necessary to identify the specific defect (see Table 10-1). Commonly used tests for PFDs are listed in Table 10-2.

THROMBASTHENIA

Measurements of platelet membrane GPs by immunochemical (Western blotting) or antibody binding techniques (flow cytometry) are necessary to confirm the diagnosis of BSS and Glanzmann's thrombasthenia. In thrombasthenia, platelet aggregation (binding of adjacent platelets to each other through linking bonds: activated GP IIb-IIIa receptors to fibrinogen) is defective although platelets may be agglutinated by ristocetin. Clot retraction is lacking (loss of binding receptors for radiating fibrin strands) in type I patients but only mildly defective or normal in type II patients. The functional importance of the GP IIb-IIIa receptor is underscored by the fact that type I patients have absent to barely detectable amounts of GP

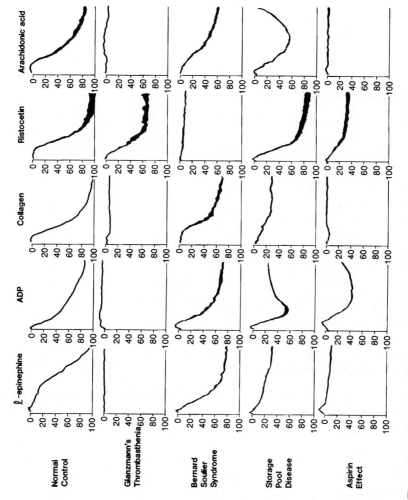

Figure 10-1 Platelet aggregation curves for various agonists. Platelet-rich plasma from a normal adult and patients with designated platelet function disorders are shown.

TABLE 10-2 Laboratory Tests Used for Evaluation of Platelet Function

Preliminary Tests
    Platelet count
    Bleeding time
    Platelet aggregation tests (Fig. 10-1)
    Prothrombin consumption
Confirmatory Tests
    Glycoprotein Ib-IX, IIB-IIIa determination
    Electron microscopy
    Thromboxane synthetase, cyclooxygenase determinations
    Platelet ADP, ATP content
    Platelet-rich plasma aggregation to ristocetin and cryoprecipitate

IIb-IIIa complexes and absent platelet fibrinogen while in type II patients GP IIb-IIIa is present in subnormal amounts (15 percent) with low but detectable platelet fibrinogen. Thrombasthenia is inherited in an autosomal recessive manner; as expected, heterozygote patients have 50 to 60 percent of IIb-IIIa complexes and are asymptomatic. The laboratory heterogeneity of the homozygous disease is illustrated by studies of Iraqi Jews and Arab patients who both have severe disease and marked IIb-IIIa complex deficiency but can be differentiated by platelet vitronectin receptor expression (Iraqi-Jewish patients have no detectable GP IIIa and decreased vitronectin receptors. Arab patients express small amounts of GP IIIa and normal vitronectin receptors).

BERNARD-SOULIER SYNDROME

Bernard-Soulier syndrome is an autosomal recessively inherited bleeding disorder characterized by mild thrombocytopenia, giant platelets and a deficiency of platelet GP Ib-IX complex. The physiologic defect is decreased platelet adhesion to subendothelium via binding to von Willebrand factor. Platelet aggregation is normal except for agglutination by ristocetin. Dysfunctional variants of BSS including reduced amounts of sialic acid on the GP receptor have been described. Heterozygotes show intermediate levels of GP Ib-IX and some large platelets but are asymptomatic.

STORAGE POOL DEFECTS

Determination of storage pool organelles by electron microscopy and measurement of platelet nucleotides and serotonin (dense granules) or β-

thromboglobulin and platelet factor 4 (a-granules) and their releasability allows confirmation of the storage pool defects. Dense body storage pool defect has been described in other inherited disorders such as Hermansky-Pudlak syndrome, Wiscott-Aldrich syndrome, Chediak-Higashi syndrome, and thrombocytopenia with absent radii (TAR) syndrome. In a few instances storage pool defects have been associated with decreased nucleotide (ADP, adenosine triphosphate [ATP]) storage or release without producing abnormal platelet aggregation curves.

OTHER PLATELET FUNCTION DISORDERS

Platelet aggregation tests may provide leads to diagnosis of other PFD. A familial impaired aggregation only to L-epinephrine has been associated with decreased a_2-adrenergic receptors (easy bruising and minimally prolonged bleeding time). Isolated impairment in responsiveness to epinephrine may be an inherited defect but is probably associated with few bleeding manifestations. An isolated receptor defect to collagen is associated with abnormal aggregation to collagen but normal responses to ADP, thrombin, and other agonists; the patient with this defect was a bleeder and had decreased platelet GP Ia. Similarly, a recently described congenital PFD is characterized by selective impairment of platelet responses to ADP possibly by decreased numbers of ADP receptors. A platelet secretion defect (normal platelet aggregation to usual agonists but impaired to thrombin and A23187, a calcium ionophore) is seen in patients with the attention deficit disorder and easy bruising. Since there are many acquired causes of abnormal platelet aggregation in normal individuals (drugs, infections; see Chap. 11), a final diagnosis of a specific PFD should be held until repeat aggregation testing and confirmatory tests can be obtained.

MANAGEMENT

Acute bleeding episodes in hereditary PFD can usually be managed with DDAVP infusions in all of the defects except thrombasthenia, Scott's syndrome, and the occasional severe form of BSS. For these latter disorders, if local measures do not secure hemostasis, platelet concentrate transfusions (as if the patient is thrombocytopenic) can be used. In some instances, thrombasthenic patients have developed antibodies against normal IIb and IIIa following transfusion. Alloimmunization against HLA antigens or platelet-specific antigens (PLA-1) also occurs and may be decreased by use of platelet matched donors when feasible. Adjunctive therapy with ε-aminocaproic acid is worth trying in mucous membrane bleeding. Corticosteroids may have a role in the preoperative shortening of the prolonged bleeding time in patients with storage pool or secretion type defects (see Miekle reference).

BIBLIOGRAPHY

Cattaneo M et al: Identification of a new congenital defect of platelet function characterized by severe impairment of platelet responses to adenosine diphosphate. *Blood* 80:2787, 1992.

Coller BS et al: Platelet vitronectin receptor expression differentiates Iraqi-Jewish from Arab patients with Glanzmann thrombasthenia in Israel. *Blood* 77:75, 1991.

George JN et al: Glanzmann's thrombasthenia: The spectrum of clinical disease. *Blood* 75:1383, 1990.

Gerrard JM et al: Biochemical studies of two patients with the gray platelet syndrome. *J Clin Invest* 66:102, 1980.

Hardisty RM et al: A new congenital defect of platelet secretion: Impaired responsiveness of the platelets to cytoplasmic free calcium. *Br J Haematol* 53:543, 1983.

Hardisty R et al: A defect of platelet aggregation associated with an abnormal distribution of glycoprotein IIb-IIIa complexed within the platelet: The cause of a lifelong bleeding disorder. *Blood* 80:696, 1992.

Horellou MH et al: Familial and constitutional bleeding disorder due to platelet cyclo-oxygenase deficiency. *Am J Hematol* 14:1, 1983.

Koike K et al: Platelet secretion defect in patients with the attention deficit disorder and easy bruising. *Blood* 63:427, 1984.

Miekle CH Jr et al: Preoperative prednisone therapy in platelet function disorders. *Thromb Res* 21:655, 1981.

Montgomery RR et al: Diagnosis of Bernard-Soulier syndrome and Glanzmann's thrombasthenia with a monoclonal assay on whole blood. *J Clin Invest* 71:385, 1983.

Rao AK et al: Differential requirements for platelet aggregation and inhibition of adenylate cyclase by epinephrine. Studies of a familial platelet alpha 2-adrenergic receptor defect. *Blood* 71:494, 1988.

Rao AK: Congenital disorders of platelet function . *Hematol Oncol Clin North Am* 4:65, 1990.

Sims PJ et al: Assembly of the platelet prothrombinase complex is linked to vesiculation of the platelet plasma membrane. Studies in Scott syndrome: An isolated defect in platelet procoagulant activity. *J Biol Chem* 264:17049, 1989.

Tracy PB et al: Factor V (Quebec): A bleeding diathesis associated with a qualitative platelet factor V deficiency. *J Clin Invest* 74:1221, 1984.

Weiss HJ et al: Isolated deficiency of platelet procoagulant activity. *Am J Med* 67:206, 1979.

Weiss HJ et al: Heterogeneity in storage pool deficiency: Studies on granule-bound substances in 18 patients including variants deficient in α-granules, platelet factor 4, β-thromboglobulin, and platelet-derived growth factor. *Blood* 54:1296, 1979.

Acquired Platelet

Function Disorders

Acquired abnormalities in the platelet, the blood vessels, the plasma milieu, and blood flow may produce deranged platelet-vessel interaction and platelet plug formation resulting in prolonged bleeding and or excessive platelet consumption and microthrombosis. The platelet function disorders (PFD) which are primarily associated with a hemorrhagic tendency are discussed here and are listed in Table 11-1.

TABLE 11-1 Acquired Platelet Function Disorders* by Proposed Mechanism or Cause

Exhausted (Storage Pool deficiency) Platelets
    Valvular heart disease (congenital, acquired)
    After cardiopulmonary bypass
    Renal allograft rejection
    Cavernous hemangioma
    Aortic aneurysm
    Transfusion reaction
    HUS, TTP, glomerulonephritis
    DIC, thrombosis
    Thermal injury
    Sickle cell anemia
    Massive splenomegaly
Activated Platelets
    Coronary artery disease
    Peripheral vascular disease
    Stroke
Antiplatelet Antibodies (IgG, IgM)
    Autoimmune disorders (ITP, SLE)
    Multiple myeloma, dysproteinemias
    Acquired platelet dysfunction with eosinophilia
Increased Fibrin-Fibrinogen Degradation Products
    Arvin, fibrinolytic therapy

TABLE 11-1 *(Continued)*

Cirrhosis
DIC
Infections
    Infectious mononucleosis
    HIV
    Septicemia
Deficiency States
    Vitamin B_{12} deficiency
    Vitamin E deficiency
    Zinc deficiency
Other Diseases
    Uremia
    Glycogen storage diseases
    Leukemia, preleukemia, myeloproliferative disorders
    Thalassemias
    Agammaglobulinemia
    Connective tissue disorders

---

*Defined as conditions with abnormal platelet aggregations (usually with prolonged bleeding time and/or clinical bleeding).
DIC, disseminated intravascular coagulation; HIV, human immunodeficiency virus; HUS, hemolytic-uremic syndrome; ITP, immune thrombocytopenic purpura; SLE, systemic lupus erythematosus; TTP, thrombotic thrombocytopenic purpura.

EXHAUSTED PLATELETS

In many PFD, disturbed platelet-vessel interaction occurs, causing activation, perturbation of membrane and release of storage pool material, and frequently consumption of the platelet. These disorders, called *platelet exhaustion* or *acquired storage pool deficiency*, are sometimes associated with evidence for consumption or change in the soluble clotting factors (fibrinogen, von Willebrand factor) and may result in prolonged bleeding time and abnormal platelet aggregation tests. Common examples include hairy cell leukemia, valvular heart disease (congenital and acquired), vascular malformations, foreign surface interactions (cardiopulmonary bypass), abnormal small vessels (renal diseases), and small vessel thrombosis (hemolytic uremic syndrome, thrombotic thrombocytopenic purpura). Evidence for platelet activation is also seen in atherosclerotic disorders.

    Evidence for activated or exhausted platelets in various clinical syndromes have been provided by three general methods: (1) platelet aggregation studies using subthreshold doses of agonists to detect activated platelets in hypercoagulable vascular disorders (increased platelet aggregation) or standard dose agonists to detect exhausted platelets (decreased platelet aggregation of the storage pool deficit pattern); (2) measurement of plasma levels of substances such as β-thromboglobulin, platelet factor 4 (PF4), thromboxane B_2 or thrombospondin to indirectly indicate platelet activation and release. Typically, following in vivo activation, there is a substantial increase in plasma β-thromboglobulin with a small increase in plasma PF4 resulting in an increased β-thromboglobulin/PF4 ratio; (3) detection of activation-induced platelet surface changes by use of monoclonal antibodies to activated receptors or granule content proteins (glycoprotein [GP] IIb-IIIa, guanosine monophosphate-140, or P-selectin, thrombospondin, Va) expressed on the activated platelet but absent from the resting platelet in a flow cytometry system. This latter technique shows promise in evaluation of platelet dysfunction (hereditary, acquired) as well as detection of activated platelets in the circulation (see reference by Abrams and Shattil).

ABNORMAL PROTEIN BINDING

Other acquired abnormalities are due to abnormal protein binding to the platelet (IgM or IgG antibodies, myeloma proteins, Waldenstrom's macroglobulins, fibrin degradation products [FDP]). Sometimes specific functional abnormalities related to membrane GP Ib or GP IIb-IIIa have been demonstrated relating the disease mechanism to the hereditary defects (Bernard-Soulier syndrome, thrombasthenia). Abnormalities of platelet function occur in infections (viral and bacterial), systemic lupus erythematosus, and hemophilia and may be related to direct platelet damage or platelet interaction with IgG or antigen-antibody complexes.

OTHER SYSTEMIC DISORDERS

Other systemic disorders that affect platelet function include uremia, glycogen storage disease, liver diseases, and myeloid disorders. A prolonged bleeding time and a tendency to clinical bleeding are frequently noted in chronic renal failure patients with uremia. Although the bleeding time prolongation correlates with the severity of renal failure, the bleeding time is a poor predictor of clinical bleeding. Patients with severe anemia of chronic renal failure frequently show a prolonged bleeding time, which improves on correction of the anemia. Platelet aggregation defects are variably present and persist in patients who are no longer anemic. The cause of the platelet dysfunction is probably multifactorial; possible mechanisms are noted in Chap. 28. Improvement in platelet function after dialysis suggests removal of a "toxic" material (urea, guanidinosuccinic or phenolic acids). The clinical significance of the platelet function deficit is unclear; invasive (renal biopsies) procedures rarely are associated with excess bleeding.

Glycogen storage diseases type Ia and Ib are associated with a mild bleeding tendency (epistaxis, mucosal bleeding) and abnormal platelet functions (increased bleeding time and decreased aggregations to collagen and adenosine diphosphate [ADP]; low von Willebrand factor in some patients). The defect is acquired since effective therapy with hyperalimentation or portacaval shunt results in correction of the platelet dysfunction.

The bleeding in the myeloproliferative disorders can be associated with hypoaggregability and a prolonged bleeding time (see Chap. 34). Qualitative platelet abnormalities include abnormal morphology, acquired storage pool defects, platelet glycoprotein abnormalities, receptor defects (a-adrenergic, Fc, prostaglandin D_2 receptors), and abnormal arachidonic acid metabolism.

DRUG-INDUCED PLATELET DYSFUNCTION

The major classes of drugs associated with abnormal platelet function are anti-inflammatory agents, antibiotics, and anticoagulants (Table 11-2). The

TABLE 11-2 Pharmacologic and other Substances Affecting Platelet Function (Abnormal Platelet Aggregation, Increased Bleeding Time, and/or Clinical Bleeding)

Agent	Mechanism	Result
Acetylsalicylic acid (aspirin)	Cyclooxygenase inhibitor	Bleeding time prolonged, clinical bleeding
Nonsteroid anti-inflammatory agents: (Ibuprofen, indomethacin, Naproxen, Diclofenac)	Prostaglandin synthesis inhibition	Bleeding time prolonged, rare clinical bleeding
β-Lactam antibiotics: (penicillin G, ampicillin, nafcillin, carbenicillin, ticarcillin, cephalosporins)	Platelet membrane binding; alteration of agonist receptors	Bleeding time prolonged, clinical bleeding
Hemostatics, antithrombotics: (ε-amino caproic acid, dextran, ticlopidine)	Membrane binding Decreased GP IIb-IIIa receptor function	Clinical bleeding Increased bleeding time
Others: (Halothane, propranolol, nitroglycerin, quinidine, ethanol, sodium valproate)		Increased bleeding time

cyclooxygenase inhibitors, of which ASA is the major example, interfere with the formation of thromboxane A_2 (a potent aggregator of platelets and vasoconstrictor) in the prostaglandin pathway of the platelet (Fig. 1-3) and inhibit the release reaction by ADP and collagen in vitro. Aspirin acts by irreversibly acetylating a serine residue at the active site of the cyclooxygenase. Other nonsteroidal anti-inflammatory drugs are reversible inhibitors. Aspirin prolongs the bleeding time in normal subjects by a mean of 4 min but has a much greater effect in subjects who already have a bleeding tendency such as von Willebrand disease, PFD, or hemophilia. The effect on bleeding time in normal subjects of as little as 1 to 2 mg/kg of ASA is noted in 2 h after oral ingestion and lasts for 2 to 4 days or up to 10 days for platelet aggregation tests. A few subjects are "hyperresponders" and prolong their bleeding time up to 11 min. The duration of effect is much less with the reversible inhibitors (6 to 24 h). In contrast, the β-lactam antibiotics are dose dependent in vivo and require high and sustained doses (up to 48 h) to achieve maximal effect on bleeding time and platelet aggregation, which can also last 7 to 10 days. Clinical bleeding (easy bruising, epistaxis, hematomas, postsurgical hemorrhage) is seen most often in patients with underlying bleeding disorders who are given these major drugs (ASA, anti-inflammatory agents, antibiotics, anticoagulants), but an occasional "hyperresponder" (no underlying defect) will display clinical bleeding after these drugs.

Many drugs such as antihistamines, local anesthetics, β-blockers, antihypertensives, and others may have an in vitro effect on platelet aggregation tests without significant effect on the bleeding time. Of commonly used drugs such as glyceryl guaiacolate, diphenhydramine, chlorpromazine, pseudoephedrine, and acetaminophen, only indomethacin and aspirin have an effect on bleeding time after oral administration. Nevertheless, when diagnostic platelet function tests are performed, the subject should be off all medications (including over-the-counter drugs, such as Alka Seltzer, which contain aspirin) and free of recent viral infections for at least 7 to 10 days (viral infections like Epstein-Barr virus may have a longer effect).

MANAGEMENT

The management of the bleeding diathesis associated with acquired PFD is related to treatment of the underlying disorder. In most instances the bleeding disorder is mild and rarely requires specific treatment or prophylaxis with platelet transfusions or DDAVP. Removal of the offending drug is usually all that is necessary in drug-related PFD. Treatment modalities used in uremia (usually to decrease the bleeding time) are dialysis, cryoprecipitate infusions or DDAVP infusion, and red blood cell transfusions or recombinant erythropoietin to correct the anemia. Recombinant erythropoitin frequently corrects the anemia and the coexisting (or secondary) bleeding time defect (see Chap. 28). DDAVP infusion has been used to correct the bleeding time or bleeding tendency in glycogen storage disease and myeloproliferative disorders.

BIBLIOGRAPHY

Abrams C, Shattil SJ: Immunologic detection of activated platelets in clinical disorders. *Thromb Haemost* 65:467, 1991.

Bick RL: Platelet function defects: A clinical review. *Semin Thromb Hemost* 18:167, 1992.

Buchanan GR et al: The effects of "anti-platelet" drugs on bleeding time and platelet aggregation in normal human subjects. *Am J Clin Pediatr* 68:355, 1977.

Burroughs SF, Johnson GJ: β-Lactam antibiotic-induced platelet dysfunction: Evidence for irreversible inhibition of platelet activation in vitro and in vivo after prolonged exposure to penicillin. *Blood* 75:1473, 1990.

Di Minno G et al: A myeloma paraprotein with specificity for platelet glycoprotein IIIa in a patient with a fatal bleeding disorder. *J Clin Invest* 77:157, 1986.

Fiore LD et al: The bleeding time response to aspirin. *Am J Clin Pathol* 94:292, 1990.

George JN, Shattil SJ: The clinical importance of acquired abnormalities of platelet function. *N Engl J Med* 324:27, 1991.

Kaplan KL: β-Thromboglobulin. *Prog Hemost Thromb* 5:153, 1980.

Marti GE et al: DDAVP infusion in five patients with type Ia glycogen storage disease and associated correction of prolonged bleeding times. *Blood* 68:180, 1986.

McLeod LJ et al: The effects of different doses of some acetylsalicylic acid formulations on platelet function and bleeding times in healthy subjects. *Scand J Haematol* 36:379, 1986.

Pareti FI et al: Acquired dysfunction due to the circulation of "exhausted" platelets. *Am J Med* 69:235, 1980.

Schafer AI: Bleeding and thrombosis in the myeloproliferative disorders. *Blood* 64:1, 1984.

Stricker RB et al: Acquired Bernard-Soulier syndrome. Evidence for the role of a 210,000-molecular weight protein in the interaction of platelets with von Willebrand factor. *J Clin Invest* 76:1274, 1985.

Suvatte V et al: Acquired platelet dysfunction with eosinophilia; study of platelet function in 62 cases. *Southeast Asian J Trop Med Public Health* 10:358, 1979.

Wenger RK et al: Loss of platelet fibrinogen receptors during clinical cardiopulmonary bypass. *J Thorac Cardiovasc Surg* 97:235, 1989.

Hereditary

---

von Willebrand

Disease

A bleeding disorder characterized by predominately mucous membrane hemorrhage (epistaxis, gastrointestinal, menorrhagia) of varying severity occurring in both males and females was investigated in a large family in the Åland Islands in 1924 by Erik von Willebrand. This genetic disorder, now known to be the most common, is called von Willebrand disease and has been extensively investigated; the pathogenesis is caused by a quantitative or qualitative deficiency of a large glycoprotein called von Willebrand factor (vWf).

vWf (present in plasma as a series of disulfide-bonded polymers of 220 kd) is synthesized in endothelial cells where it is stored in the Weibel-Palade bodies as polymers of 0.5 to 20 million d, and in megakaryocytes where it is stored in the a-granules of platelets. The gene encoding for vWf is located on chromosome 12, producing a protein of 2813 amino acid residues, pre-pro-vWf. During processing (removal of signal peptide, glycosylation), a large polypeptide (741 residues) is cleaved. This cleaved pro-polypeptide is found in the platelet a-granules and was formerly called von Willebrand antigen II (function unknown). The mature vWf subunit of 2050 residues is assembled into multimers (polymers). The larger multimers are required for normal biologic function probably because of increased numbers of ligand-binding sites and the physical properties of extended polymers during high shear in the microcirculation.

Many of the other functions of vWf have been localized to discrete regions of the subunit. Binding sites for collagen and heparin coincide with the sites for platelet glycoprotein (GP) Ib binding; discrete segments of domain A1 also mediate ristocetin-induced vWf binding to platelets (similar binding is induced by the venom protein, botrocetin, at a different site). A second

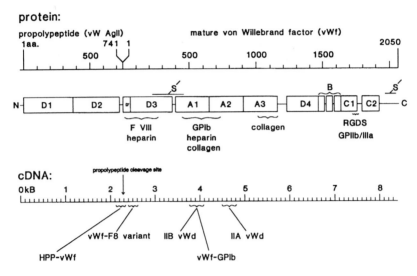

Figure 12-1 Model of the protein and cDNA domains of von Willebrand factor. The areas identified at the bottom of the figure represent the areas containing some of the known molecular variants of vWf. Abbreviations: HPP-vWf, hereditary persistence of pro-vWf; vWf-F8, variant with abnormal binding of FVIII to vWf; vWf-GPIb, variant of vWf that doesn't bind to platelet glycoprotein Ib; IIA and IIB vWd, type II variants of vWd. (Used with permission of R. Montgomery.)

collagen binding site has been localized to domain A3. The factor VIII binding site is localized to domain D3 (the amino terminal portion of the mature vWf).

vWf functions in hemostasis by mediating adhesion of platelets to exposed subendothelium through binding at the platelet GP Ib and IIb/IIIa sites, forming the basis for the hemostatic plug. In addition, vWf forms a noncovalent complex with factor VIII, thus stabilizing and protecting it from rapid removal from the circulation. These structure-function relationships are shown in Fig. 12-1 and provide a partial understanding of the multitude of mutations that could occur, resulting in the heterogeneous disorder von Willebrand disease.

CLASSIFICATION OF VON WILLEBRAND DISEASE

Most patients with von Willebrand disease have the heterozygous type (autosomal dominant) with mild bleeding manifestations; less frequently, the homozygous or doubly heterozygous types can occur and cause severe bleeding. Although the classification is constantly changing, a working approach based on the analysis of the multimeric structure of vWf in plasma and platelets has proven useful (Table 12-1 and Fig. 12-2) particularly in deciding which patients may respond to therapy with the vasopressin

TABLE 12-1 Classification of von Willebrand Disease Based on Measurements of Factor VIII, Plasma and Platelet von Willebrand Factor, and Ristocetin Cofactor and Multimers

Type I. Quantitative deficiency of vWf (low vWf antigen, factor VIII and ristocetin cofactor activity)

  IA. All plasma vWf multimers present in normal proportion

  IB. Plasma large vWf multimers relatively decreased

  IC. All plasma vWf multimers present but structural abnormality in individual multimers

  Platelet content of vWf ristocetin cofactor activity may be normal (IA), low (IA), or discordant (IB; vWf normal but ristocetin cofactor decreased)

Type II. Qualitative deficiency of vWf (decreased large multimers, vWf antigen, and ristocetin cofactor; factor VIII normal or decreased)

  IIA. Large and intermediate multimers absent in plasma and platelets

  IIA-1. Normal amount vWf antigen (plasma, platelets)

  IIA-2. Decreased amount vWf antigen (plasma, platelets)

  IIA-3. Decreased amount vWf antigen (plasma only)

  IIB. Large multimers absent in plasma, all multimers present in platelets, platelets **hyperresponsive** to ristocetin

  IIC, D, E, etc. Unique structural abnormality of individual multimers

Type III. Severe form, often homozygous, levels of vWf < 1%; low factor VIII (2–10%); all multimers absent.

Platelet Type. Findings similar to IIB except positive patient platelet aggregation to cryoprecipitate; pseudo von Willebrand disease.

*vWf, von Willebrand factor.

analogue DDAVP. Patients with the most common type I (all multimers present) respond to DDAVP administration by raising their levels of vWf and factor VIII. Many subtypes of type II (large multimers absent) do not respond to DDAVP clinically; DDAVP is contraindicated in the rare patient with type IIB because of the increased platelet binding of the abnormal vWf with subsequent platelet clumping and thrombocytopenia; disease in type III patients (homozygous) is too severe to be stimulated by DDAVP (Table 12-2).

GENETICS

Approximately 1 percent of the population may have some type of inherited defect of vWf; however, the majority of these defects are mild or asymptomatic clinically. Type I, the partial quantitative deficiency of vWf, is inherited as an autosomal dominant trait and accounts for about 80 percent

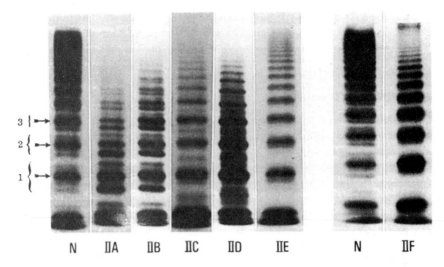

Figure 12-2 Examples of vWf multimeric analysis. A normal individual (N) is compared with various subtypes (IIA, IIB, IIC, IID, IIE, IIF). The three smallest individual oligomers are indicated by brackets. In types IIC, IID, IIE, and IIF, either some normal bands are missing or other bands are present. (Reproduced with permission from Berkowitz SD et al: von Willebrand disease. In: Zimmerman TS, Ruggeri ZM (eds): Coagulation and Bleeding Disorders. The Role of the Factor VIII and von Willebrand Factor. New York, Marcel Dekker, 1989, p 222.)

TABLE 12-2 Guidelines for Use of DDAVP in von Willebrand Disease

Usually Effective	Sometimes Effective*	Ineffective	Contraindicated
Type IA (normal platelet vWf)	Type IA (low platelet vWf)	Type III	Type IIB
Type IC	Type IB (platelet discordant)	Normandy variant	Platelet type von Willebrand disease
Variant with larger than normal multimers	Subtypes of Type II		
Variant with persistence of pro-vWf			

SOURCE: Adapted from Ruggeri ZM, Zimmerman TS: von Willebrand factor and von Willebrand disease. *Blood* 70:895, 1987.

* Trial of DDAVP is indicated.

vWf, von Willebrand factor.

of all von Willebrand disease. No consistent genetic abnormality at the molecular level has been determined for this group except for missense and nonsense mutations associated with reduced levels of vWf messenger RNA in a few patients. The qualitative deficiency or type II patients are less common (15 to 20 percent) and localized to exon 28 (amino acid residues 463 to 921; GP Ib binding domain) of the von Willebrand's disease gene (see Fig. 12-1), which facilitates the diagnosis of these disorders. A subset of patients with the uncommon (0.5 to 5/million) homozygous type III defect have total or partial deletions of the vWf gene (these deletions can predispose to formation of alloantibody inhibitors). The parents of type III patients are obligate heterozygotes occasionally with moderate decreases in plasma vWf and are usually asymptomatic.

Other variants in whom the molecular defect is known include hereditary persistence of circulating pro-vWf (incomplete cleavage with persistent extracellular pro-vWf multimers) and von Willebrand disease "Normandy." The latter patients have factor VIII deficiency that mimics hemophilia A (factor VIII levels of 0.02 to 0.08 U/mL) with normal vWf antigen, ristocetin cofactor, and multimeric patterns, but is inherited on an autosomal basis. The gene defect resulting in abnormal binding of factor VIII to vWf has been produced by at least three different mutations involving the factor VIII binding site. The latter defect was previously reported from our laboratory as a variant form of von Willebrand disease (coinheritance of type I disease) and displayed the discrepancy in one and two stage factor VIII assays shown in Table 14-2. These and similar defects should be considered in investigation of "autosomal" or sporadic hemophilia or in females with hemophilia A.

DIAGNOSIS OF VON WILLEBRAND DISEASE

von Willebrand disease is typically suspected in a patient with clinical evidence of membrane (epistaxis, gastrointestinal hemorrhage, menorrhagia) or postsurgical bleeding who has a prolonged bleeding time with a normal platelet count; the bleeding time is variable and may be frequently normal in mild patients. The family history is frequently positive. In addition to the routine screening tests (platelet count is decreased in IIB and pseudo von Willebrand disease; the APTT is variable and may be normal) plasma vWf antigen, ristocetin cofactor activity, factor VIII, and multimeric analysis should be performed and family studies done as appropriate (Table 12-3). These studies will allow classification into types I, II, or III (see Table 12-1).

In type II, ristocetin-induced platelet aggregation of patient platelet-rich plasma (ristocetin-induced platelet aggregation), if increased, indicates type IIB. Alternatively, increased reactivity of fixed normal platelets with risto-

TABLE 12-3 Measurements Used to Classify von Willebrand Disease (see Table 12-1)

Test	Method	Interpretation
vWf	Immunologic (Laurell, ELISA)	Quantitation of protein in plasma or platelet lysate
Ristocetin cofactor	Ristocetin-induced platelet agglutination (patient sample plus normal platelets)	vWf activity (plasma or platelet lysate)
Factor VIII	Factor VIII assay	Factor VIII coagulant activity
Ristocetin-induced platelet aggregation	Ristocetin-induced platelet aggregation (patient platelet-rich plasma plus ristocetin 0.5 mg/mL)	Decreased in type I, IIa, III vWD; increased in type IIB and platelet type* vWD
Multimers	Agarose gel electrophoresis	vWf multimeric structure

*Platelet type vWD can be distinguished from IIB by positive aggregation of patient platelet-rich plasma by cryoprecipitate.
vWD, von Willebrand disease; vWF, von Willebrand factor.

cetin in presence of patient plasma indicates the IIB defect. Further subtyping and classification require multimeric analysis in different gel systems (low concentration agarose best for quantitating high molecular weight multimers, high concentration agarose best for triplet structure) and determination of platelet vWf binding or content.

In diagnosing mild type I patients with borderline test values, it is important to keep in mind that vWf increases with stress (acute phase reactant), pregnancy, and age, and varies during the menstrual cycle (lowest in the follicular phase). Term infants have higher levels than normal adults in the first few weeks of life. Also, ABO blood groups influence the levels (group O: vWf:Ag; mean = 0.75, lower limit 0.36 U/mL; group A: mean = 1.06, lower limit 0.49 U/mL; group B: mean = 1.17, lower limit 0.57 U/mL). The best single test for vWf detection is the ristocetin cofactor assay, but frequently the vWf:Ag plasma and multimers are needed to be more certain of the diagnosis. Because of these confounding variables, it is frequently necessary to repeat the diagnostic studies more than once and study family members to make a diagnosis. Molecular studies of the difficult patient hold promise for the future. For instance, currently many patients (especially type II) can be classified by use of cDNA derived from the reverse transcription of platelet RNA.

Reports of the association of factor XII deficiency (heterozygote levels) in von Willebrand disease have appeared and may be due to the simultaneous occurrence of two genetic defects or an acquired deficiency of factor XII from undetermined causes. This association should be considered when APTT prolongation cannot be explained by a low factor VIII level.

MANAGEMENT

The most important step in the management of a patient suspected to have von Willebrand disease is to confirm the diagnosis and classification as securely as possible. As noted in Table 12-2, the choice of therapeutic agent to halt hemorrhage depends on the classification. Since mild disease is difficult to diagnose precisely and because of the variable response to DDAVP in type II, it is frequently useful to perform a trial DDAVP infusion soon after diagnosis. The bleeding time, platelet count, factor VIII, and vWf ristocetin cofactor levels are measured before and 30 min after a standard dose of DDAVP. The information obtained is mainly used for planning therapy of emergency bleeding episodes, since many patients with mild and moderate disease do not bleed excessively even at time of surgery (i.e., prophylactic therapy is not needed as often as it is in hemophilic patients).

For patients in whom DDAVP is not indicated, the use of viral-free vWf concentrate is recommended. (Currently in the United States the most useful product is Humate P; most other factor VIII concentrates do not contain enough functional vWf to be effective.) Cryoprecipitate may also be used when an effective viral-free concentrate is not available. Because these concentrates will correct the bleeding time for only a few hours (4 to 6) even though the ristocetin cofactor activity and factor VIII activity are corrected for longer periods, the products are usually given every 12 h in the seriously bleeding patient or after surgical procedures. In patients with von Willebrand disease, infusions of functioning vWf (plasma, cryoprecipitate, concentrate) will correct the factor VIII level to a greater extent and for a longer half-disappearance time than the same dose will in hemophilia A patients (pseudosynthesis). Therefore, concentrates of pure vWf without factor VIII preclude the need for factor VIII administration. For example, when human von Willebrand factor concentrate, Biotransfusion, containing low factor VIII activity, is used in diseased patients, the vWf recovery was 77.3 percent at 1 h and the factor VIII recovery was 87.6 percent.

Bleeding episodes and some surgical procedures are amenable to treatment with estrogens in women with type I disease; even women with type III von Willebrand disease may decrease bleeding tendency in general when taking oral contraceptive agents. Antifibrinolytic agents (ε-aminocaproic acid, tranexamic acid) are useful adjuncts in treating mucous membrane bleeding (dental extractions).

Precipitating antibodies to vWf can develop in severe homozygous von Willebrand disease patients following multiple transfusions with blood derivatives. Adverse effects include decreased survival of transfused vWf and occasional severe anaphylactoid reactions.

BIBLIOGRAPHY

Barthels M et al: Additional factor XII (Hageman factor) deficiency in hemophilia A and in von Willebrand syndrome. *Klin Wochenschr* 60:303, 1982.

Blombach M et al: On laboratory problems in diagnosing mild von Willebrand's disease. *Am J Hematol* 40:117, 1992.

Duray PH et al: Gastrointestinal angiodysplasia: A possible component of von Willebrand's disease. *Human Path* 15:529, 1984.

Eikenboom JCJ et al: Mutations in severe type III von Willebrand disease in the Dutch population: Candidate missense and nonsense mutations associated with reduced levels of von Willebrand factor messenger RNA. *Thromb Haemost* 68:448, 1992.

Fay PJ et al: Propolypeptide of vWf circulates in blood and is identical to von Willebrand antigen II. *Science* 232:995, 1986.

Federici AB et al: Type II H von Willebrand disease: New structural abnormality of plasma and platelet vWf in a patient with prolonged bleeding time and borderline levels of ristocetin cofactor activity. *Am J Hematol* 32:287, 1989.

Gill JC et al: The effect of ABO blood group on the diagnosis of von Willebrand disease. *Blood* 69:1691, 1987.

Ginsburg D, Bowie EJW: Molecular genetics of von Willebrand disease. *Blood* 79:2507, 1991.

Goudemand J et al: Clinical and biological evaluation in von Willebrand's disease of a vWf concentrate with low factor VIII activity. *Br J Haematol* 80:214, 1991.

Holmberg L, Nilsson IM: von Willebrand's disease. *Eur J Haematol* 48:127, 1992.

Mannucci PM et al: Precipitating antibodies to factor VIII/vWf in von Willebrand's disease: Effects on replacement therapy. *Blood* 57:25, 1981.

Kroner PA et al: Abnormal binding of factor VIII is linked with the substitution of glutamine for arginine 91 in vWf in a variant form of von Willebrand disease. *J Biol Chem* 266:19146, 1991.

Mazurier C: von Willebrand disease masquerading as haemophilia A. *Thromb Haemost* 67:391, 1992.

Miller JL: Sorting out heightened interactions between platelets and vWf: "IIB or not IIB?" is becoming an increasingly answerable question in the molecular era. *Am J Clin Pathol* 96:681, 1991.

Ruggeri ZM, Zimmerman TS: von Willebrand factor and von Willebrand disease. *Blood* 70:895, 1987.

Sadler JE: von Willebrand factor. *J Biol Chem* 266:22777, 1991.

Zimmerman TS, Ruggeri ZM: *Coagulation and Bleeding Disorders. The Role of Factor VIII and von Willebrand Factor.* New York and Basel, Marcel Dekker, 1989.

Acquired

von Willebrand

Disease

Alterations in the amount and function of von Willebrand factor (vWf) have been noted in many physiologic and pathologic states. As noted in Chap. 3, this factor is an acute phase reactant; raised levels are observed in inflammatory and other disease states as well as after stress (exercise, fever) and administration of adrenaline and DDAVP. Plasma concentrations of vWf are increased in disorders that affect the vascular system (increased release from damaged endothelial cells) such as systemic lupus erythematosus (SLE), pregnancy-induced hypertension, diabetes mellitus, cerebrovascular disease, mitral stenosis, pulmonary hypertension, and deep venous thrombosis (DVT); a high concentration of vWf is a risk factor for reinfarction in survivors of myocardial infarction.

The oligomers range in mass from 1 to 15 to 20×10^6 d as demonstrated by multimeric analysis (see Chap. 12). These and even larger oligomers along with the propolypeptide (vW:AgII) are synthesized by endothelial cells where they are stored in the Weibel-Palade bodies and in megakaryocytes where they are stored in the a-granules (Fig. 13-1). The "super large" multimers, which are associated with increased platelet adhesion and clumping, do not usually appear in the plasma except in the fetus and newborn where they are physiologic and gradually disappear with age (over a few weeks) and after administration of DDAVP. The unusually large multimers are also seen in the pathologic conditions hemolytic uremic syndrome (HUS) and thrombocytic thrombocytopenic purpura (TTP; see Chap. 29), and scleroderma. Quantitative or qualitative deficiencies (or both) of vWf can be associated with a bleeding tendency and is called acquired von Willebrand disease.

Acquired von Willebrand disease can be diagnosed (Table 13-1) in children and adults as a bleeding tendency characterized by easy bruising,

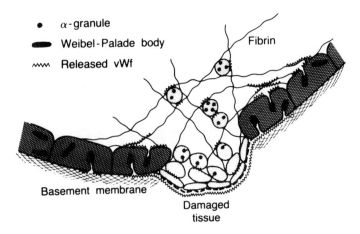

Figure 13-1 Representation of the storage compartments for vWf (α-granule and Weibel-Palade body) and their involvement after vascular injury. Released vWf from the platelets and the Weibel-Palade bodies stabilize the interaction of the platelets with the vessel wall endothelial cells, and promote platelet-fibrin interaction and platelet aggregation. (Used with permission from Wagner DD: Storage and secretion of von Willebrand factor. In: Zimmerman TS, Ruggeri ZM (eds): Coagulation and Bleeding Disorders. The Role of Factor VIII and von Willebrand Factor, New York, Marcel-Dekker, 1989, p. 174.)

mucous membrane bleeding (gastrointestinal, epistaxis), surgical- or dental-induced bleeding, or occasionally in asymptomatic individuals during the investigation of a prolonged bleeding time. In particular, bleeding patients with myeloproliferative or lymphoproliferative diseases, gammopathies, and tumors should alert the clinician to acquired disease. The screening laboratory tests may be normal but usually show prolongation of the bleeding time with or without an abnormal APTT. Past history and family history are frequently negative except for symptoms related to an underlying disorder.

TABLE 13-1 Diagnostic Approach to Patient Suspected of Acquired von Willebrand Disease

Basic hemostatic screen including bleeding time.
Assays for factor VIII, vWf:Ag, and ristocetin cofactor activity in plasma of patient and patient mixed with pooled normal plasma 1:1 at 0 and 2 h at 37°C.
Plasma vWf multimers.
Assay for immune complexes (IgG:vWf) using staphylococcal protein A sepharose (see reference Fricke et al).
Ristocetin-induced platelet aggregation (normal platelet-rich plasma plus patient plasma).
Determination of half-disappearance time of factor VIII and ristocetin cofactor activities after DDAVP or vWf concentrate.

*vWf:Ag, von Willebrand factor antigen.

TABLE 13-2 Acquired von Willebrand Disease

Immunologic (usually evidence for antibody)
 Waldenstrom's macroglobulinemia
 Benign monoclonal gammopathy
 Multiple myeloma
 Lymphoproliferative disorders (CLL, lymphoma)
 Autoimmune (SLE, scleroderma, carcinoma)
Other (usually no evidence for antibody)
 Myeloproliferative disorders (CML, PV)
 Hypothyroidism
 Cardiac defects (valvular disease, congenital and acquired)
 Glycogen storage disease
 EBV infection
 Uremia
 Mesenchymal defects (mitral valve prolapse, angiodysplasias)
 Ehlers-Danlos syndrome
 Hemangioma of spleen
 Wilms tumor
 Carcinoma
 Drugs: hydroxyethyl starch, dextran, heparin, L-asparaginase, thrombolytic
  therapy

---

*Quantitative and/or qualitative deficiencies of von Willebrand factor associated with a bleeding tendency.
CLL, chronic lymphocytic leukemia; CML, chronic myelocytic leukemia; EBV, Epstein-Barr virus; PV, polycythemia vera; SLE, systemic lupus erythematosus.

As noted in Table 13-2, the associated causes for acquired von Willebrand disease may be divided into two groups: disorders associated with an immunologic etiology (circulating antibody or inhibitor to vWf, or selective adsorption of vWf to abnormal lymphocytic clones) and disorders without antibody where defective synthesis, increased absorption (drugs or tumor cells), or defective release of vWf occurs.

ACQUIRED VON WILLEBRAND DISEASE (WITH AUTOANTIBODIES)

Circulating inhibitors, usually IgG antibodies, directed against the vWf molecule may be associated with a von Willebrand syndrome in patients with benign monoclonal gammopathy, macroglobulinemia, multiple myeloma, lymphoproliferative diseases (lymphoma, acute lymphocytic leukemia), or autoimmune disorders such as SLE, scleroderma or idiopathic. Assay of vWf antigen, factor VIII, and ristocetin cofactor activity shows low levels of all three or, occasionally, only low vWf activity. Multimeric analysis is of type I or II pattern. Mixing studies with patient and normal plasma characteristically show inhibition of ristocetin cofactor activity or defective ristocetin-induced platelet aggregation. Some patients (lymphoproliferative disorder) may not exhibit a circulating inhibitor by in vitro mixing studies. The inhibitor can be entirely complexed with vWf and only demonstrated by heating or by means of an antibody-binding assay using staphylococcal protein A to absorb the antibody and show inhibition in the ristocetin cofactor assay. Factor VIII activity and inhibitor (Bethesda assay) can be normal.

Plasma half-disappearance times of vWf activity after DDAVP stimulation are decreased as compared to type I von Willebrand disease patients. Bleeding episodes in these patients may be managed by infusions of DDAVP or vWf concentrate (Humate-P) in large doses (an anamnestic rise in vWf antibody is infrequent). Immunosuppressive therapy (prednisone) or treatment of the underlying diseases may also be effective. Severe bleeding due to circulating inhibitor (Waldenstrom's macroglobulinemia) has been effectively managed by intensive plasma exchange. High-dose intravenous immunoglobulin has been helpful in some cases of acquired disease with autoantibodies.

ACQUIRED VON WILLEBRAND DISEASE (WITHOUT AUTOANTIBODIES)

Several disorders have been associated with decreased vWf antigen and activity, variable vWf multimeric pattern, alterations in factor VIII activity at times, and an acquired bleeding tendency or prolonged bleeding time on occasion. These acquired syndromes are usually mild but have occasionally been associated with a significant bleeding tendency. Circulating inhibitors have not been detected usually. The proposed mechanisms vary with the disorder. A type II multimeric pattern (decrease in large multimers) has occurred in patients with myeloproliferative syndromes (thrombocythemia, thrombocytosis, polycythemia vera); some of these patients have had a bleeding tendency which has responded to DDAVP.

A similar decrease in largest vWf multimers associated with reduced vWf (antigen and ristocetin cofactor activity) has been reported in children with acyanotic congenital heart disease (ventricular septal defects, atrial septal defect, aortic stenosis); the defect was normalized with correction of the abnormal hemodynamic state. Acquired disease with a type II multimeric pattern was observed in one child after Epstein-Barr virus infection. The mechanism for these acquired type II defects may be increased turnover or destruction of the large multimers (increased adsorption to platelets, lymphocytes [as in chronic lymphocytic leukemia] or other cells).

Acquired von Willebrand disease has been described in certain mesenchymal dysplasias and vascular disorders such as mitral valve prolapse, connective tissue disorders, and intestinal angiodysplasia or telangiectasia. Decreased synthesis may produce a type I syndrome associated with bleeding in hypothyroidism. Other causes of acquired disease include tumors (Wilms, adrenal cortical carcinoma) and splenic hemangioma. The latter disorder was the cause of acquired disease in a 30-month-old child and was cured by splenectomy. Of interest, even though multimeric analysis indicated a type I pattern, the plasma vWf before splenectomy displayed decreased binding to collagen as seen in type II patients. Qualitative abnormalities of vWf have also been described in diabetes mellitus (poor glycemic control) and in uremia.

Pharmacologic agents associated with decreased levels of vWf antigen or activity include heparin (reduces ristocetin cofactor activity by interfering with vWf-GP Ib binding), hydroxyethyl starch and dextran, and L-asparaginase. Thrombolytic therapy is associated with a reduction of plasma high molecular weight multimers.

BIBLIOGRAPHY

Ball J et al: Demonstration of abnormal factor VIII multimers in acquired von Willebrand's disease associated with a circulating inhibitor. *Br J Haematol* 65:95, 1987.

Budde U et al: Acquired von Willebrand's disease in the myeloproliferative syndrome. *Blood* 64:981, 1984.

Dalton RG et al: Hypothyroidism as a cause of acquired von Willebrand's disease. *Lancet* 1:1007, 1987.

DiMichele DM et al: von Willebrand factor (vWf) collagen-binding (CB) defect in acquired von Willebrand's disease (vWd) associated with splenic hemangioma. *Blood* 68:331a, 1986.

Fricke WA et al: Comparison of inhibitory and binding characteristics of an antibody causing acquired von Willebrand syndrome: An assay for von Willebrand factor binding by antibody. *Blood* 66:562, 1985.

Gill JC et al: Loss of the largest von Willebrand factor multimers from the plasma of patients with congenital cardiac defects. *Blood* 67:758, 1986.

Goudemand J et al: Acquired type II von Willebrand's disease: Demonstration of a complexed inhibitor of the von Willebrand factor-platelet interaction and response to treatment. *Br J Haematol* 68:227, 1988.

Jakeway JL: Acquired von Willebrand disease. *Hematol Oncol Clin North Am* 6:1409, 1992.

Kinoshita S et al: Acquired von Willebrand disease after Epstein-Barr infection. *J Pediatr* 119:595, 1991.

Macik BG et al: The use of high-dose intravenous gamma-globulin in acquired von Willebrand syndrome. *Arch Pathol Lab Med* 112:143, 1988.

Mannucci PM et al: Studies of the pathophysiology of acquired von Willebrand's disease in seven patients with lymphoproliferative disorders or benign monoclonal gammopathies. *Blood* 64:614, 1984.

Pasi KJ et al: Qualitative and quantitative abnormalities of von Willebrand antigen in patients with diabetes mellitus. *Thromb Res* 59:581, 1990.

Sanfelippo MJ et al: Development of a von Willebrand-like syndrome after prolonged use of hydroxyethyl starch. *Am J Clin Pathol* 88:653, 1987.

Silberstein LE et al: The efficacy of intensive plasma exchange in acquired von Willebrand's disease. *Transfusion* 27:234, 1987.

Sobel M et al: Heparin inhibition of von Willebrand factor-dependent platelet function in vitro and in vivo. *J Clin Invest* 87:1787, 1991.

Weinstein MJ et al: Fetal and neonatal von Willebrand factor (vWF) is unusually large and similar to the vWF in patients with thrombotic thrombocytopenic purpura. *Br J Haematol* 72:68, 1989.

Hemophilia A
(Factor VIII Deficiency)

Factor VIII (antihemophilic factor, AHF) is a 320-kd glycoprotein, synthesized mainly in the hepatocyte, which circulates in the plasma in a concentration of 0.1 to 0.2 μg/mL in a stable complex with another glycoprotein, von Willebrand factor. When proteolytically activated by factor Xa or thrombin, VIIIa acts as a cofactor to accelerate the activation of factor X by factor IXa; the coagulant activity is termed factor VIII activity while the immunologic quantitation of factor VIII is factor VIII antigen or VIII:Ag. The genetic deficiency of factor VIII is classic hemophilia or hemophilia A, which with factor IX deficiency, occurs in a frequency of 1/10,000 of the whole population (factor VIII, 85 percent; factor IX, 14 percent, others 1 percent).

STRUCTURE-FUNCTION RELATIONSHIP

When factor VIII is activated by thrombin or Xa in the presence of metal ions on a phospholipid surface (platelets), factor X activation by IXa is enhanced 10,000-fold. This important cofactor activity is derived by limited proteolysis of the native molecule factor VIII to VIIIa as depicted in Fig. 14-1. The polypeptide structure of the protein is composed of domains in the order of A1:A2:B:A3:C1:C2. The A domains occur in both the heavy and light chains and have a 30 percent homology with ceruloplasmin and factor V. The second and third A domains are separated by a large connecting region containing most of the N-linked glycosylation sites (B domain), followed by two C domains of 150 amino acids each, which have a homology with lectin-binding proteins.

Activation of factor VIII results in a calcium-dependent heterodimer that consists of a fragment of 50 kd containing the first A domain and a fragment of 73 kd containing the third A domain and two C domains. During this activation process the light chain is released from the stabilizing

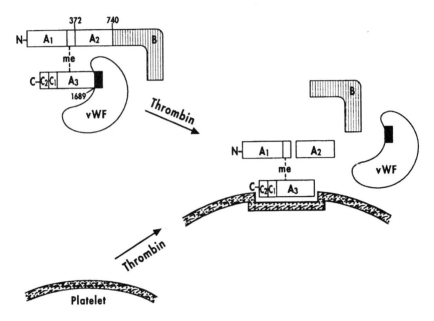

Figure 14-1 Thrombin activation of factor VIII and assembly on activated platelet surface. Me, metal ion, probably Ca^{++}. The domain structure of factor is designated (A_1, A_2, B_1,, A_3, C_1, C_2). The numbers refer to amino acids cleavage sites. Note that after thrombin activation, von Willebrand factor and the B domain are disassociated and not included in the molecular assembly on the platelet surface. (Adapted with permission from Nesheim M et al: The effect of plasma von Willebrand factor on the binding of human factor VIII to thrombin-activated human platelets. J Biol Chem 266:17815, 1991.)

effect of von Willebrand factor followed by further degradation and inactivation by activated protein C, thrombin, Xa, and possibly plasmin. Factor VIII activity is dependent on formation of the heterodimer (VIIIa) and is measured in plasma by three types of assays: one-stage, two-stage, and chromogenic substrate assay. Comparison of these assay techniques is shown in Table 14-1. All three methods give comparable results when assaying hemophilic patients, before and after treatment, suspected carriers, normal controls, and most variants of von Willebrand disease and hemophilia.

A subset of mild hemophilia A patients shows definitely lower levels of factor VIII measured by the two-stage assay as compared with the one-stage assay; some patients with von Willebrand disease may rarely show the same phenomenon attributed to increased aluminum hydroxide adsorption of von Willebrand factor in the two-stage assay system. Patients with acquired changes in factor VIII due in part to activation (chronic disseminated intravascular coagulation [DIC], preeclampsia, leukemias, liver disease, etc.) may exhibit normal or higher levels by the one-stage

TABLE 14-1 Comparison of Factor VIII Assays

One-Stage	Two-Stage	Chromogenic
Methods		
Diluted subject plasma	Diluted subject plasma	Diluted subject plasma
+	(adsorbed to remove	+
VIII-def substrate plasma	vit K factors)	Reagent mixture (IXa, Pl,
+	+	Ca^{++})
APTT reagent	Reagent mixture	↓
↓	(serum, factor V	Incubate
Add Ca^{++}	plasma)	Add to synthetic substrate
↓	+	↓
Fibrin end point	Ca^{++}	Measure color change
	↓	
	Incubate	
	Subsample	
	+	
	Ca^{++}, substrate plasma	
	↓	
	Fibrin end point	
Advantages		
Simplicity	Precision (especially	Precision
Readily automated	at low levels)	Not sensitive to activation
Widely used for	Not sensitive to	No requirement for VIII-
monitoring concentrate	activation	def plasma
usage	No requirement for	Readily automated
	VIII-def plasma	
Disadvantages		
Need for VIII-def plasma	Complex	Requires specific
Sensitive to activation	Difficult to standardize	instrumentation
APTT reagent variability	reagents	Questionable accuracy in
	Not easily automated	presence of inhibitors

SOURCE: Adapted from Brandt JT, Triplett DA: Laboratory assays for factor VIII:C. In: Zimmerman TS, Ruggeri ZM (eds): *Coagulation and Bleeding Disorders. The Role of Factor VIII and von Willebrand Factor*, New York, Marcel Dekker, 1989, pp. 343–357.

assay. Table 14-2 indicates these differences in a group of patients studied in our laboratory. Interestingly, the variants of hemophilia A and von Willebrand disease (single family members shown) frequently had normal or only slightly increased APTTs. Factor VIII:Ag is quantitated by immunoradiometric or ELISA assays using human anti-factor VIII or monoclonal antibodies.

TABLE 14-2 Differences in the One-Stage and Two-Stage Assays in Patients Studied in Our Laboratory

Disorder	Factor VIII, One Stage (U/mL)	Factor VIII, Two Stage (U/mL)
Normal adults (20)	1.03	1.02
Sickle cell disease (crisis)	6.0	3.0
DVT, vena cava	3.36	1.4
Metastatic neuroblastoma	2.4	1.35
Ulcerative colitis	3.0	1.5
SLE—vasculitis	2.75	1.8
Hemophilia A, mild (15)	0.15	0.14
Hemophilia A, mild (variant)	0.18	0.01

*DVT, deep venous thrombosis; SLE, systemic lupus erythematosus.

GENETICS OF HEMOPHILIA A

The gene responsible for hemophilia A is located on the long arm of the X chromosome at Xq28. Females (heterozygotes) with two X chromosomes can carry a mutation on one chromosome and remain unaffected because of the compensating normal gene. A male (hemizygote) will have hemophilia if his X chromosome carries the mutant gene. In a mating between a female carrier and an unaffected male, 50 percent of daughters will be heterozygous for the hemophilia mutation (carriers) and 50 percent of the sons will be hemophiliacs. Conversely, a mating between a hemophilic male and a normal female, no sons will be affected (paternal Y and maternal X chromosomes), but all daughters will be obligate carriers. Hemophilia A has remained a relatively common bleeding disorder since biblical times because of high sporadic occurrence of the disorder (high mutation rate) and the X-linked inheritance.

The gene for human factor VIII is unusually large and spans 186 kilobases (kb) of DNA. Discovery of hemophilia-producing mutations in the factor VIII gene is progressing steadily. Gene deletions from two base pairs to greater than 186 kb have been determined in about 5 percent of patients with severe hemophilia. Point mutations (stop codons, "nonsense," or a different amino acid code, "missense") have been discovered in more than 80 reported patients with both severe or mild hemophilia. Almost all of these patients have concordant levels of factor VIII and VIII:Ag but a rare family will have low factor VIII activity but normal VIII:Ag (cross-reacting material, CRM positive). For example, factor VIII-East Hartford is a CRM-positive hemophilia A variant in which reduced factor VIII activity is due to substitution of cysteine for arginine 1689 abolishing an essential thrombin cleavage site and a site for von Willebrand factor binding. The in vitro procoagulant activity of the mutant molecule is partially restored when treated with a reducing agent (cysteamine) which disassociates the VIII from von Willebrand factor.

A recent study suggests, however, that half the mutations are not within the coding regions and splice junctions of the gene and may be due to mutations in DNA sequences outside the regions studied (introns or outside the gene). An unusual cluster of mutations involving intron 22 leading to defective joining of exons 22 and 23 in the mRNA has been reported. In one compilation, inhibitors to factor VIII were observed in 9 of 36 patients with gene deletions and 10 of 25 patients with point mutations. Thus, these mutations which often result in no factor VIII protein may predispose to inhibitors but do not ensure their development.

Female Hemophilia

Severe hemophilia due to factor VIII or factor IX deficiency may rarely be seen in females. The possible causes include homozygosity for the gene (consanguinity in hemophilic family, postzygotic mutation, germ line mutation in parent marrying into hemophilic family), chance inactivation of X chromosome with normal gene (extreme lyonization), genetic abnormality in a phenotypic female with abnormal gene (Turner's syndrome, testicular feminization, mosaicism), abnormalities involving X chromosome (deletion, inversion, translocation) and von Willebrand disease Normandy (see Chap. 12). Family and detailed molecular biologic studies should provide the diagnosis.

Carrier Detection and Prenatal Diagnosis

All newly diagnosed patients and/or their families should have genetic counseling to include appropriate testing and identification of carriers in the pedigree. Because only a small percentage of hemophilic families display a specific gene defect (deletion or point mutation), other methods are frequently used to identify carriers within a family. The ratio of factor VIII activity to von Willebrand factor antigen (vWf:Ag) is indicative of the obligate carrier (low ratio) in approximately 90 percent of instances. When careful duplicate assays indicate a ratio < 2 standard deviations from the mean of a group of normal age-matched control women studied in the same laboratory, there is a high probability that the woman is a carrier. If the factor VIII activity is below the normal range, that is, < 40 percent, the carrier may also be a mild bleeder (especially with trauma or surgery) and should be advised accordingly.

Several intragenic polymorphisms (usually in the introns) with restriction endonuclease sites (restriction fragment length polymorphism, RFLPs) can be used in some instances to predict the carrier state with an accuracy limited only by the possibility of crossing over between the genetic defect and the polymorphism. With these RFLP markers for the factor VIII gene (both intragenic and closely linked extragenic) and the clotting assay ratio, almost all carriers can be identified if informative family members are available.

Prenatal diagnosis may be performed early in pregnancy (8 to 11 weeks' gestation) by chorionic villus sampling if prior evaluation has indicated informative DNA analysis for the genetic defect; if DNA markers are not available, fetoscopy and sampling of fetal blood with coagulation factor analysis (factor VIII activity and VIII:Ag) may be performed at 20 weeks' gestation. Optimal evaluation and genetic counseling for potential carriers should be done by the comprehensive hemophilia center as soon as the diagnosis is established in a new patient or family. Efforts should be made to obtain cord blood samples for factor VIII assays on male infants whose mothers are carriers so that potential venipuncture-related bleeding may be avoided.

CLINICAL MANIFESTATIONS OF HEMOPHILIA A

Patients with classical hemophilia display a spectrum of bleeding manifestations (deep muscle and joint hemorrhage, hematomas, easy bruising, posttraumatic deep bleeding, postsurgery and laceration wound bleeding, postoral injury and tooth extraction [molars] oozing, intracranial hemorrhage [ICH], intra- and retroperitoneal bleeding, and gastrointestinal and renal bleeding (Table 14-3). The propensity to musculoskeletal hemorrhage can lead to recurrent hemarthroses (target joints) and chronic muscle injury and fibrosis. Even the patient with mild disease can develop permanent damage to a particular muscle group or joint with a trauma-induced bleed if not properly treated.

The diagnosis of hemophilia A is first suspected in one of several clinical situations: a pregnancy with or the birth of an infant to a mother with a family history of hemophilia or a pedigree of X-linked bleeders; or in the absence of a positive family history, the appearance of bleeding in the neonatal period (postcircumcision or puncture wound bleeding, large hematomas, unexplained ICH) or a pattern of easy bruising and deep muscle-joint or posttrauma bleeding later in life. Severe hemophilia is routinely diagnosed within the first year of life but mild hemophilia may be unsuspected until a traumatic or surgical challenge in the second or third decade or later. The basic hemostatic screen is usually normal except for a prolonged APTT. The diagnosis is confirmed by a plasma assay for factor VIII. Suspected hemophilia must be confirmed by carefully performed assays which often include factor IX and XI and not by the APTT alone.

TABLE 14-3 Clinical Manifestations in Hemophilia A

Factor VIII Assay	Severe (0–0.01 U/mL)	Moderate (0.02–0.05 U/mL)	Mild (0.06–0.4 U/mL)
Age at onset of bleeding	Within first year	Usually before 2 y	3–14 y or older
Musculoskeletal bleeding	"Spontaneous" joint and muscle bleeding, frequent "target joints"	Joint and muscle bleeding with minor trauma, may have "target joints"	Unusual except with significant trauma
CNS bleeding	Prevalence—3% Mean age 14 y (1 wk–53 y)	Less prevalent than severe	Rare; with significant trauma
Postsurgical bleeding	Usually frank bleeding	Wound hematomas and oozing, rarely none	Hematomas and oozing or none
Inhibitor development	15–20% prevalence	< 3%	Very rare
Trauma-induced bleeding	Common with contact sports	Muscle and joint bleeding with contact sports	Significant hematomas; deep bleeding only with significant trauma
Bleeding with tooth extraction	Usual	Common	Often, can be persistent
Response of level to exercise	None	None	Slight increase (5%)
Response to DDAVP	None	Usually < 10%	Usually 2–3 fold
Neonatal manifestations	Postcircumcision bleeding, occasional ICH	Usual post circumcision bleeding Rare ICH	None
Renal bleeding (hematuria)	Common, may be severe	Not unusual	Can occur, usually mild

*ICH, intracranial hemorrhage.

The Bleeding Time in Hemophilia

A prolonged bleeding time (10 to 20 min), not related to anti-inflammatory medications, abnormal platelet aggregation tests, or during concentrate infusions, has been documented in 15 to 84 percent of several series of patients with hemophilia A. The prolonged bleeding time is more often seen when the Simplate device is used and is correlated with severity of bleeding manifestations, platelet IgG levels, circulating immune complexes, and vascular injury. However, the role of unrecognized viral infections (HIV, hepatitis) was not adequately evaluated in these groups of patients.

ACQUIRED ALTERATION IN FACTOR VIII

As noted in Chap. 3, physiologic alterations in factor VIII include elevated (1.5 times normal) levels at birth in term infants, increased levels in pregnancy (1.5 to 2 times normal in third trimester), and gradually increasing levels in the adult with aging up to 68 years after which the level falls slightly. Factor VIII is raised acutely after strenuous exercise, epinephrine or DDAVP administration, and acute stress. Both factor VIII and von Willebrand factor are acute phase reactants and are elevated in febrile states, postoperatively, and in most inflammatory conditions. Estrogen-progestin steroids raise the level while corticosteroids do not. In addition, both proteins (von Willebrand factor was called VIII-related antigen in older literature) are elevated in disease states such as carcinoma (usually disseminated), leukemia, liver diseases, renal diseases, hemolytic anemias (sickle cell disease), diabetes mellitus, deep vein thrombosis, and myocardial infarction. In some disorders where intravascular activation of coagulation may occur, the factor VIII level as measured by the one-stage assay is higher than the von Willebrand factor measurement. Examples are preeclampsia, chronic DIC, acute leukemia, and disseminated cancer. Low levels of factor VIII are noted in hypothyroidism and acute DIC (consumption coagulopathy).

TREATMENT AND COMPLICATIONS

The key to successful treatment of patients with hemophilia is the prompt correction of their factor deficiency to hemostatic levels for acute bleeding or potential bleeding episodes. For factor VIII-deficient patients this means giving DDAVP (desmopressin) for mild defects and administration of factor VIII concentrates for moderate and severe deficiencies. Extended periods of prophylactic therapy to prevent recurrent bleeding may be part of the regimen. Details of transfusion therapy are given in Chap. 56. The overall goal in management is to minimize disability and facilitate social and physical well-being while helping the patient achieve full potential—all this without causing any harm. This goal is best achieved by a team approach in a comprehensive hemophilia center which provides current recommendations to the primary caregiver regarding treatment regimens, which include monitoring for complications; orthopedic, physical, medical and dental problems; genetic counseling; and psychosocial support.

The complications of hemophilia may be divided into two general categories: those associated with inadequate or no clotting factor replacement and those related to the factor replacement itself. The first category includes life-threatening hemorrhages (especially ICH, dissecting hematomas in vital areas, and uncontrolled posttrauma or surgical bleeding), formation of pseudotumors, debilitating and progressive musculoskeletal lesions resulting in crippling deformities, neurologic sequelae of CNS and peripheral nerve injury, limited lifestyle and productivity, drug dependency, and mental depression. All of these complications may be prevented by optimal transfusion therapy and effective comprehensive care.

The complications of transfusion therapy have been significant in the hemophilia population. The most serious of these complications are related to the hepatitis viruses (hepatitis B, hepatitis C [HCV], and non-A, non-B viruses) and HIV-1. Cumulative data in hemophilia patients exposed to clotting factor concentrates over the past 20 years and prior to recent viral inactivation techniques suggest that the majority have chronic liver disease (chronic persistent hepatitis with variable progression to cirrhosis) caused by HCV. Rare patients develop hepatocellular carcinoma.

Fortunately, recent viral inactivation methods and the routine use of hepatitis B vaccine have virtually eliminated these complications; however, human parvovirus B19 and, rarely, hepatitis A virus, may still be transmitted. Patients can now be monitored with serologic and virologic (viral RNA by polymerase chain reaction) techniques to determine infection in virtually 100 percent of cases. Likewise, the viral-inactivated products are free of HIV. Prior to the heat-treated concentrates (1984), more than 70 percent of hemophiliacs exposed to factor VIII concentrates and 48 percent exposed to factor IX concentrates have become HIV antibody positive. Infectivity in patients exposed only to volunteer donor cryoprecipitate was only 15 percent. Although the number continues to increase, upward of 40 percent of these HIV-positive older adults had developed AIDS by 1988. A lower incidence is noted in younger adults and children. Hemophiliacs with HIV antibody are actively infected and may transmit HIV to sexual partners. In addition, many of these patients show deteriorating T-cell function (CD4 lymphocyte estimation) and increased susceptibility to infection and other hematologic changes (thrombocytopenia, leukopenia). Other recently reported complications may be related to HIV seroconversion, that is, pulmonary hypertension and septic arthritis.

The other major complication of therapy is the development of a factor VIII inhibitor. The prevalence of inhibitor development in the hemophilia A population is approximately 15 percent. For details of this complication and its management see Chap. 21.

PROGNOSIS

After an improvement in survival in the 1970s where the leading causes of death were liver disease, cerebral hemorrhages, and malignancies, the relative mortality (in the 1980s) is increasing primarily due to the deaths from AIDS. The 1990s, in which patients will be treated with viral-free products, should again show a decline in mortality and, hopefully, the morbidity of chronic arthropathy and other bleeding complications.

BIBLIOGRAPHY

Aly AM et al: Cysteamine enhances the procoagulant activity of factor VIII-East Hartford, a dysfunctional protein due to a light chain thrombin cleavage site mutation (arginine-1689 to cysteine). *J Clin Invest* 89:1375, 1992.

Blanchette VS et al: Hepatitis C infection in children with hemophilia A and B. *Blood* 78:285, 1991.

Bloom AL: Progress in the clinical management of haemophilia. *Thromb Haemost* 66:166, 1991.

Brandt JT, Triplett DA: Laboratory assays for factor VIII:C. In: Zimmerman TS, Ruggeri ZM (eds): *Coagulation and Bleeding Disorders. The Role of Factor VIII and von Willebrand Factor*. New York, Marcel Dekker, 1989, pp 343–357.

Gjerset GF et al: Treatment type and amount influenced human immunodeficiency virus seroprevalence of patients with congenital bleeding disorders. *Blood* 78:1623, 1991.

Goedert JJ et al: A prospective study of human immunodeficiency virus type 1 infection and the development of AIDS in subjects with hemophilia. *N Engl J Med* 321:1141, 1989.

Higuchi M et al: Molecular characterization of severe hemophilia A suggests that about half the mutations are not within the coding regions and splice junctions of the factor VIII gene. *Genetics* 88:7405, 1991.

Johnson SS et al: Newborn factor VIII complex: Elevated activities in term infants and alterations in electrophoretic mobility related to illness and activated coagulation. *Br J Haematol* 47:597, 1981.

Jones PK, Ratnoff OD: The changing prognosis of classic hemophilia (factor VIII "deficiency"). *Ann Intern Med* 114:641, 1991.

Kane WH, Davie EW: Blood coagulation factors V and VIII: Structure and functional similarities and their relationship to hemorrhage and thrombotic disorders. *Blood* 71:539, 1988.

Lusher JM, McMillan CW: Severe factor VIII and factor IX deficiency in females. *Am J Med* 65:637, 1978.

Naylor JA et al: Factor VIII gene explains all cases of hemophilia A. *Lancet* 340:1066, 1992.

Stuart MJ et al: Bleeding time in hemophilia A: Potential mechanisms for prolongation. *J Pediatr* 108:215, 1986.

Thompson AR: Molecular biology of the hemophilias. *Prog Hemost Thromb* 10:175, 1991.

Triger DR, Preston FE: Chronic liver disease in haemophiliacs. *Br J Haematol* 74:241, 1990.

Troisi CL et al: A multicenter study of viral hepatitis in a United States hemophilic population. *Blood* 81:412, 1993.

Tuddenham EG et al: Haemophilia A: Database of nucleotide substitutions, deletions, insertions, and rearrangements of the factor VIII gene. *Nucleic Acids Res* 19:4821, 1991.

Yoffe G, Buchanan GR: Intracranial hemorrhage in newborn and young infants with hemophilia. *J Pediatr* 113:333, 1988.

Hemophilia B
(Factor IX Deficiency)

The existence of factor IX as a separate clotting factor was recognized over 40 years ago from studies of patients with hemophilic bleeding manifestations. The factor was called plasma thromboplastin component (PTC) or "Christmas" factor in the original reports, which resulted in the synonyms for congenital factor IX deficiency: Christmas disease, PTC deficiency, and hemophilia B. Factor IX, a vitamin K-dependent factor with a molecular weight of 57,000, circulates as a single chain glycoprotein proenzyme in the concentration of 3 to 5 μg/mL. Factor IX, when activated by factor XIa or factor VIIa-tissue factor in the presence of cofactors (factor VIII, calcium, phospholipid), rapidly converts factor X to Xa. The hereditary deficiency of factor IX results in a bleeding diathesis whose clinical characteristics are indistinguishable from factor VIII-deficient hemophilia.

STRUCTURE-FUNCTION RELATIONSHIP

The gene for factor IX codes for a signal peptide, a propeptide (promoter region), and the mature 415-amino acid protein that is present in the plasma. The processing steps removing the signal peptide and propeptide occur in the hepatocyte prior to secretion. As shown in Fig. 15-1, the domain structure includes the Gla region containing 12 γ-carboxylglutamyl residues dependent on the vitamin K carboxylase system and the propeptide for posttranslational modification of Glu to Gla. The resulting calcium binding sites anchor the protein to phospholipids. The next two domains, epidermal growth factorlike or EGF, are cysteine rich, share homology with protein C and factor X, and may function as binding sites for platelet membranes. The next domains are taken by the activation peptide (AP) and its flanking sequences; the AP is formed by peptide bond cleavage at Arg 145-Ala 146 and Arg 180-Val 181.

134

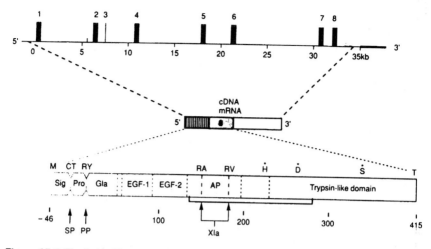

Figure 15-1 The factor IX gene and protein. The gene (upper portion) consists of eight exons and the seven intervening sequences totaling 34 kb. Protein is in lower portion with amino terminus at left and carboxy terminus at right. Sig, signal peptide; the CT (cys-Thr) bond is cleaved by a single peptidase (SP). A second intracellular cleavage by a propeptidase (PP) occurs at RY (Arg-Tyr) removing propeptide (Pro) before secretion. Domains: Gla; EGF (epidermal growth factorlike regions); AP (activation peptide). Factor XIa cleaves RA (Arg-Ala) and RV (Arg-Val) to yield factor IXa. Active site residues for serine protease activity are His 221 (H), Asp 269 (D), and Ser 365 (S). (Used with permission from Thompson AR. Structure and biology of factor IX. In: Hoffman R, Benz EJ Jr, Shattil S, Furie B, Cohen HJ. Hematology Basic Principles and Practice. New York, Churchill Livingstone, 1991, p 1308.)

Once cleaved, the AP remains bound to factor IXa forming disulfide-bonded light and heavy chains. The remainder of the molecule, "trypsin-like" domain (heavy chain), contains the active center, Ser 365, which is directly involved in cleavage of its substrate, factor X, thus fulfilling its function as a serine protease.

Factor IX is activated by the cleavage of the two bonds (above) by factor XIa or factor VIIa-tissue factor or from Russell viper venom cleavage at the Arg 180-Val 181 bond. Except for calcium, no other cofactors are needed for the activation. However, the activation of factor IX by factor VIIa-tissue factor complex is more rapid in the presence of factor X. Factor IXa is inactivated by antithrombin-III (AT-III), which forms a stable complex at the Asp 359 substrate-binding pocket.

Factor IX coagulant activity is measured by a one-stage APTT assay using IX-deficient plasma as substrate; the molecule can be measured quantitatively by immunologic assays using heterologous or monoclonal antibodies (IX:Ag). Immunoradiometric assay procedures using monoclonal antibodies may be influenced by genetic variants (allotypes) of normal human factor IX. No direct chromogenic assay is available for factor IX (factor IXa has only factor X as its substrate). Other chemical assay procedures for factor IX are not suitable for determination in plasma samples.

GENETICS

Like hemophilia A, factor IX-deficient hemophilia or hemophilia B is an X-linked recessive bleeding disorder. The gene encoding for factor IX is located near the terminus of the long arm (q) of the X chromosome. The 34-kb gene contains eight exons and seven introns (Fig. 15-1); the number of exons and splice junction types are highly conserved in homologous vitamin K-dependent proteins.

Hemophilia B is a markedly heterogeneous disorder with a wide range of baseline factor IX and IX:Ag levels and a variety of specific gene defects. Approximately 1 in 30,000 males are affected, with most of the families showing a unique mutation. Examples of the over 220 reported defects are shown in Table 15-1. Deletions of the gene and some point mutations are sometimes associated with inhibitor formation (antigen is often negative or absent). Point mutations, the most common defect, can be associated with mild and severe hemophilia B. The Leyden phenotype (severe hemophilia as a child which becomes mild after puberty) has been described in five separate families who have defects in the promoter region of the gene. If the promoter defect is at the -26 mutation site, disruption of the androgen-sensitive element occurs and the patient fails to recover (Hemophilia B Branderburg). Antigen-positive (cross-reacting material positive) defects, with clinical severity that is both severe and mild, are also known. These patients have levels of factor IX:Ag which are near normal or discrepantly higher than their factor IX activity levels. Most of these families display point mutations affecting various regions of the gene ranging from the Gla region to defects in the 180 to 182 and 390 to 397 trypsinlike (catalytic) domain. The latter defects, when associated with a dysfunctional protein which prolongs the PT when ox brain but not human brain is used as the source of thromboplastin, are called "BM" phenotype, most of whom have clinically severe disease. The finding of the BM phenotype in only one of two variants with the same molecular defect (Long Beach, Los Angeles, see Table 15-1) suggested that the prolonged ox brain PT is related to increased amounts of IX antigen and not a structural defect.

An interesting type of mild to moderate hemophilia B has been reported in at least 20 hemophiliacs residing in the midwestern and western United States, Ontario, and France. All have identical haplotypes, an isoleucine 397-threonine mutation, and perhaps share a common ancestor. The original factor IX-deficient patient, Mr. Christmas, is a severely deficient patient (IX:C, IX:Ag < 0.01 U/mL) whose mutation is Cys 206-Ser.

TABLE 15-1 Examples of the Heterogeneity of Hemophilia B

Mutation	Defect	Phenotype	Coagulation Tests (U/mL)
Antigen Negative			
FIX-Manchester	Deletion, entire gene	Severe; inhibitor-yes	IX:C=<0.01
FIX-Rheine	Deletion, entire gene	Severe; inhibitor-no	IX:C and IX:Ag= <0.01
FIX-London 8	Point mutation Cys 336-Arg	Severe; inhibitor-no	IX:C=0.02 IX:Ag=0.02
FIX-Leyden	Promotor region defects	Severe as child; mild to normal as adult	IX:C=<0.01 as child; rise with puberty or androgens to 0.3–0.6
Antigen Positive			
FIX-Seattle-3	Point mutation (Glu27-Lys) affecting γ-carboxylation	Severe; inhibitor-no	IX:C=<0.01 IX:Ag=0.30
FIX-Zutphen	Point mutation (Cys 18-Arg) Decreased Ca^{++} binding	Severe	IX:C=<0.01 IX:Ag=1.0
FIX-Chapel Hill	Point mutation (Arg 145–His) affecting zymogen activation	Mild-moderate; inhibitor-no	IX:C=0.05 IX:Ag=1.01
FIX-Long Beach	Point mutation (Ile 397-Thr) affecting catalytic activity	Moderate severe	IX:C=<0.01 IX:Ag-1.0 BM phenotype (Increase ox brain PT)
FIX-Los Angeles	Point mutation (Ile 397-Thr) affecting catalytic activity	Moderate severe	IX:C=<0.01 IX:Ag=0.32 (Nl ox brain PT)

*FIX, factor IX; IX:Ag, factor IX antigen; IX:C, factor IX activity; Nl, normal.

Carrier Detection and Prenatal Diagnosis

Carrier detection using IX activity and IX:Ag assays is possible in only about a third of families because of increased number of mutations with low IX:Ag and the effects of lyonization. At least 50 percent of obligate carriers will have a factor IX activity level < 60 percent; often the level will be in the range where bleeding may occur at time of trauma or surgery (< 30 percent activity). Currently, the most effective method to detect the carrier state is direct sequencing of an amplified DNA fragment to demonstrate heterozygosity (after the defect has been identified in the patient). Intragenic polymorphisms which can be detected both immunochemically and with nucleotide probes may also be used in selected cases keeping in mind that striking differences occur in these polymorphisms among different ethnic groups. DNA techniques, which are able to determine the gene defect in almost all cases, must be used for attempts at prenatal diagnosis because levels of IX:Ag and IX activity are not discriminating from the normal fetal levels in most instances (overlap of normal range, contamination by thromboplastic material).

CLINICAL MANIFESTATIONS

The clinical manifestations of mild, moderate, and severe hemophilia B are the same as for hemophilia A. Mild hemophilia B patients may have normal or near normal APTTs. Therefore, in undiagnosed mild bleeding disorders, a factor IX assay should be performed even if the APTT is reported as normal. Markedly low levels of factor IX are sometimes observed in hemophilia B carriers (extreme lyonization) or from other causes of female hemophilia (see Chap. 14).

ACQUIRED ALTERATIONS OF FACTOR IX

Physiologically low levels of factor IX are found in the fetus (0.05 to 0.15 U/mL at 20 weeks) and term newborn infant (0.15 to 0.50 U/mL); these levels reach the normal adult range by 6 months of age. Acquired low factor IX has been observed in liver disease, vitamin K deficiency, warfarin therapy, nephrotic syndrome, Gaucher's disease, and in acquired factor IX inhibitor states.

Although factor IX has been reported to rise about 1.5 times in normal pregnancy, levels do not change appreciably in women with genetic defects and may require replacement therapy at delivery. Oral estrogen-progestin agents do not appreciably alter factor IX levels.

TREATMENT AND COMPLICATIONS

The principles of treatment and discussion of complications of hemophilia B are essentially the same as noted for hemophilia A. The specific treatment of hemophilia B has consisted of the administration of prothrombin-complex concentrates (PCC) to achieve hemostatic levels of factor IX. Fresh frozen plasma can also be used but therapeutically useful factor IX levels are difficult to obtain without overloading the patient's vascular system. Currently available PCCs also contain the other vitamin K-dependent clotting factors in varying amounts including activated forms (VIIa, Xa) which cause the products to be thrombogenic during surgery or infected states. Thrombotic complications (deep venous thrombosis, disseminated intravascular coagulation, and myocardial infarction) after intense use of the PCCs (prophylaxis, surgery) still occur; the prophylactic use of heparin (added by the manufacturer or treater) has therefore been recommended. Modern virucidal processes have rendered the newer products free of HIV and the hepatitis viruses. Highly purified (monoclonally or chromatographically derived) products containing only factor IX and free of hepatitis and HIV viruses are now available and probably will become the products of choice in all transfusion therapy (see Chap. 56 for further discussion).

Inhibitors to factor IX develop in approximately 2.5 to 3 percent of hemophilia B patients (see Chap. 21). Of 23 patients who have inhibitors and whose genes have been characterized, 14 had gross gene deletion but the remaining 9 did not. Gene deletion is not the sole explanation for inhibitor development.

BIBLIOGRAPHY

Boklan BP, Sawitsky A: Factor IX deficiency in Gaucher disease. *Arch Intern Med* 136:489, 1976.

Briet E et al: Hemophilia B Leyden. A sex linked hereditary disorder that improves after puberty. *N Engl J Med* 306:788, 1982.

Chung KS et al: Purification and characterization of an abnormal factor IX (Christmas factor) molecule. Factor IX Chapel Hill. *J Clin Invest* 62:1078, 1978.

Crossley M et al: Recovery from hemophilia B Leyden: An androgen responsive element in the factor IX promoter. *Science* 257:377, 1992.

Diuguid DL, Furie B: Molecular genetics of hemophilia B. In: Hoffman R, Benz EJ Jr, Shattil S, Furie B, Cohen HJ. *Hematology Basic Principles and Practice,* New York, Churchill Livingston, 1991, pp 1316–1324.

Giannelli F et al: Haemophilia B: Database of point mutations and short additions and deletions. *Nucleic Acids Res* 18:4053, 1990.

Guy GP et al: An unusual complication in a gravida with factor IX deficiency: Case report with review of the literature. *Obstet Gynecol* 80:502, 1992.

Ketterling RP et al: T296–M, a common mutation causing mild hemophilia B in the Amish and others: Founder effect, variability in factor IX activity assays, and rapid carrier detection. *Hum Genet* 87:333, 1991.

Ludwig M et al: Hemophilia B caused by five different nondeletion mutations in the protease domain of factor IX. *Blood* 79:1225, 1992.

Poon MC: Patients with hemophilia B (Christmas disease) who have anti-factor IX: Genetic heterogeneity. *J Lab Clin Med* 112:283, 1988.

Spitzer SG et al: Replacement of isoleucine-397 by threonine in the clotting protein-ase factor IXa (Los Angeles and Long Beach variants) affects macromolecular catalysis but not L-tosylarginine methyl ester hydrolysis. Lack of correlation between the ox brain prothrombin time and the mutation site in the variant proteins. *Biochem J* 265:219, 1990.

Taylor SAM et al: Characterization of the original Christmas disease mutation (cysteine 206→serine): From clinical recognition to molecular pathogenesis. *Thromb Haemost* 67:63, 1992.

Hereditary
Factor XI Deficiency

Hereditary factor XI (plasma thromboplastin antecedent [PTA]) deficiency was first described by Rosenthal and others in 1955 as a hemophilia-like bleeding disorder that could be treated satisfactorily with stored plasma. The disorder is inherited in an autosomal manner with heterozygotes showing a factor XI coagulant activity level of 25 to 60 percent of normal while homozygotes have levels < 15 percent. Both heterozygotes and homozygotes may exhibit bleeding manifestations (usually mucous membrane or postsurgical hemorrhage) of variable severity which is not necessarily correlated with the plasma factor XI coagulant activity. Over half the reported cases have occurred in the Jewish race; the Ashkenazi Jewish population in Israel has a heterozygote frequency of 1:8.

STRUCTURE-FUNCTION RELATIONSHIP

Factor XI circulates in the plasma as a glycoprotein zymogen of the trypsin group of serine proteases and is complexed to high molecular weight kininogen (HMWK). The 160-kd molecule is a homodimer composed of two identical 83-kd polypeptides connected by a disulfide bond. The liver is the only site of factor XI production. Factor XI monomer is activated by factor XIIa by cleavage at the Arg 369-Ile 370 bond, resulting in a 47-kd heavy chain and a 35-kd light (contains catalytic site) chain. Recent evidence indicates that factor XI may also be cleaved by thrombin at the same site, aided by dextran sulfate in vitro; whether this happens in plasma has been questioned. Activated platelets bind and promote the activation of factor XI in the presence of HMWK; activated platelets also secrete a factor XIa inhibitor which is similar or identical to the Alzheimer amyloid precursor protein. Factor XIa activates factor IX in the presence of calcium ions and also hydrolyzes the chromogenic substrate S-2366, which is the basis for a factor XI activity assay. Under physiologic conditions, factor XIa is inhibited mainly by a-1-antitrypsin but also by antithrombin III (AT III) and the platelet-specific anti-XIa.

GENETICS

The gene coding for factor XI is 23 kb long and is found on the long arm of chromosome 4 (4q35). Factor XI deficiency is inherited as an autosomal recessive trait. The majority of patients have a parallel reduction in factor XI activity and antigen; only three cases of cross-reacting material (CRM)-positive disease have been reported (genetic lesion unknown). To date, three point mutations in the gene have been identified: type I, a splice junction abnormality between Lys 185-Gly 186; type II, a nonsense mutation, Glu 117-stop; and type III, a missense mutation, Phe 283-Leu. Type II and III mutations are the predominant causes of factor XI deficiency among Ashkenazi Jews. Factor levels and bleeding tendency for these defects are shown in Table 16-1. The heterozygous state is more difficult to define by coagulant assays in the Askenazi population (Table 16-2) but in other studies almost all heterozygotes displayed levels below the normal range with a cutoff of 0.6 to 0.7 u/mL.

TABLE 16-1 Clinical and Laboratory Manifestations in Homozygous Factor XI Deficiency

Deficiency	APTT	Factor XI Activity u/mL	Clinical Findings
Genotype II/II (16)	108/32	0.012	Bleeding after NP-oral trauma Injury bleeding increased
Genotype II/III (23)	85/32	0.033	Bleeding after NP-oral trauma Injury bleeding
Genotype III/III (13)	67/32	0.097	Bleeding after NP-oral trauma Rare injury bleeding
Genotype, unknown (1)	85/32	0.015	No bleeding after childbirth, gynecologic surgery, or NP-oral trauma

SOURCE: Modified from Asakai R et al: Factor XI deficiency in Ashkenazi Jews in Israel. *N Engl J Med* 325:153, 1991.

*Number of subjects are in parentheses; APTT values are mean patient/control; NP, nasopharyngeal; injury bleeding, events after tooth extraction, surgery, and childbirth; genotype, unknown is author patient.

CLINICAL MANIFESTATIONS

The diagnosis of hereditary factor XI deficiency is usually considered in the evaluation of a mild to moderate bleeder or in the evaluation of a prolonged APTT. As illustrated in Table 16-2, homozygous or heterozygous states can often be separated from the normal adult range by the factor XI activity assay performed on a freshly drawn plasma sample (frozen samples may increase activity). As reviewed in the Kitchens reference, the lower limits of normal used to separate possible heterozygotes may be as high as 0.7 U/mL for factor XI activity. Recent family studies in Askenzai Jews showed a greater overlap between heterozygotes and normal and suggested the need for molecular studies in borderline cases. When factor XI antigen has been measured, a close correlation with activity assays was seen with rare exception of a homozygote positive for cross-reacting antigen. The bleeding time is prolonged in some cases, possibly indicating a factor XI-platelet interaction defect. As many as 50 percent of heterozygotes may have mildly prolonged bleeding times (personal data).

The frequency and severity of bleeding manifestations have not correlated with the clotting factor level (heterozygote or homozygote) in several large series. Some homozygotes do not bleed even after surgical stress, whereas heterozygotes are sometimes severe bleeders. The possible causes of bleeding that may be associated with or part of hereditary factor XI deficiency are listed in Table 16-3. Bleeding tendency is usually consistent within a kindred but is not determined exclusively by either factor XI:C or factor XI:Ag levels. Associated defects (hemophilia A, platelet function

TABLE 16-2 Classification of Subjects into Normal, Heterozygote, or Homozygote by Use of Plasma Factor XI Assays

Study	Normal Adult Range (U/dL)	Heterozygotes (U/dL)	Homozygotes (U/dL)
Kitchens (Summary 5 studies)	75–127	25–69	0–13
Asakai et al. (both II and III genotypes)	45–205	28–126	0.2–17
Present data (Denver)	58–130 (n=48)	20–56 (n=51)	1–16 (n=6)

*The Kitchens summary and the Asakai data are taken from the references given. In our data, heterozygotes were defined by family studies or by assay level with abnormal APTT in subjects in whom no other explanation for abnormality was found.

TABLE 16-3 Possible Causes of Variation in Severity of Bleeding Tendency in Hereditary Factor XI Deficiency

A. Inheritance of associated hemostatic defect
   von Willebrand disease
   Platelet function defect (storage pool disease, Bernard-Soulier disease)
   Other coagulopathy (factor VIII deficiency)
   Noonan's syndrome
B. Drug ingestion (ASA)
C. Quantitative/qualitative defect in factor XI molecule
D. Quantitative/qualitative abnormality in platelet-associated factor XI

defects, von Willebrand disease) can occur and may be associated with increased bleeding. Noonan's syndrome (dysmorphic facies, short stature, congenital heart disease, easy bruising) is often associated with partial factor XI deficiency. Severe bleeding occurs in heterozygotes as well. As shown in Table 16-4, possible platelet-factor XI interaction defects could result in abnormal bleeding times and a greater hemorrhagic tendency. This example and others in the literature suggest that normal platelet

TABLE 16-4 Hereditary Factor XI Deficiency with Prolonged Bleeding Time[*]— Effect of Treatment on Hemorrhagic Tendency

Age	Bleeding Episode	Treatment	Response
22	Postpartum hemorrhage	Curettage	Cessation
29	Cervical biopsy	RBC transfusion	Gradual cessation
30	Cone biopsy of cervix	FFP, 15–20 U/kg × 3: RBCs	Minimal effect
		10 packs platelets + DDAVP	Cessation
31	Exploratory laparotomy	5 packs platelets + DDAVP	No response
		10 packs platelets + FFP × 2	Cessation

[*]Both patient and her son have factor XI levels of 0.25–0.40 U/mL and prolonged bleeding times (often > 20 min); von Willebrand factor and platelet aggregation studies were normal except for decreased response to L-epinephrine.
Note that patient bleeding did not respond to FFP alone in dose which raised factor XI level to 0.6 U/mL.
FFP, fresh frozen plasma; RBC, red blood cells.

transfusions are sometimes needed to correct the bleeding defect in these patients.

TREATMENT

Infusions of fresh frozen plasma into hereditary XI-deficient patients have shown the factor XI half-disappearance time to be 55 h. Frequent infusions (12 to 24 h) are necessary to maintain levels of 40 to 60 percent. A new factor XI plasma-derived concentrate is now available in Europe for clinical trials (Bio-Products, Oxford, UK) and levels > 100 percent of normal were achieved after single infusions. Mucous membrane and dental bleeding, frequently seen in factor XI-deficient patients, may respond nicely to adjunctive therapy with antifibrinolytic agents. An acquired factor XI inhibitor may rarely develop in the transfused patient and may be detected by APTT mixing studies or by a Bethesda-type assay (see Chap. 21).

BIBLIOGRAPHY

Asakai R et al: Factor XI deficiency in Ashkenazi Jews in Israel. *N Engl J Med* 325:153, 1991.

Bolton-Maggs PH et al: Inheritance and bleeding in factor XI deficiency. *Br J Haematol* 69:521, 1988.

Bolton-Maggs PH et al: Production and therapeutic use of a factor XI concentrate from plasma. *Thromb Haemost* 67:314, 1992.

Brunnée T et al: Activation of factor XI in plasma is dependent on factor XII. *Blood* 81:580, 1993.

Kitchens CS: Factor XI: A review of its biochemistry and deficiency. *Semin Thromb Hemost* 17:55, 1991.

Mannhalter C et al: Identification of a defective factor XI cross-reacting material in a factor XI-deficient patient. *Blood* 70:31, 1987.

Novakova IRO et al: Factor XI kinetics after plasma exchange in severe factor XI deficiency. *Haemostasis* 16:51, 1986.

Ragni MV et al: Comparison of bleeding tendency, factor XI coagulant activity, and factor XI antigen in 25 factor XI-deficient kindreds. *Blood* 65:719, 1985.

Rosenthal RL et al: Plasma thromboplastin antecedent (PTA) deficiency: Clinical, coagulation, therapeutic and hereditary aspects of a new hemophilia-like disease. *Blood* 10:120, 1955.

Schnall SF et al: Acquired factor XI inhibitors in congenitally deficient patients. *Am J Hematol* 26:323, 1987.

Sharland M et al: Coagulation-factor deficiencies and abnormal bleeding in Noonan's syndrome. *Lancet* 339:19, 1992.

Smith RP et al: Platelet coagulation factor XIa-inhibitor, a form of Alzheimer amyloid precursor protein. *Science* 248:1126, 1990.

Tavori S et al: The effect of combined factor XI deficiency with von Willebrand factor abnormalities on haemorrhagic diatheses. *Thromb Haemost* 63:36, 1990.

Walsh PN: Factor XI: A renaissance. *Semin Hematol* 29:189, 1992.

Walsh PN et al: Regulation of factor XIa activity by platelets and α_1-protease inhibitor. *J Clin Invest* 80:1578, 1987.

Winter M et al: Factor XI deficiency and a platelet defect. *Haemostasis* 13:83, 1983.

Contact Factor
Deficiencies

Hereditary deficiencies of factor XII (Hageman factor), prekallikrein (PK, Fletcher factor), and high molecular weight kininogen (HMWK, Fitzgerald, Flaujeac, Williams factors), are coagulation curiosities; all three are associated with a strikingly prolonged APTT without a bleeding diathesis. These coagulation factors along with factor XI (see Chap. 16) are responsible for the initiation of coagulation through the intrinsic pathway by means of activation by surface contact. In essence, factor XII binds directly to a negatively charged surface and is "autoactivated"; circulating complexes of PK-HMWK and XI-HMWK bind to the surface through the HMWK molecule. Factor XIIa activates PK to kallikrein which produces reciprocal activation of factor XII (2000 times more rapid than autoactivation). Factor XIIa then activates factor XI to XIa. In addition, kallikrein cleaves bradykinin from HMWK and is partly responsible for intrinsic plasma fibrinolysis by converting plasminogen to plasmin via activation of urokinase. The biologic consequences and differential diagnosis of the contact factor deficiencies are discussed below.

FACTOR XII DEFICIENCY

Factor XII (Hageman factor) is a serine protease glycoprotein with a molecular weight of approximately 84,000 d and a plasma concentration of 30 μg/mL. Surface-mediated (glass, kaolin, cellite, dextran sulfate, endotoxin, urates, crude collagen, sulfatides) autoactivation and reciprocal kallikrein activation produce a series of proteolytic cleavages of factor XII resulting in a-factor XIIa and β-factor XIIa. Both a-factor XIIa and β-factor XIIa activate PK, whereas a-factor XIIa is a better activator of factor XI than β-factor XIIa. Both a-factor XIIa and β-factor XIIa activate other proenzymes including factor VII, plasminogen, and complement, C1. With generation of Hageman factor fragments and kallikrein, the contact system is linked to the kinin system, the intrinsic fibrinolytic system, and the complement system in addition to liberating renin from prorennin and priming neutrophils for chemotactic activity. The major inhibitor of factor XIIa is C1 esterase inhibitor; other inhibitors are antithrombin III (AT-III), a_2-antiplasmin (a_2-AP), and a_2-macroglobulin.

Hageman factor deficiency is inherited in an autosomal recessive manner with homozygotes (or double heterozygotes) having < 0.01 U/mL factor XII. Heterozygotes show plasma levels ranging from 0.17 to 0.83 U/mL in various studies; about half the heterozygotes show levels less than the normal range. Indeed, in several reports, several individuals in the normal control group with levels < 50 to 60 percent are noted. In our experience the most common cause of an isolated prolongation of the APTT in a nonbleeding child or adult (without a lupus anticoagulant) is mild factor XII deficiency. Most of homozygous factor XII subjects are cross-reacting material (CRM) negative; only 2 of 81 cases tested showed factor XII:Ag levels of 0.39 and 0.80 U/mL. The dysproteinemic molecule of one of these individuals has an amino acid substitution (Cys 571-Ser) which could give rise to an altered active site or secondary substrate binding site (factor XII, Washington, DC). Documentation of a kallikrein cleavage site defect in another CRM-positive healthy woman with < 1 percent factor XII clotting activity is called factor XII Locarno. Hageman factor deficiency is not associated with a bleeding tendency even at major surgery or pregnancy; however, some individuals with factor XII deficiency have had a thrombotic tendency (see Chap. 42). One review of 121 cases showed an incidence of 8.2 percent of deep venous thrombosis or pulmonary embolism. In another series of 103 patients with recurrent thromboembolic disease, 15 percent had low factor XII levels in the heterozygous range. Activation of the contact system and plasminogen activation after DDAVP infusion occurred in healthy volunteers and was absent in factor XII-deficient subjects.

Acquired alterations of the Hageman factor pathway (factor XII, PK, HMWK) have been noted in many disease states, but proof for pathogenetic significance is lacking for most of these. Evidence for activation and decreased contact factor levels are seen in endotoxin-induced sepsis and shock, disseminated intravascular coagulation (DIC), adult respiratory distress syndrome, polycythemia vera, nephrotic syndrome, and hepatic cirrhosis. Further evidence for the activation of the contact system may be found in the precise measurement (radioimmunoassay) of plasma factor XIIa-C1-inhibitor and kallikrein-C1-inhibitor complexes. Spontaneous increase in factor VII activity after cold storage of plasma (cold-promoted activation) depends on factor XII and increased kallikrein activity and is seen in pregnancy and oral contraceptive users with elevated levels of factor XII.

PREKALLIKREIN (FLETCHER FACTOR) DEFICIENCY

Prekallikrein is a single chain γ-globulin with two forms at molecular weight 85,000 and 88,000; it circulates in a concentration of 35 to 45 μg/mL as an equimolar complex with HMWK. PK is converted to a-kallikrein by a-factor XIIa most efficiently in the presence of HMWK and a surface. The cleavage (Fig. 17-1) produces a heavy chain which binds to HMWK and interacts with a surface and a light chain with the enzymatic active site. As a protease, a-kallikrein liberates kinins from kininogens, activates factor XII, activates plasminogen, converts prorennin to renin, interacts with human leukocytes, and destroys C1 components. Prolonged incubation with β-factor XIIa converts a-kallikrein to β-kallikrein, which has much less activity. The major circulating inhibitor of kallikrein is C1 inhibitor plus a_2-macroglobulin and

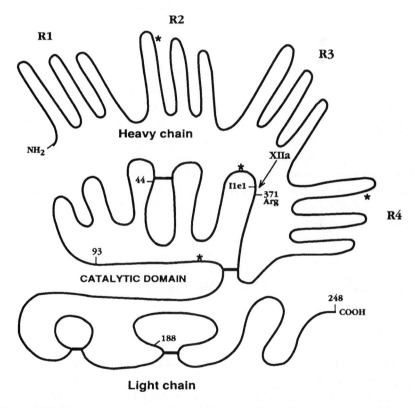

Figure 17-1 Diagrammatic representation of plasma prekallikrein. The cleavage site by factor XIIa is depicted by the arrow; (Arg 371-Ile 1) note the heavy chain with four tandem repeats (R1 to R4) and the light chain containing the catalytic triad located at His-44, Asp-93, and Ser-188. N-linked glycosylation sites are shown by asterisk. (Adapted from Fujikawa K, Saito H: Chap. 88. In: Scriver CR, Beaudet AL, Sly WS, Valle D (eds): The Metabolic Basis of Inherited Disease, 6th ed., New York, McGraw-Hill, 1988.)

AT III. PK may be measured in plasma by amidolytic (substrate PPAN, S-2302), esterolytic, coagulation, and immunochemical assays; the coagulation assay using Fletcher factor-deficient plasma has limited accuracy due to the need for high plasma dilutions and critical incubation times.

The hereditary deficiency of PK or Fletcher factor deficiency is a rare disorder with few clinical or laboratory consequences except a markedly prolonged APTT without a bleeding tendency like Hageman factor deficiency. Inheritance is autosomal recessive with the heterozygotes displaying intermediate to normal levels of prekallikrein. Evidence that 5 of 18 homozygotes have CRM has been reported. A dysfunctional molecule (PK activity =0; PK:Ag=0.35) with substitution of an amino acid which hinders cleavage by β-factor XIIa has been described. Although the homozygotes' plasma may show in vitro impaired intrinsic fibrinolysis, decreased chemotactic activity and decreased kinin generation, physiologic observations in man have failed to reveal any significant impairment in hemostasis, fibrinolysis. or inflammatory responses. Reported clinical associations with the homozygous condition include myocardial infarction, cerebral thrombosis, hyperthyroidism (2 cases) and systemic lupus erythematosus (SLE).

Gestationally dependent decreased levels of PK as well as factor XII have been observed in preterm and term infants and are known to rise to adult levels by 6 months of age. Moderately low levels of PK (15 to 75 percent) are seen in most homozygous HMWK-deficient subjects. Decreased PK occurs in hereditary angioneurotic edema (C1 esterase inhibitor deficiency), infections (bacterial sepsis, typhoid fever, Rocky Mountain spotted fever, dengue), DIC, liver disease, nephrosis, sickle cell disease, chronic renal failure, type II hyperlipoproteinemia, renal allograft rejection, and adult and infant respiratory distress syndrome. These alterations of PK are usually interpreted to mean activation of the contact system.

HIGH MOLECULAR WEIGHT KININOGEN DEFICIENCY

Kininogens occur in human plasma in two forms: HMWK (120 kd) and a low molecular weight form, LMWK (68 kd). Both are single chain glycoproteins which on proteolytic cleavage give rise to bradykinin, a mediator of vasodilation, smooth muscle contraction, and increased vascular permeability; in addition, both are potent inhibitors of cysteine proteases (cathepsins, calpain). HMWK, and not LMWK, also plays an important role in the contact phase of coagulation as a carrier and cell surface receptor for factor XI and PK; HMWK facilitates as a cofactor enzyme-substrate interactions on the surface since neither factor XI nor PK binds directly to the surface. These structure-function relationships are shown in Fig. 17-2.

When activated (cleaved) by kallikrein, HMWK binds to anionic surfaces

Heavy chain

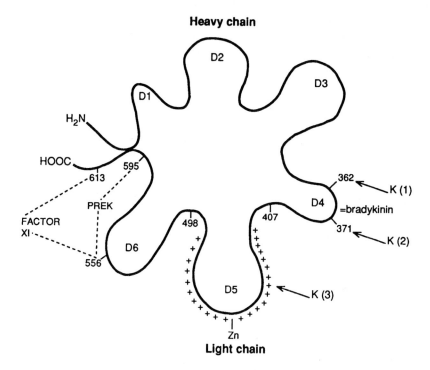

Light chain

Figure 17-2 Diagrammatic representation of high molecular weight kininogen. Domains are indicated (D1 to D6). The sites and order of cleavage by kallikrein (K) are shown by the arrows. The nonapeptide (bradykinin) is released by cleavages K(1) and K(2). Key amino acids are numbered. The + symbols indicate the histidine and glycine-rich region (D5) responsible for interaction with negatively charged surfaces and Zn^{++} ions. The binding regions for factor XI and prekallikrein are indicated on D6. (Adapted from Schmaier AH: Modulation of the cell-membrane expression of the kininogens regulates the rate of bradykinin delivery to cells. In press.)

(platelets, neutrophils, endothelial cells) in the presence of zinc ions and thus acts as a bridging molecule between cell surfaces and factor XI and PK to allow more rapid proteolytic activation by factor XIIa. Therefore, a deficiency of HMWK interferes with optimal activation of the contact factor pathway and results in deficient intrinsic activation of factor XI and subsequently factor IX, deficient intrinsic fibrinolysis, as well as decreased kinin system functions. These deficiencies have been demonstrated in the plasma of the rare individuals with hereditary deficiencies of HMWK (Fitzgerald, Williams, Flaujeac traits); since both HMWK and LMWK are the result of alternative mRNA splicing of the same gene, most of the dozen or so reported individuals have deficiencies of both the kininogens. Nevertheless, no clinical evidence of hemostatic or other defect has been noted in either the homozygotes (HMWK usually < 0.01 U/mL) or heterozygotes (HMWK approximately 0.5 U/mL).

Acquired alterations in the kininogens have been observed in several disease entities where they may have a pathogenetic role: hypotensive septicemia (man and experimental animal models), adult respiratory distress syndrome, and cardiopulmonary bypass morbidity.

DIAGNOSIS OF CONTACT FACTOR DISORDERS

The diagnosis of a hereditary deficiency of factor XII, PK, or HMWK is usually considered when evaluating a prolonged APTT in situations where the other screening tests and the clinical history are noncontributory, that is, the diagnosis of the "isolated" prolonged APTT in a nonbleeder. Consideration of Table 17-1 and Fig. 17-3 allow several generalizations to be made.

If the APTT is *greatly prolonged* (usually greater than twofold the APTT of a severe factor VIII-deficient hemophiliac) and corrects to the normal range with 1:1 mixing with normal plasma, the homozygous deficiency state (factor XII, PK, or HMWK) is suspect (factor XII deficiency is more common). If a 10-min incubation of the patient's plasma (as compared to the usual 3 min) "corrects" to near normal (using kaolin or micronized silica as the activator in an APTT), the deficiency state is due to PK; this is the so-called "Fletcher factor" screening test which is only applicable to possible homozygotes. Specific coagulation factor activity assays using congenitally deficient plasmas and the APTT system are necessary for confirmation and differentiation of factor XII from HMWK deficiency. The use of potent activators like ellagic acid in the APTT system or long incubation times may not allow these differentiations to be made precisely.

TABLE 17-1 Coagulation Studies in Hereditary Deficiencies of Contact System

Deficiency		Usual Factor Assay* U/mL	Screening APTT (s)	Percent NP corrects PTT	Correction of KPTT, 10 min inc at 37°C
Factor XII	Ho	<0.01	Greatly↑	50	No
(Hageman)	He	0.25–0.55	Slight↑		Yes
Prekallikrein	Ho	<0.01	Greatly↑	>2	Yes
(Fletcher)	He	≈0.5	Normal		
HMWK	Ho	<0.01	Greatly↑	>12.5	No
(Flaujeac,	He	0.3–0.6	Normal		
Fitzgerald,					
Williams)					

*Some heterozygotes will have factor levels in the normal range and normal screening APTT.
He, heterozygote; Ho, homozygote; KPTT, kaolin PPT; NP, normal plasma; Inc, incubation.

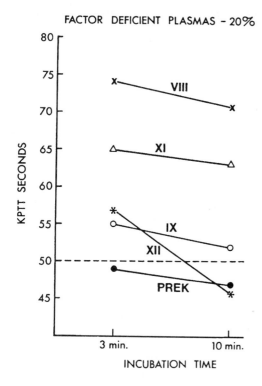

FACTOR DEFICIENT PLASMAS – 20%

Figure 17-3 The results of kaolin PTTs are shown for hereditary deficiencies of various clotting factors (severely deficient plasmas mixed with normal plasma to yield a 0.20 U/mL factor level) at 3-min and 10-min incubation times.

Heterozygous Deficiency States

In our and others' laboratories the cause of an "isolated" *mildly prolonged* APTT (if due to contact factor deficiency) is almost always moderate to mild factor XII deficiency. See Fig. 17-3 and note that only factor XII-deficient plasma corrects into the normal range on 10-min incubation, the major "slow-activator." The original APTT in heterozygotes of PK and HMWK is usually normal; plasmas contain much greater levels of PK (over 2 percent) and HMWK (over 12.5 percent) than necessary for the normalization of the APTT. Remember that HMWK-deficient plasmas usually have a low levels of PK as well. A rare patient may have mild deficiencies of all three factors. Family members (potential heterozygotes) of a diagnosed homozygous contact factor-deficiency patient should be identified to prevent future expensive evaluations of a possible mildly prolonged APTT (see Chap. 4).

BIBLIOGRAPHY

Bouma BN, Griffin JH: Initiation mechanisms; the contact activation system in plasma. In: Zwaal RFA, Hemker HC (eds): *Blood Coagulation*, Amsterdam, Elsevier, 1986, pp 103–128.

Carvalho AC et al: Activation of the contact system of plasma proteolysis in the adult respiratory distress syndrome. *J Lab Clin Med* 112:270, 1988.

Fuhrer G et al: FXII. *Blut* 61:258, 1990.

Fujikawa K, Saito H: Contact activation. In: Scriver CR, Beaudet AL, Sly WS, Valle D (eds): *The Metabolic Basis of Inherited Disease*, 6th ed., New York, McGraw-Hill, 1988, pp 2189–2206.

Gordon EM et al: Reduced titers of Hageman factor (factor XII) in Orientals. *Ann Intern Med* 95:697, 1981.

Gordon EM et al: The role of augmented Hageman factor (factor XII) titers in the cold-promoted activation of factor VII and spontaneous shortening of the prothrombin time in women using oral contraceptives. *J Lab Clin Med* 99:363, 1982.

Halbmayer WM et al: The prevalence of factor XII deficiency in 103 orally anticoagulated outpatients suffering from recurrent venous and/or arterial thromboembolism. *Thromb Haemost* 68:285, 1992.

Hathaway WE et al: Clinical and physiologic studies of two siblings with prekallikrein (Fletcher factor) deficiency. *Am J Med* 60:654, 1976.

Kaplan AP, Silverberg M: The coagulation-kinin pathway of human plasma. *Blood* 70:1, 1987.

Lämmle B et al: Thromboembolism and bleeding tendency in congenital factor XII deficiency—a study on 74 subjects from 14 Swiss families. *Thromb Haemost* 65:117, 1991.

Levi M et al: Reduction of contact activation related fibrinolytic activity in factor XII deficient patients. Further evidence for the role of the contact system in fibrinolysis in vivo. *J Clin Invest* 88:1155, 1991.

Saito H et al: Human plasma prekallikrein (Fletcher factor) clotting activity and antigen in health and disease. *J Lab Clin Med* 92:84, 1978.

Schapira M et al: Prekallikrein activation and high molecular-weight kininogen consumption in hereditary angioedema. *N Engl J Med* 308:1050, 1983.

Soulier JP, Gozin D: Present knowledge on contact factors; theoretical and practical aspects. *Blood Trans Immunohaematol* 6:785, 1984.

Stormorken H et al: A new case of total kininogen deficiency. *Thromb Res* 60:457, 1990.

Prothrombin, Factor V, Factor VII, Factor X, and Combined Factor Deficiencies

Quantitative and qualitative deficiencies of factor II (prothrombin), factor V (proaccelerin, labile factor), factor VII (proconvertin), and factor X (Stuart-Prower factor) can result in a moderately severe bleeding disorder. All of these factor deficiencies are inherited as an autosomal recessive trait (bleeding is noted primarily in the homozygote or compound heterozygotes). These disorders are rare: factor II deficiency, fewer than 30 families reported; factor V deficiency, one person per million; factor VII deficiency, 1/500,000; factor X deficiency, 1/500,000. Combined coagulation factor deficiencies will also be discussed below.

PROTHROMBIN DEFICIENCY

Prothrombin (factor II) is a vitamin K-dependent single chain glycoprotein with a molecular weight of 72,000 and a plasma concentration of about 100 μg/mL. Prothrombin is converted to thrombin by factor Xa in the presence of Ca^{++}, factor Va, and phospholipids; this complex is called prothrombinase (Fig. 18-1). The activation of prothrombin results in several well-defined products: Xa cleavage at Arg 274-Thr 275 yields fragment 1-2 (used as a marker of intravascular coagulation) plus prethrombin 2 which produces a-thrombin; Xa or thrombin itself cleaves at Arg 286-Thr 287 which yields thrombin and a fragment 1·2·3. In addition, the venom of *Echis carinatus* and prothrombinase cleave Arg 323-Ile 324 to produce a species (meizothrom-

II:Ag levels averaging about 0.10 U/mL and display easy bruising and hematoma formation, epistaxis, menorrhagia, and bleeding after trauma or surgery. Bleeding symptoms (postcircumcision oozing, gastrointestinal bleeding, hematomas) in the neonatal period may be initially diagnosed as hemorrhagic disease of the newborn. Hemarthroses are rare. Severe deficiencies (< 0.01 U/mL) have not been reported and may be incompatible with life. Heterozygotes show intermediate prothrombin levels and are asymptomatic.

Hemorrhagic manifestations in the dys- or hypodysprothrombinemic families are variable and range from severe bleeding manifestations to no symptoms. Part of the explanation for this variability may be due to the characteristics of the molecular lesion and whether homozygous or compound heterozygous (see Table 18-1). Laboratory manifestations show a normal hemostatic screen except for slight to moderate prolongation of the APTT and PT; Echis venom clotting time is often abnormal.

Therapy of acute bleeding episodes may be accomplished by achieving a plasma level of 25 percent with fresh frozen plasma. Repeat transfusions are usually not necessary because of the long half-life of prothrombin (3 days). More intense therapy (major surgery) may require prothrombin-complex concentrates (PCCs) that usually contain adequate prothrombin but thromboembolic complications and viral contamination must be considered.

FACTOR V DEFICIENCY

Factor V is a large glycoprotein with a molecular weight of 330,000; it circulates in a single chain form with a concentration of 7 μg/mL. The structure of factor V is similar to factor VIII with a 40 percent amino acid sequence identity; the gene is located on chromosome 1. Factor V is synthesized in megakaryocytes, vascular endothelial cells, and possibly hepatocytes; 20 percent of the circulating factor V is found in the a-granules of platelets. Factor V can be activated by thrombin, Xa, and platelet proteases; the activated factor V or Va binds to the phospholipid bilayer of cell membranes (platelets, endothelial cells, monocytes) forming a receptor for factor Xa and prothrombin; this complex (termed prothrombinase) is responsible for the conversion of prothrombin to thrombin and is much more efficient than Xa alone (see Fig. 18-1). Like factor VIIIa, Va is rapidly inactivated by activated protein C (APC) which destroys the binding sites for Xa and prothrombin. Plasmin also produces proteolytic degradation of Va after first enhancing the procoagulant effect.

Hereditary factor V deficiency or parahemophilia is a mild to moderately severe bleeding disorder inherited in an autosomal recessive mode. The bleeding disorder is variable, with some patients showing surgical- and trauma-induced hemorrhage, menorrhagia, postpartum hemorrhage, neonatal intracranial hemorrhage (ICH), epistaxis, and rare deep hematoma or joint bleeding while other patients with similar factor V levels have little or no bleeding. The platelet content of factor V appears to be correlated with these observations. An increased incidence of anomalies (especially cardiovascular lesions) with homozygous factor V deficiency is of particular interest.

The homozygotes display coagulant activity levels of < 10 percent of normal usually with comparable factor V antigen levels. A few patients (4 of 14 and 2 of 21 in two series) will have increased factor V antigen indicating a dysproteinemia. Factor V levels are lower in patients' platelets than in normals and an occasional patient will show a prolonged bleeding time. As expected, the APTT and PT will be prolonged. The evaluation of a new patient should include a factor VIII assay because combined deficiencies of factor V and factor VIII can occur. All other hemostatic tests are normal.

Heterozygotes do not have a bleeding tendency; their factor V levels will range from 40 to 60 percent of normal; occasionally the PT will be prolonged by 1 to 2 s. An interesting family with a bleeding disorder and plasma factor V levels of 36 to 40 percent had a qualitative factor V defect in their platelets in association with mild thrombocytopenia and a slightly prolonged bleeding time (factor V Quebec).

Acquired factor V deficiency has been noted in acute and chronic liver disease, disseminated intravascular coagulation (DIC) syndromes, and due to acquired inhibitors. Mild deficiencies (0.23 to 0.66 U/mL) were also reported in children with Ph1-positive chronic myelogenous leukemia; these patients consumed transfused factor V rapidly and the levels were corrected after effective chemotherapy; no evidence for DIC was present.

Bleeding episodes are treated with infusions of fresh frozen plasma in a dose to raise the level by 20 to 25 percent. No concentrated products are available. Successful management of surgical procedures has been accomplished with daily infusions of fresh frozen plasma. Platelet concentrates are effective in therapy but should be reserved for more serious bleeding or inhibitor patients to prevent platelet alloimmunization.

FACTOR VII DEFICIENCY

Factor VII (proconvertin), a vitamin K-dependent and liver-produced single chain glycoprotein (molecular weight 47,000), circulates in a concentration of 0.5 μg/mL. Several enzymes may activate (cleavage of Arg 152-Ile 153 bond) factor VII to the two chain form VIIa: thrombin, plasmin, factor XIIa, factor IXa, and factor Xa (factor IXa and Xa are probably the most important in vivo). Via the extrinsic pathway, coagulation is initiated when VII/VIIa binds to tissue thromboplastin (TF) exposed on disrupted cells forming a complex which generates the active forms of Xa (and subsequently IXa); these enzymes proteolytically activate factor VII to the 40- to 120-fold more active VIIa. Since native factor VII and VIIa have the same affinity for TF, the excess amount of factor VII that is available competes for the thromboplastin and prevents full expression of the VIIa. In addition to this feedback mechanism, the pathway is inhibited by a lipoprotein complex called tissue factor pathway inhibitor (TFPI; see Chaps. 1 and 45).

An autosomal recessively inherited bleeding diatheses due to a deficiency of factor VII has been recognized since 1951. Heterozygous patients are usually asymptomatic (factor VII:C levels of approximately 40 to 50 percent) but homozygous or double heterozygous patients have a severe bleeding disorder with manifestations like those of classical hemophilia (factor VII:C levels < 0.01 U/mL; usually < 0.03 U/mL). A rare individual may have no history of bleeding or even have a thrombotic tendency. Clinical onset is frequently as an infant with umbilical cord stump bleeding, cephalohematoma, or ICH. Over all ages, the prevalence of ICH of 16 percent has been observed.

Other common hemorrhagic manifestations include oral mucosal bleeding, epistaxis, hemarthroses, gastrointestinal bleeding, severe menstrual bleeding, postpartum and postsurgical hemorrhage. Since 1971 cross-reacting material (CRM)-positive variants (factor VII:Ag > factor VII:C) have been recognized and compose up to 50 percent of the 100 or so reported families. Following the report of factor VII Padua (mild bleeding disorder, factor VII:C, 0.09 U/mL with normal factor VII:Ag) in which variable activation by different thromboplastins (rabbit brain and lung, ox brain thromboplastin) was demonstrated, other "variants" according to thromboplastin reactivity have been described.

Molecular genetic analysis will hopefully prove a better way to study the heterogeneity of factor VII deficiency. The gene for factor VII is on chromosome 13 near the gene for factor X; the factor VII molecule has eight exons which code for the Gla region, two epidermal growth factor domains, an activation peptide region, and a catalytic domain. A preliminary report indicates two missense mutations in a patient with severe factor VII deficiency; one mutation produced Arg-Gln change at the cleavage site for activation (Arg 152-Ile 153).

The diagnosis of factor VII deficiency is suspected when the only abnormal screening test is the PT, thus prompting a factor VII activity assay. In severe factor VII deficiency, the PT is prolonged upward of 20 to 30 s while heterozygotes show only a prolongation of 1 to 3 s. In fact, the isolated mildly prolonged PT in an asymptomatic patient often represents mild factor VII deficiency (heterozygote); the normotest may be even more sensitive to carrier detection.

The half-life of factor VII is 4 to 6 h (Fig. 18-2); therefore, it is difficult to maintain hemostatic levels with fresh frozen plasma alone. However, for single episode bleeding, a level of 15 percent can be achieved by a fresh frozen plasma transfusion of 10 to 15 mL/kg. Most available PCCs contain relatively little factor VII; a new concentrate (Immuno) containing only factor VII will

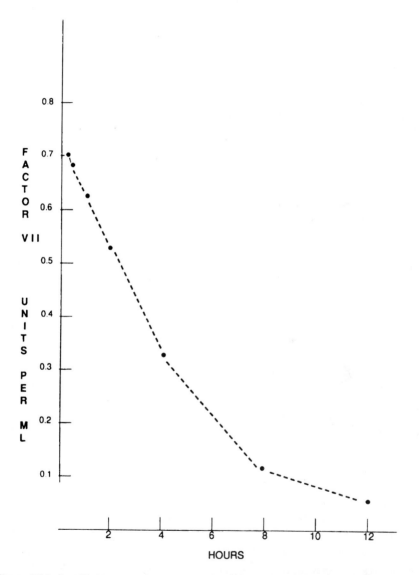

Figure 18-2 A purified concentrate of factor VII (Immuno) was infused into a young adult woman with severe factor VII deficiency in a steady (nonbleeding) state. The resulting plasma levels are plotted over time; the half-disappearance time is estimated at approximately 4 h. Previous half-disappearance times for factor VII given as prothrombin complex concentrates (Konyne) were < 2 h.

soon be available and will probably become the treatment of choice for these rare patients.

FACTOR X DEFICIENCY

Factor X zymogen is a glycoprotein synthesized in the hepatocyte as a single polypeptide chain (488 amino acids); after posttranslational changes including vitamin K-dependent γ-carboxylation of the first 11 glutamic acid residues, cleavage of the leader sequence and glycosylation (15 percent carbohydrate), the mature protein is secreted and circulates as a two chain disulfide bonded molecule (light chain, Mr 16,200, heavy chain Mr 42,000) in a concentration of 10 μg/mL. Activation of factor X occurs at the point of convergence of the intrinsic system (via the IXa-VIIIa-phospholipid complex) and the extrinsic system (via the VIIa-TF-phospholipid complex) in presence of Ca^{++}. The cleavage of Arg 194-Ile 195 bond in the heavy chain produces Xa and an activation peptide of Mr 14,000 which has been used as a marker for intravascular coagulation. Factor X may also be activated by RVV and a cancer procoagulant (cysteine protease). Factor Xa is the key serine protease in the prothrombinase complex (see Fig. 18-1).

The gene for factor X is on chromosome 13 where it spans 24 kb, consists of seven introns and eight exons and shows homology with other vitamin K-dependent proteins. A congenital bleeding disorder is inherited as an autosomal recessive trait. Within a few years after the report of the "Stuart clotting defect" in 1957, it was recognized that factor X deficiency was a markedly heterogeneous group of patients who could be classified by measurements of antigen (CRM+, CRM−) and by activation defects using extrinsic (PT) and intrinsic (PTT) and direct (RVV, no cofactor) systems. Examples of the variation are given in Table 18-2. In several of these families, the genetic mutation has been defined.

Clinically the homozygotes or double heterozygotes exhibit moderate to severe bleeding tendencies which include hemarthroses, deep hematomas, menorrhagia, and postsurgical hemorrhage. Infants have presented with ICH antenatally and in the neonatal period. Most commonly both the PT and APTT are prolonged; however, variant factor X deficiencies have been reported in which only the PT or only the APTT are abnormal (see Table 18-2). The Stypven time (RVV time) is prolonged; other screening tests including the bleeding time are normal. Heterozygotes are usually asymptomatic and have normal laboratory screening tests except for a slightly prolonged PT occasionally.

Acquired factor X deficiency may occur in patients with primary amyloidosis and paraproteinemia and has been attributed to being secondary to interaction of factor X with amyloid fibrils or the paraprotein. The bleeding ten-

TABLE 18-2 Examples of Factor X Variants

Variant	FX:Ag U/mL	F:X activity U/mL (assay)	PT (s)	APTT (s)	Other Characteristics
Stuart (Ho)	<0.01	<0.01 by all assays	85/12	510/66	Severe bleeding
Stuart (He)		0.21–0.52	—	—	
Prower (Ho)	0.85	0.08 (Ext) 0.07 (RVV)	Inc	170/50	Bleeding
Friuli (Ho)	1.0	0.07 (Ext) 0.90 (RVV)	33/13	68/45	Point mutation Bleeding
Vorarlberg (Ho)	0.20	0.05 (Ext) 0.254 (Int)	106/14	64/38	Point mutation No bleeding
San Antonio (He + He)	0.36	0.14 (Ext)	20/14	Nl	Postsurgical bleeding
Melbourne	1.2	1.0 (Ext) 0.09 (Int) 1.05 (RVV)	12/13	50/40	No bleeding
Santo Domingo (Ho)	0.05	<0.01	30/12	75/32	Severe bleeding Point mutation

Ho, homozygote; He, heterozygote; (Assay), type of assay used; Ext, extrinsic (PT); Int, intrinsic (APTT). Values for PT and APTT are given in s/control; RVV, Russell viper venom.

dency may be life threatening. Other coagulation changes (decreased factor IX, fibrinolysis, prolonged thrombin time) can be seen. The half-life of transfused factor X is very short and often ineffective. Selective factor X deficiency has also been reported in leukemia while combined deficiencies with other vitamin K-dependent factors are seen in vitamin K deficiency and liver disease.

Treatment of acute bleeding episodes in hereditary factor X deficiency is effectively achieved by transfusions of fresh frozen plasma. A level of 10 to 20 percent is sufficient for hemostasis except for complicated surgical procedures where the use of PCCs may be needed. The hereditary deficiency can improve during pregnancy and has been amenable to therapy with estrogen therapy at other times. The treatment of the acquired deficiency in amyloidosis is more complicated and is discussed in Chap. 33.

COMBINED HEREDITARY COAGULATION FACTOR DEFICIENCIES

Hereditary multiple coagulation factor deficiencies occurring in the same individual are of two general types: those deficiencies with an established association on a genetic basis (factor V and factor VIII deficiency; vitamin K-dependent factor deficiencies, combined factor VIII and IX deficiency, factor VII and factor VIII deficiency and deletion of chromosome 13 (VII and X deficiency); *and* those multiple deficiencies inherited coincidentally (all of the above plus other combinations).

Combined factor V and VIII deficiency (familial multiple factor deficiency I, see Soff and Levin reference) is a well-documented autosomal recessively inherited condition reported in a number of families (particularly around the Mediterranean basin). Homozygotes display excessive bleeding after surgical trauma, abortions, and childbirth; women have menorrhagia; hemarthroses are rarely seen. Factor VIII and V levels are from 5 to 20 percent of normal. Heterozygotes show intermediate levels of factor V and factor VIII and may have a mild bleeding tendency. The specific gene defect is unknown although it was earlier proposed that the combined deficiency was from uncontrolled proteolysis due to a deficiency of protein C inhibitor. Subsequent studies of protein C inhibitor were normal. Newly diagnosed sporadic cases of mild or moderate hemophilia A or factor V deficiency should have both factor V and VIII assayed to not overlook the combined disorder. Treatment of bleeding episodes includes use of DDAVP to increase level of factor VIII or fresh frozen plasma or both depending on severity of bleeding tendency.

Combined deficiencies of factors II, VII, IX, and X have occurred (mild hemorrhagic symptoms with coagulation factor levels of 15 to 20 percent of normal). Parents of affected individuals have often been normal. The defect has been associated with pseudoxanthoma elasticum, as well as the pheno-type of warfarin embryopathy. Vitamin K therapy has increased the factor levels temporarily in some cases, raising the possibility that the defect is a genetic abnormality affecting vitamin K reductase or carboxylase or defects in vitamin K transport and utilization. Abnormal carboxylation was demon-strated in a child with hereditary deficiency of factors II, VII, IX, X, and protein C and S.

Intermediate levels of factors VII and X (40 to 50 percent) were observed in two patients with chromosome 13 deletion syndrome (mental retardation, craniofacial dysmorphy, hypospadias, congenital heart disease) which sug-gested hemizygosity for the genetic loci for the clotting factors. Other familial multiple coagulation factor deficiencies associated on a genetic basis include factor VIII, IX, XI and factor IX, XI. Coincidental combinations include various possibilities and have been reviewed in the reference by Soff and Levin.

BIBLIOGRAPHY

Brenner B et al: Hereditary deficiency of all vitamin K-dependent procoagulants and anticoagulants. *Br J Haematol* 75:537, 1990.

Canfield WM, Kisiel W: Evidence of normal functional levels of activated protein

C inhibitor in combined factor V/VIII deficiency disease. *J Clin Invest* 70:1260, 1982.

Chediak J et al: Successful management of bleeding in a patient with factor V inhibitor by platelet transfusions. *Blood* 56:835, 1980.

Chiu HC et al: Heterogeneity of human factor V deficiency. Evidence for the existence of antigen-positive variants. *J Clin Invest* 72:493, 1983.

Fair DS et al: Isolation and characterization of the factor X Friuli variant. *Blood* 73:2108, 1989.

Girolami A et al: Factor VII Padua$_2$: Another factor VII abnormality with defective ox brain thromboplastin activation and a complex hereditary pattern. *Blood* 54:46, 1979.

Goodnight SH et al: Factor VII antibody-neutralizing material in hereditary and acquired factor VII deficiency. *Blood* 38:1, 1971.

Greipp PR et al: Factor X deficiency in amyloidosis: A critical review. *Am J Hematol* 11:443, 1981.

Haber S: Norethynodrel in the treatment of factor X deficiency. *Arch Intern Med* 114:89, 1964.

Hasegawa DK et al: Factor V deficiency in Philadelphia-positive chronic myelogenous leukemia. *Blood* 56:585, 1980.

Henriksen RA, Mann KG: Substitution of valine for glycine-558 in the congenital dysthrombin thrombin Quick II alters primary substrate specificity. *Biochemistry* 28:2078, 1989.

Knight RD et al: Replacement therapy for congenital factor X deficiency. *Transfusion* 25:78, 1985.

Mann KG et al: Nonenzymatic cofactors: Factor V. In: Zwaal RFA, Hemker HC (eds): *Blood Coagulation*, Amsterdam, Elsevier, 1986, pp 15–34.

Mazzucconi MG et al: Evaluation of the nature of mildly prolonged prothrombin times. *Am J Hematol* 24:37, 1987.

Montgomery RR et al: Prothrombin Denver—A new dysprothrombinemia. *Circulation* 62(suppl 111): 279, 1980.

Negrier C et al: Increased thrombin generation in a child with combined factor IX and protein C deficiency. *Blood* 81:690, 1993.

Osterud B: Initiation mechanisms: Activation induced by thromboplastin. In: Zwaal RFA, Hemker HC (eds): *Blood Coagulation*, Amsterdam, Elsevier, 1986, pp 122–139.

Pfeiffer RA et al: Deficiency of coagulation factors VII and X associated with deletion of a chromosome 13 (q34). *Hum Genet* 62:358, 1982.

Rabiet MJ et al: Molecular defect of prothrombin Barcelona. Substitution of cysteine for arginine at residue 273. *J Biol Chem* 261:15045, 1986.

Ragni MV et al: Factor VII deficiency. *Am J Hematol* 10:79, 1981.

Reddy SV et al: Molecular characterization of human factor X San Antonio. *Blood* 74:1486, 1989.

Shapiro SS, McCord S: Prothrombin. *Prog Hemost Thromb* 4:177, 1978.

Soff GA, Levin J: Familial multiple coagulation factor deficiencies. Review of the literature: Differentiation of single hereditary disorders asssociated with multiple factor deficiencies from coincidental concurrence of single factor deficiency states. *Semin Thromb Hemost* 7:112, 1981.

Tracy PB, Mann KG: Abnormal formation of the prothrombinase complex: Factor V deficiency and related disorders. *Hum Pathol* 18:162, 1987.

Triplett DA et al: Hereditary factor VII deficiency: Heterogenity defined by combined functional and immunochemical analysis. *Blood* 66:1284, 1985.

Tsuda H et al: A case of congenital factor V deficiency combined with multiple congenital anomalies: Successful management of palatoplasty. *Acta Haematol* 83:49, 1990.

Watzke HH et al: Molecular defect (Gla+14–Lys) and its functional consequences in a hereditary factor X deficiency (Factor X "Vorarlberg"). *J Biol Chem* 265:11982, 1990.

Abnormalities

# of Fibrinogen

The hereditary abnormalities of fibrinogen include afibrinogenemia, hypofibrinogenemia, dysfibrinogenemia, and hypodysfibrinogenemia. These disorders result from genetically controlled quantitative or qualitative changes in the fibrinogen molecule and are described below. Acquired abnormalities of fibrinogen are common because the glycoprotein is a major acute phase reactant and the major substrate of the key enzymes of the coagulation system, thrombin and plasmin. Intravascular coagulation syndromes are discussed in Chap. 25.

STRUCTURE-FUNCTION RELATIONSHIP

Fibrinogen is a 340,000 d glycoprotein synthesized in the hepatocyte and megakaryocyte; it circulates in the plasma in a concentration of 200 to 400 mg/dL. Figure 19-1 indicates the structure-function relationships of the fibrinogen molecule. Cleavage of fibrinopeptides A and B (FPA, FPB; hydrolysis of Arg-Gly bonds) by thrombin exposes a site that binds to the C terminus of the γ-chain and initiates polymerization of the fibrin monomers. This soluble fibrin clot is stabilized by the amidolytic action of activated factor XIII which forms a covalent bond by the condensation of lysine and glutamine side chains with the removal of an ammonia group. The formation of a fibrin clot is the principal but not exclusive function of the molecule. Early proteolytic alterations of fibrinogen occur physiologically leading to fibrinogens with lower molecular mass (305,000 and 270,000). Other later, and part of the degradation process, plasmin cleavage sites include regions between D and E domains in all three chains producing fragments Y, D, and E. These fragments have several biologic functions including stimulation of human hemopoietic cell lines, vasoactive properties, and bacteria clumping. Many specific binding sites and interactions are known for the fibrinogen molecule including those with thrombin, calcium, platelets (C terminal of Aα- and

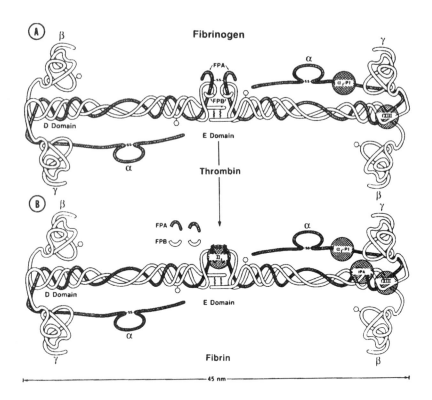

Figure 19-1 Fibrinogen consists of three pairs of polypeptide chains, Aα, Bβ, and γ, joined by disulfide bonds to form a symmetric dimetric structure (A). The NH2-terminal regions of all six chains form the central domain (E domain) of the molecule containing FPA and FPB sequences that are cleaved by thrombin during enzymatic conversion to fibrin. Carbohydrate moieties (♀) are located at one site on each of the γ- and Bβ-chains. Enzymatic conversion of fibrinogen to fibrin (B) by thrombin cleavage results in release of FPA and FPB. A nonsubstrate (secondary) binding site for thrombin (IIa) is present in the central domain of α,β-fibrin, and depends on the presence of the β15 to 42 sequence. Binding sites for IIa, t-PA, factor XIII, and α2-plasmin inhibitor, respectively, are indicated on the fibrinogen or fibrin molecule. (Used with permission from Mosesson MW: Fibrin polymerization and its regulatory role in hemostasis. J Lab Clin Med 116:8, 1990.)

γ-chain), fibronectin, factor XIII, plasminogen, tissue plasminogen activator (t-PA), a₂-antiplasmin, collagen, thrombospondin, and other cell interactions (erythrocytes, monocytes). Posttranslational amino acid modifications carry carbohydrate, phosphate, and sulfate and play a role in fibrin formation. Carbohydrate clusters containing sialic acid are present on the Bβ- and γ-chains.

Fibrinogen assay methods are usually based on one of the following principles: (1) coagulation time or velocity (Clauss or thrombin clotting method); (2) amount of coagulable protein (tyrosine content or Biuret colorimetrically or ultraviolet adsorption); (3) amount of precipitable protein (heat, 52° to 58°C [126° to 136°F], or salt) and (4) immunoreactive protein (antifibrinogen antibodies). The most popular and reproducible method used in the United States is a modification of the Clauss method (Dade) using a pooled human plasma standard. Because diluted plasma is tested and excess thrombin is used, the effect of heparin or fibrinogen degradation products (FDP) in the sample is negligible. It has been observed that hereditary and physiologic (newborn) dysfibrinogens may give a spuriously lower value as compared to immunologic quantitation. Indeed, this observation is used to indicate a dysfibrinogen when investigating a prolonged thrombin time if one realizes that the ratio of antigenic to functional fibrinogen is slightly elevated in normal controls (see Rodgers and Garr reference).

GENETICS

The three genes responsible for the synthesis of the a-, β- and γ-chains of fibrinogen are located close to each other on chromosomes 4, band 4q32. Each gene is 6500 to 7500 base pairs in length and is regulated in part by a monocyte-derived hepatocyte stimulating factor or interleukin-6. Several genetic defects result in phenotypes which display either bleeding tendencies, thrombotic complications, difficulties in wound healing, or no symptoms. Congenital afibrinogenemia is a rare autosomal recessively inherited defect with severe bleeding manifestations (like hemophilia) in the homozygote. Consanguinity is common and one or both parents may show hypofibrinogenemia. No molecular defects such as gene deletion or rearrangements have been reported. Hypofibrinogenemia with both recessive and dominant modes of transmission are known. Some of these cases may be examples of a dysfibrinogenemia in which the detection of low fibrinogen was due to functional abnormalities measured by a thrombin clotting assay. Some cases of hypofibrinogenemia may be due to an inability to assemble and secrete fibrinogen normally; liver histology shows globules of fibrinogen within cells.

The most frequent genetic abnormality is dysfibrinogenemia, which is usually due to a point mutation inherited in an autosomal dominant manner (both heterozygotes and homozygotes are abnormal). At least half of the nearly 300 families reported are asymptomatic. Table 19-1 lists examples of these abnormal fibrinogens which have had the molecular defect defined. In general, the defects with delayed fibrinopeptide release have amino acid substitutions at position 7, 12, 16, or 19 of the a chain (thrombin cleaves between 16 and 17). These defects are associated with mild to moderate bleeding symptoms or are asymptomatic. Defects in the Bβ-chain are less frequent and can be associated with decreased thrombin binding (more free

TABLE 19-1 Examples of Hereditary Dysfibrinogenemias

Name	Molecular Defect	Functional Defect	Clinical Manifestation
Detroit	Aα-Arg 19-Ser	Defective polymerization	Bleeding (Ho)
Lima	Aα-Arg 141-Ser	Defective polymerization ↑glycosylation	None (Ho)
Chapel Hill II, Milano IV, and others	Aα 16-His	Defective FPA release	Bleeding and thrombosis (He, Ho)
Metz	Aα-Arg 16-Cys	Defective FPA release	Bleeding (Ho)
Ledyard		Abnormal polymerization	Bleeding (He)
New York I	Bβ deletion from 9-72 (exon 2)	↓Thrombin binding; defective FPB release	Recurrent thrombosis (He)
Naples	Bβ-Ala 68-Thr	↓Thrombin binding	Thrombosis (Ho)
Seattle I or Christchurch II	Bβ-Arg 14-Cys	Defective FPB release	None
Osaka II	γ-Arg 275-Cys	Abnormal polymerization	None
Asahi	γ-Met 310-Thr Extra oligosaccharide	Severely impaired polymerization; ↓XIIIa crosslinking	Bleeding (He) Poor wound healing
Vlissengen	γ-deletion of dipeptide (Asn 319 and Asp 320)	Impaired polymerization ↓Ca++ binding	Massive pulmonary embolism
Dusart	Aα554-Cys	Slow polymerization Lysis-resistant fibrin	Thrombosis (He)
Haifa	γ-Arg 275-His	Polymerization defect Plasmin-binding defect	Thrombosis (He)

*FPA, fibrinopeptide A; FPB, fibrinopeptide B; He, heterozygote; He, homozygote.

thrombin) and a thrombotic tendency. The γ-chain defects result in abnormally delayed fibrin polymerization. Delayed wound healing due to abnormal XIIIa cross-linking has been described in a few variants (Paris I with elongation of the γ-chain); urea solubility test is abnormal.

CLINICAL MANIFESTATIONS

Table 19-2 shows the clinical and laboratory signs which lead to the diagnosis of an hereditary disorder of fibrinogen. The parents of afibrinogenemic patients are either normal or have hypofibrinogenemia. Family members with dysfibrinogenemia may show positive signs (dominant inheritance) or may be asymptomatic; therefore, immediate family members should be screened with the abnormal test (TCT or reptilase time). In complicated or unusual cases, other causes of a prolonged thrombin time should be excluded (see Chap. 4) including heparin effect. Some patients have both qualitative and quantitative defects in fibrinogen with levels ranging from 50 to 120 mg/dL. The TCT is usually markedly prolonged and fibrinopeptide release and polymerization abnormalities may be found. Sometimes these hypodysfibrinogenemia patients will show rapid turnover of the abnormal fibrinogen as well as an inhibitory effect on the normal TCT in mixing studies. These patients can have a bleeding disorder and a history of frequent spontaneous abortions (Bethesda III).

ACQUIRED ALTERATIONS IN FIBRINOGEN

Fibrinogen is the prime example of an acute phase reactant protein. As noted above, the synthesis of fibrinogen is keyed to stimulation by interleukins or hepatocyte-stimulating factor derived from monocyte-macrophages during inflammation, infection, or malignancy. During severe stress or fibrinogen breakdown, the turnover rate (normally 3 to 5 days) may increase 25-fold. In addition to elevations of the fibrinogen level with acute phase reaction, other physiologic alterations are known. During pregnancy, plasma fibrinogen rises as early as the third month and increases gradually to values at term of 350 to 650 mg/dL; a similar estrogen dose-dependent rise is seen during oral contraceptive agent therapy. Hyperfibrinogenemia is a risk factor in stroke and coronary heart disease. A variation at the β-fibrinogen gene locus is associated with an increased risk of peripheral atherosclerosis.

Causes of acquired hypofibrinogenemia include liver disease, ascites, disseminated intravascular coagulation (DIC) states, and L-asparaginase therapy. Other drugs decreasing the plasma fibrinogen level (possibly by affecting monocyte-cytokine interactions) include N-3 fatty acids, ticlopidine, alcohol,

TABLE 19-2 Clinical and Laboratory Manifestations of Congenital Fibrinogen Disorders

	Clinical	Laboratory
Afibrinogenemia	Severe lifelong (often cord bleeding) hemorrhagic diathesis as in moderate to severe hemophilia	No clotting is seen in all screening tests (APTT, PT, TCT). Bleeding time is prolonged; all fibrinogen assays are zero or trace.
Hypofibrinogenemia	Mild bleeding disorder; menorrhagia, recurrent abortions, postsurgery bleeding on occasion, placental abruption	APTT usually normal; PT slightly prolonged or normal*; TCT and reptilase time mildly prolonged. Decrease in fibrinogen to < 100–150 mg/dL by thrombin clotting and immunoassay.
Dysfibrinogenemia	Chronic history of bleeding tendency after surgery and trauma; possible poor wound healing. Positive family history (or) Thrombotic tendency (recurrent deep venous thrombosis, pulmonary embolism, etc.) Positive family history (or) Asymptomatic	All screening tests can be normal except prolonged TCT and reptilase time (ranging from a few seconds to > 100 s) with normal fibrinogen level. (APTT and PT may be slightly prolonged). Higher fibrinogen level by immunologic test than thrombin clotting method.

*The APTT and PT usually are normal until fibrinogen is < 100 mg/dL.

fibrates, and pentoxifylline. Posttranslational modifications of the fibrinogen molecule affecting phosphorus or carbohydrate content may occur in the fetus and newborn infant (increased phosphorus and sialic acid) and in liver disease (increased sialic acid). These changes result in a mildly prolonged thrombin time which can be "corrected" by calcium ions. Therefore, the calcium thrombin time will often fail to detect these changes. Similar thrombin time prolongations may be seen in the nephrotic syndrome (dysfibrinogen).

Other causes of acquired "dysfibrinogenemia" include inhibitor or antibodies (rarely) or incipient or early DIC (commonly). A clinically silent dysfibrinogenemia caused by an antibody that delayed FPB release markedly prolonged the thrombin time in a 50-year-old man with a γ-globulin paraprotein.

TREATMENT AND COMPLICATIONS

The rare patient with afibrinogenemia requires replacement transfusion therapy (usually with cryoprecipitate) for acute bleeding episodes as well as comprehensive care as provided for hemophilic patients. The prolonged bleeding time has shortened after DDAVP. A few of these patients may develop antibodies to fibrinogen, complicating their therapy. Prophylactic cryoprecipitate every 7 to 10 days has been used successfully in children. Patients with bleeding tendencies due to hypo- or dysfibrinogenemias rarely require replacement therapy; when necessary, cryoprecipitates have been useful.

BIBLIOGRAPHY

Bogli C et al: Fibrinogen Milano IV, another case of congenital dysfibrinogenemia with an abnormal fibrinopeptide A release (Aa 16 Arg → His). *Haemostasis* 22:7, 1992.

Dang CV et al: The normal and morbid biology of fibrinogen. *Am J Med* 87:567, 1989.

De Marco L et al: von Willebrand factor interaction with the glycoprotein IIb/IIIa complex: Its role in platelet function as demonstrated in patients with congenital afibrinogenemia. *J Clin Invest* 77:1272, 1986.

Ebert R: *Index of Variant Fibrinogens*, Rockville, Md, RF Ebert, 1990.

Fowkes FG et al: Fibrinogen genotype and risk of peripheral atherosclerosis. *Lancet* 339:693, 1992.

Galanakis DK: Fibrinogen anomalies and disease. A clinical update. *Hematol Oncol Clin North Am* 5:1171, 1992.

Gandrille S et al: A study of fibrinogen and fibrinolysis in 10 adults with nephrotic syndrome. *Thromb Haemost* 59:445, 1988.

Henschen A, McDonagh J: Fibrinogen, fibrin and factor XIII. In: Zwaal RFA, Henker HC (eds): *Blood Coagulation*. Amsterdam, Elsevier, 1986, pp 171–242.

Huber P et al: Human beta-fibrinogen gene expression: Upstream sequences involved in its tissue specific expression and its dexamethasone and interleukin 6 stimulation. *J Biol Chem* 265:5695, 1990.

Koepke JA: Standardization of fibrinogen assays. *Scand J Haematol*, Suppl 37:130, 1980.

Lee MH et al: Fibrinogen Ledyard (AαArg16–Cys): Biochemical and physiologic characterization. *Blood* 78:1744, 1991.

Matsuda M: Abnormal fibrinogens: The present status of structure elucidation. *Biomed Prog* 4:51, 1991.

Marciniak E, Greenwood MF: Acquired coagulation inhibitor delaying fibrinopeptide release. *Blood* 53:81, 1979.

Menache D: Congenital fibrinogen abnormalities. *Ann NY Acad Sci* 408:121, 1983.

Nawarawong W et al: The rate of fibrinopeptide B release modulates the rate of clot formation: A study with an acquired inhibitor to fibrinopeptide B release. *Br J Haematol* 79:296, 1991.

Rodgers GM, Garr SB: Comparison of functional and antigenic fibrinogen values from a normal population. *Thromb Res* 68:207, 1992.

Seydewitz HH, Witt I: The fraction of high molecular weight (HMW) fibrinogen and phosphorylated fibrinopeptide A in fetal fibrinogen. *Thromb Res* 55:785, 1989.

Factor XIII,

α_2-Antiplasmin and

Plasminogen Activator

Inhibitor-1 Deficiencies

Hereditary deficiencies of factor XIII (fibrin-stabilizing factor, FSF), α_2-antiplasmin (α_2-AP or α_2-plasmin inhibitor) and plasminogen activator inhibitor-1 (PAI-1) cause a lifelong bleeding diathesis with several features in common. All three are rare disorders inherited in an autosomal recessive manner. Laboratory hemostatic screening tests including platelet count, bleeding time, APTT, PT, thrombin time, and fibrinogen levels are normal. Specific factor assays must be performed to indicate the diagnosis. The mechanism of bleeding in each condition is due to defects occurring after the fibrin clot is formed, that is, lack of cross-linking of the clot by factor XIII and the excessive lysis of the clot due to deficiencies of major physiologic inhibitors of fibrinolysis, α_2-AP and PAI-1 (Fig. 20-1). Additional information regarding these three clotting factors may be found in Chaps. 26 and 42.

FACTOR XIII DEFICIENCY

Factor XIII (plasma glutaminase, FSF) is a cysteine enzyme which circulates in the plasma (bound to fibrinogen); the plasma zymogen (30 μg/mL) occurs as a tetramer of paired α- and β-chains with a molecular mass of 309,000 d. An intracellular form (platelets, megakaryocytes, monocytes, placenta, prostate, uterus) is a dimer of two α-chains. Activation of factor XIII is by thrombin in the presence of Ca^{++}, which results in exposure of

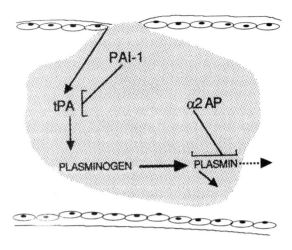

Figure 20-1 Excessive plasmin formation in hemostatic plug producing clot lysis and hemorrhage can be due to a deficiency of PAI-1 or α_2-AP.

the active center cysteine. The activation peptide, active center, and calcium binding sites are in the a-chain protein; the β-chain protein probably serves a carrier or protective function. When activated, XIIIa catalyzes the formation of a covalent bond between glutamine and lysine residues and accomplishes a cross-linked trimolecular complex. Several cross-linked complexes formed by XIIIa are fibrin-fibrin, fibrin-fibrinogen, fibrin-a_2-AP, fibrin-von Willebrand factor, fibrin-thrombospondin, fibrin-fibronectin, and fibronectin-collagen. These substrates have many features in common such as being adhesive proteins, platelet a-granule proteins, and participation in macromolecular complexes on cell or subendothelial surfaces which suggests they have a role in wound healing, tissue repair, tumor growth, and atherosclerosis.

The factor XIII cross-linking activity may be precisely quantitated by measuring fluorescent dansylcadaverine or labeled putrescine incorporation into casein (a surrogate system). The a- and β-proteins may be quantitated by immunoassay. A screening test demonstrating that patient's plasma clot dissolves in 5 M urea or 1 percent monochloroacetic acid is indicative of a severe (< 1 to 2 percent) deficiency of factor XIII. The screening test is clinically useful since only severe deficiencies exhibit hemorrhagic tendencies.

The genes for factor XIII a- and β-proteins are located on autosomal chromosomes (chromosome 6 for a-protein) and are transmitted in a recessive manner. The homozygotes have the bleeding disorder which is variously expressed according to transmission of genes for a- and β-proteins. The heterozygotes are not bleeders but show intermediate levels of a- or β-proteins and 50 to 60 percent levels of factor XIII activity. A classification of hereditary factor XIII deficiency has been proposed and is given in Table 20-1. The

TABLE 20-1 A Classification of Hereditary Factor XIII Deficiency

Type	Relative Incidence	Factor XIII Activity	β-Protein	α-Protein
I	Rare	Low to absent	Low to absent	Low to absent
II	Frequent	Low to absent	Normal or slightly low	Low to absent
III	Rare	Low	Absent	Low

SOURCE: Girolami A, Sartori MT, Simoni P: An updated classification of factor XIII defect. *Br J Haematol* 77:565, 1991.

common type (II) usually shows no α-protein in plasma or platelets and < 1 percent factor XIII; type I, also severe, has low to absent α- and β-protein; type III, a much less severe phenotype (XIII activity of 24 percent, normal clot stability) has absent β-protein but detectable low protein α in plasma; the patients displayed only obstetric hemorrhage.

More than 200 cases of factor XIII deficiency have been reported since 1960. The most common sites of hemorrhage are umbilical cord stump in > 80 percent of cases (1 to 19 days of age) and intracranial (30 percent of cases), which is often spontaneous or after mild trauma. Other sites of bleeding include subcutaneous hematomas, joint bleeding (uncommon), and muscle hematomas. Defective wound healing, delayed bleeding episodes, and habitual abortion are often seen. Menorrhagia is sometimes observed. Treatment of acute bleeding episodes is easily accomplished using plasma or concentrates. The hemostatic level is low (approximately 2 to 3 percent) and the half-disappearance time after infusions is long (9 to 10 days). As illustrated by the following case, prophylaxis is relatively easily achieved.

Case Report—Factor XIII Deficiency, Type II

A female infant, born at term in 1984, was noted to have persistent bleeding from the umbilical stump. The infant's plasma clot dissolved readily in 5 M urea solution, and the bleeding ceased after an infusion of fresh frozen plasma. Detailed studies revealed:

	Factor XIII (U/mL)	α-chains (U/mL)	β-chains (U/mL)
Infant	0.02*	0	0.47
Mother	0.53	0.58	0.80
Father	0.72	0.66	0.7

*Performed 3 weeks after a plasma infusion.

The infant was placed on prophylactic transfusions of fresh frozen plasma (10 mL/kg) every 3 weeks and has remained free of hemorrhage except for a 2-month trial off plasma. At that time increased bruising and a large subcutaneous hematoma appeared, leading to reinstitution of plasma therapy. Growth and development have been normal. A brother born in 1988 also has the disorder.

Acquired low levels of factor XIII are observed in the following situations: newborn infant (approximately 50 percent of adult), liver diseases, leukemias, disseminated intravascular coagulation (DIC), various malignant diseases, rheumatoid arthritis, and Henoch-Schönlein purpura. Autoimmune (IgG antibodies) inhibitors of factor XIII activity have been noted as the cause of severe bleeding in adults (abnormal urea solubility tests were noted which did not correct on 1:1 mixing); the majority of reported cases were taking isoniazid or procainamide. Successful treatment included plasmapheresis and immunoadsorption.

α_2-ANTIPLASMIN DEFICIENCY

α_2-Antiplasmin is a single chain glycoprotein with a molecular weight of 51,000 and a plasma concentration of 7 mg/dL. α_2-AP is synthesized in the liver and is bound to plasminogen (70 percent) or occurs as a free form which is a less effective plasmin inhibitor. As noted in the section on fibrinolysis, α_2-AP regulates the system at three levels: (1) α_2-AP blocks the activity of plasmin by forming an instantaneous complex; this fast inhibition is backed up by α_2-macroglobulin; (2) α_2-AP inhibits the adsorption of plasminogen to fibrin; and (3) α_2-AP is cross-linked to fibrin by XIIIa, making the fibrin more resistant to local plasmin. The plasma half-life of the bound form is approximately 2.3 to 2.8 days. The plasma concentration of α_2-AP can be measured by functional (usually a chromogenic assay with the tripeptide S-2251) and by immunologic assays with specific antisera. α_2-AP-plasmin complexes can be measured by sensitive immunologic techniques and are indicators of in vivo activation of the fibrinolytic system.

Inherited α_2-AP deficiency is associated with a severe bleeding disorder (as in hemophilia) in the homozygous state and a mild or asymptomatic disorder in the heterozygous state (Table 20-2). The level of α_2-AP activity ranges from 0.02 to 0.15 U/mL in the homozygote to 0.35 to 0.70 U/mL in the heterozygote. The molecular defect in one of the first reported homozygotes is due to a deletion of Glu 137 causing a block in intracellular transport (α_2-AP, Okinawa). In most reported families immunoreactive α_2-AP was reduced in proportion to the functional activity (type 1 deficiency). However, normal amounts of immunoreactive α_2-AP were found in two members of a Dutch family who have activity levels < 0.04 U/mL. The dysfunctional

TABLE 20-2 Clinical Manifestations of Hereditary a_2-Antiplasmin Deficiency

Disorder	Plasma Levels (Chromogenic Substrate S-2251)	Euglobulin Lysis Time	Bleeding Manifestations
Homozygous deficiency	0.02–0.15 U/mL	Normal or decreased	Umbilical cord stump Postsurgical bleeding Hemarthroses Soft tissue hematomas Prolonged laceration bleeding Muscle bleeding Epistaxis
Heterozygous deficiency	0.35–0.70 U/mL	Normal; occasionally decreased	None (or) Postsurgical bleeding Bleeding after tooth extraction Easy bruising Menorrhagia

molecule has been named a_2-AP Enschede and is due to an alanine insertion adjacent to the reactive site. All hemostatic tests and coagulation assays are normal in the 15 families with a_2-AP deficiency reported, except for occasionally shortened euglobulin lysis times (ELT); no evidence of a hyperfibrinolytic state (increased fibrin degradation products, etc.) can be detected.

Acquired deficiencies of a_2-AP are seen in liver disease (decreased synthesis), nephrotic syndrome (urinary loss), systemic amyloidosis (complex formation and amyloid binding), DIC states and thrombolytic therapy (complex formation with plasmin), and cardiopulmonary bypass (hemodilution and consumption). Although many of these disorders have other hemostatic abnormalities in association with low a_2-AP, bleeding manifestations are apt to be more severe when the level is < 25 to 50 percent of normal.

Fortunately, the bleeding episodes in the hereditary disorder respond well to oral administration of ε-aminocaproic acid (Amicar) or tranexamic acid. The drug may also be useful in selected cases of acquired deficiency (amyloidosis, cardiopulmonary bypass).

PLASMINOGEN ACTIVATOR INHIBITOR-1 DEFICIENCY

Plasminogen activator inhibitor-1 is a serine protease inhibitor (serpin; molecular weight 52,000, 379 amino acids) which has a 30 to 50 percent homology with other members of the serpin family. The 12.2 kb gene for PAI-1 is located on chromosome 7 closely linked to the gene for cystic fibrosis. PAI-1 is found in plasma and extracellular sites where it is in complex with vitronectin and in platelets (a-granules). PAI-1 is stored or synthesized in the endothelial cells and hepatocytes and is the major fast-acting inhibitor for tissue plasminogen activator (t-PA). Two types of assays have been used for detection of PAI-1 in plasma. An activity assay performed by titration with single chain t-PA and immunologic assays (ELISA, IRMA) have indicated a wide normal range of 0.5 to 68 U/mL for activity and 6 to 600 ng/mL for antigen. The wide range suggests that PAI-1 is an acute phase reactant. Plasma for assay should be collected in a low pH buffer to eliminate the effect of other inhibitors and at an uniform time of day to control for diurnal variations.

Recent case reports indicate that a congenital deficiency of PAI-1 results in a lifelong bleeding diathesis (epistaxis, postsurgical hemorrhage, delayed onset hematomas after injury, and gastrointestinal bleeding) associated with normal routine hemostatic screening tests but with hyperfibrinolysis as evidenced by short ELTs. One patient exhibited plasma PAI-1 antigen and activity levels near zero but with normal PAI-1 in platelets. Amicar was effective in preventing bleeding after dental extractions. Another patient showed low PAI-1 activity in serum and platelet lysates but normal antigen in serum. The third patient, a 9-year-old girl with injury-related hematomas and bleeding after surgery, had entirely normal screening tests except for a 12-min bleeding time. PAI-1 antigen and activity were undetectable. The patient displayed a homozygous, two base pair insertion in exon 4 of the PAI-1 gene. Both parents were heterozygous for the mutant sequence. An acquired deficiency of PAI-1 due to an autoantibody in amyloidosis has been associated with a bleeding tendency. Low PAI-1 associated with increased levels of t-PA has resulted in severe postoperative bleeding in at least one patient (Stankiewicz reference).

BIBLIOGRAPHY

Dieval J et al: A lifelong bleeding disorder associated with a deficiency of plasminogen activator inhibitor type 1. *Blood* 77:528, 1991.

Fay WP et al: Brief report: Complete deficiency of plasminogen-activator inhibitor type 1 due to a frame-shift mutation. *N Eng J Med* 327:1729, 1992.

Girolami A et al: An updated classification of factor XIII defect. *Br J Haematol* 77:565, 1991.

Henschen A, McDonagh J: Fibrinogen, fibrin and factor XIII. In: Zwaal RFA, Hemker HC (eds): *Blood Coagulation*, Amsterdam, Elsevier, 1986, pp 219–230.

Holmes WE et al: Alpha-2-antiplasmin Enschede: Alanine insertion and abolition of plasmin inhibitory activity. *Science* 238:209, 1987.

Kluft C et al: A familial hemorrhagic diathesis in a Dutch family: An inherited deficiency of a_2-antiplasmin. *Blood* 59:1169, 1982.

Kruithof EKO et al: Plasminogen activator inhibitor 1 and plasminogen activator inhibitor 2 in various disease states. *Thromb Haemost* 59:7, 1988.

Larsen PD et al: Factor XIII deficiency and intracranial hemorrhages in infancy. *Pediatr Neurol* 6:277, 1990.

Lorand L et al: Human factor XIII: Fibrin-stabilizing factor. In: Spaet TH (ed): *Progress in Hemostasis and Thrombosis*, New York, Grune and Stratton, 1980, pp 245–290.

Loskutoff DJ et al: Type 1 plasminogen activator inhibitor. In: Coller BS (ed): *Progress in Hemostasis and Thrombosis*, New York, Saunders, 1989, pp 87–115.

Miura O et al: Hereditary a_2-plasmin inhibitor deficiency caused by a transport-deficient mutation (a_2-PI-Okinawa); deletion of Glu 137 by a trinucleotide deletion blocks intracelluilar transport. *J Biol Chem* 264:18213, 1989.

Nishida Y et al: A new rapid and simple assay for factor XIII activity using dansylcadaverine incorporation and gel filtration. *Thromb Res* 36:123, 1984.

Saito H: Alpha-2-plasmin inhibitor and its deficiency states. *J Lab Clin Med* 112:671, 1988.

Schleef RR et al: Bleeding diathesis due to decreased functional activity of type 1 plasminogen activator inhibitor. *J Clin Invest* 83:1747, 1989.

Stankiewicz AJ et al: Increased levels of tissue plasminogen activator with a low plasminogen activator inhibitor-1 in a patient with postoperative bleeding. *Am J Hematol* 38:226, 1991.

Williams EC: Plasma a_2-antiplasmin activity, role in the evaluation and management of fibrinolytic states and other bleeding disorders. *Arch Intern Med* 149:1769, 1989.

Acquired Coagulation
Factor Inhibitors

Acquired coagulation factor inhibitors are circulating antibodies that specifically neutralize the procoagulant activity of the various coagulation factors and result in a deficiency state frequently associated with a bleeding tendency. These inhibitors, which are different from the antiphospholipid antibodies or lupus anticoagulant (see Chap. 43), arise as alloantibodies in patients with hereditary factor deficiencies or as autoantibodies in patients with and without an underlying immune disorder. The most common and well-characterized inhibitor is directed against factor VIII and occurs in at least 15 percent of hemophilia A patients (alloantibody) and much less commonly in postpartum women, elderly individuals, patients with autoimmune disorders, and apparently normal individuals (autoantibodies). Management of these patients is difficult and costly; the attention of an experienced consultant is required.

FACTOR VIII INHIBITORS

In a multicenter study (United States Inhibitor Study Group) of 1522 patients with hemophilia A, a prevalence of 14.2 percent inhibitor patients was noted at time of entry. Twenty-eight percent had developed an inhibitor by age 5 years, 46 percent by age 10 years, and 66 percent by age 20 years. During the 4-year study, 31 patients developed new inhibitors, 29 of whom had factor VIII levels < 0.03 U/mL and 17 of whom developed the inhibitor within 75 exposure days to factor VIII (mostly high titer inhibitors). Of interest, 7 of 31 had transient low titer inhibitors which disappeared despite continued factor VIII usage.

Like the United States group, other studies have indicated a prevalence of 5 to 20 percent with an increased risk of inhibitor formation under the age of 5 to 7 years. A recent prospective study from Germany indicated that inhibitors developed in 24 percent (15 of 63) of hemophilia A patients followed from early childhood; almost all had occurred by age 5 years; 8 patients had a transient inhibitor. Thus frequent assessment of the inhibitor status indicates a higher incidence of antibodies (frequently transient) in newly transfused children. Inhibitors arise more often in black than white hemophiliacs in the United States, and concordance of inhibitors in siblings has been observed. These clinical and epidemiologic observations suggest a genetic predisposition to the development of a factor VIII inhibitor. Studies of HLA antigens in hemophilia patients with inhibitors have been conflicting and inconclusive except for decreased HLA-A1 and absence of HLA-Cw5, suggesting a potential genetic marker for inhibitor formation.

Over 95 percent of inhibitors occur in severe factor VIII deficiency. Analysis of the factor VIII gene has revealed a greater incidence of inhibitor formation in patients with deletions or missense mutations; restriction fragment length polymorphism analysis of the major histocompatibility complex (MHC) gene provided data (increased restriction fragments in the inhibitor patients) supporting a MHC-related basis for antibody formation. Additional indirect evidence for genetic control is suggested by the classification of VIII inhibitor patients into low responders (usually < 5 Bethesda units, BU) and high responders (> 10 BU); about 25 percent of patients are low responders regardless of the transfusion intensity, whereas more than 60 percent of patients will show brisk anamnestic rises of titer (to BU titers in the hundreds or rarely thousands in some cases). In summary, our current state of knowledge does not allow prediction of inhibitor formation in individuals with classic hemophilia.

Much more rarely, factor VIII inhibitors may arise spontaneously in "autoimmune" disorders such as rheumatoid arthritis, systemic lupus erythematosus (SLE), asthma, inflammatory bowel disease, erythema multiforme, drug reactions (penicillin), and pemphigus. Other underlying conditions include monoclonal gammopathies, malignancies, and pregnancy. However, about half the cases of spontaneous factor VIII inhibitors occur in disease-free individuals, in particular, in the first few months postpartum or in elderly individuals. Major bleeding is frequently present and the mortality rate is high (Table 21-1).

Factor VIII Antibody Characteristics

Although occasionally IgM antibodies have been reported, most factor VIII antibodies are of the IgG immunoglobulin class. In both hemophilic and spontaneous inhibitor patients, both IgG1 and IgG4 subclasses are seen. IgG4, which is associated with repeated or prolonged immunization and which does not fix complement, predominates. Light chains have been most frequently of κ or mixed κ and λ type and less frequently only λ. Taken

TABLE 21-1 Classification of Factor VIII Inhibitor Patients

Type	Underlying Disorder	Antibody Characteristics	Relative Occurrence	Laboratory Measurements	Response to Treatment
Alloantibody	Factor VIII deficient hemophilia, usually severe	IgG (rarely IgM); IgG1, IgG4 subclass; usually κ light chain; type 1 kinetics	15–20% of all hemophilia A	VIII:C usually <0.01 U/mL; Bethesda titer 1 to > 1000	Majority are high responders with brisk increase in antibody after factor VIII stimulation; 25% low responders—antibodies can be saturated with transfusion factor VIII; variable response to immunosuppressive drugs
Autoantibody	None or autoimmune disorder (SLE, rheumatoid arthritis); allergic reactions; leukemias; malignancy; or postpartum state	IgG IgG1, IgG4 subclass; usually λ light chain; type 2 kinetics	Extremely rare (1/million)	VIII:C is variable but usually low measurable level; Bethesda titer highly variable	Majority are low responders but still difficult to achieve hemostatic level of factor VIII; anamnestic response less frequent; usually good response to immunosuppressive drugs

together, these findings support an oligoclonal origin for the antibodies. Most antibodies to factor VIII react with discrete regions of the factor VIII light chain (within the C2 domain, phospholipid-binding sites) or the factor VIII heavy chain within the A2 domain.

The reaction between factor VIII and its antibodies is time dependent and displays two kinetic patterns. The simple or type 1 pattern (in antibody excess) results in neutralization of VIII:C completely; the antibody reacts with the specific sites with great affinity until all antibody is bound. Type 2 or complex kinetics is rapid at first but does not result in irreversible binding (less affinity, more easily dissociated); antibody often coexists with measurable factor VIII. The type 1 kinetics is usually seen in transfused hemophilic patients with inhibitors. In some cases large amounts of factor VIII can completely neutralize existing antibody, resulting in hemostatic levels of factor VIII. The type 2 pattern is usually observed in spontaneously acquired autoantibody disorders. Measurable levels of factor VIII can coexist with antibody available to destroy transfused factor VIII. Both allo- and autoantibodies react with the same regions on the factor VIII molecule so that a molecular explanation for the different kinetic patterns is not obvious.

Clinical and Laboratory Manifestations

Hemophilia

The existence of an alloantibody in a hemophiliac patient is suspected when bleeding manifestations become more severe or response to usual therapy is less than expected or when detected by a routine inhibitor screening test (usually prolongation of the APTT of normal plasma when mixed 1:1 with patient plasma and incubated at 37°C for 2 h; modifications of this test increase sensitivity). The factor VIII assay is usually < 1 percent. The confirmatory test for a factor VIII inhibitor is the Bethesda assay (Fig. 21-1). A similar assay, using factor VIII concentrate, is used in Europe ("new" Oxford units); one BU is equal to 1.21 new Oxford units. Once an inhibitor is recognized in a hemophiliac patient, serial assays should be done to establish persistence of the inhibitor, severity, and response to antigenic stimulation (transfusion) so that a classification of low versus high responder can be made.

Autoimmune

The spontaneous occurrence of an autoantibody type factor VIII inhibitor has been noted at any age but most frequently occurs in postpartum women or in older (55 to 75 years) individuals. Major bleeding including hemarthroses, melena, deep hematomas, hematuria, and intracranial or retroperitoneal hemorrhage requiring transfusions occurs in over half the patients. Laboratory evaluation reveals normal hemostatic screening tests except for a pro-

immune tolerance treatment (ITT), it is better to use bypassing products which do not stimulate factor VIII antibody rises and allow the antibody titer to fall to low or negative levels before starting ITT, or, if a sustained period of treatment is anticipated (surgery), the institution of ITT can be done with large doses of factor VIII concentrate. An occasional high titer patient will require multiple plasmaphereses or use of extracorporeal absorption columns to lower the antibody before specific hemostatic treatment. The use of intravenous immunoglobulin (IVIG) to provide anti-idiotype modulation of the immune response has been advocated with limited success.

Following the pioneer work of Brackmann and others (the Bonn protocol) in the late 1970s, many centers have reported successful establishment of immune tolerance in hemophilia A inhibitor patients by giving large doses of factor VIII with or without pharmacologic immunosuppression. Although costly to accomplish, the current success rate (upward of 50 percent, see Fig. 21-2) with ITT suggests that this approach should be considered for all patients; the most success has been in younger patients who are low responders and who are given large doses of factor VIII concentrate during the ITT.

Various ITT regimens have been used; these include high dose factor VIII concentrates (100 to 200 U/kg) or low dose (50 U/kg) daily with and without immunosuppression (prednisone, cyclophosphamide) and occasionally with IVIG. The most intensive immunosuppression protocol used successfully includes combined factor VIII, cytoxan, high-dose IVIG preceded by immunoadsorption of antibody in high titer patients (Malmo protocol). Prolonged treatment (for > 1 year in some instances) is associated with a reduction in antibody titer to unmeasurable levels and a normal half-life of transfused factor VIII; frequently this state of "immune tolerance" may require ongoing but less frequent administration of factor VIII to prevent relapse. After induction of tolerance, patients still have circulating IgG4 antibodies which differ in specificity, lack inhibitory clotting activity, and do not increase rate of factor VIII elimination.

Autoimmune Inhibitors

From 60 to 90 percent of patients with autoantibodies to factor VIII (uncontrolled reports) benefit from treatment with immunosuppressive drugs (corticosteroids, cyclophosphamides, azathioprine, cyclosporine, vincristine). In an ongoing controlled study over half the patients responded to prednisone therapy alone; some required the addition of cyclophosphamide. Therefore, immunosuppression should be instituted soon after the diagnosis of spontaneous factor VIII inhibitors in most patients. Intravenous γ-globulin, which apparently works by long-term suppression and short-term neutralization (anti-idiotypic antibodies), may have a role in treatment of these patients. Low titer patients occasionally show a hemostatic response to intravenous DDAVP. Even though measurable levels of factor VIII may be achieved by use of factor VIII concentrates, the hemostatic effect is often inadequate in moderately high titer patients. Often it is necessary to use porcine factor VIII with or without plasmapheresis to lower the antibody titer to achieve hemostasis. A patient with a high titer postpartum factor VIII antibody showed normalization of factor VIII after a 7-week course of human interferon-α2a, an immune response modifier.

FACTOR IX INHIBITORS

The overall incidence of factor IX inhibitors in hemophilia B is approximately 3 percent. The inhibitors tend to occur in severe factor IX deficiency; some but not all of these patients have deletions of the factor IX gene. The antibodies are usually IgG1 and IgG4 but a rare patient with IgA antibody has been described. The antibodies are less time dependent in their reactions with factor IX and can usually be detected by APTT mixing tests (1:1 with normal plasma). A modification of the Bethesda assay is used to quantitate the antibody. Both high and low responders have been described and therapy is similar to that described for factor VIII alloantibodies including the use of the bypassing products (consider rVIIa product) and immune tolerance treatment (Malmo protocol using factor IX instead of factor VIII).

Spontaneously acquired factor IX autoantibodies are also known (even in children) but are quite rare. These are usually more complex (type II) antibodies and have occurred most often in patients with an underlying autoimmune disorder. The mainstay of treatment is immunosuppression.

FACTOR XI INHIBITORS

Acquired factor XI inhibitors in hereditary factor XI deficiency are extremely rare, a finding possibly due to the paucity of transfusions in the congenitally deficient patients. A few patients have been reported with antibody titers ranging from 0.75 to 12 BU and no or occasional postoperative bleeding to 6000 BU in a patient with a severe thigh hematoma. The antibody is usually IgG4 (when determined), which acts by binding to multiple sites (activation and cleavage), and is frequently time dependent for destruction of factor XI clotting activity. Anamnestic response to transfusion is variable. Bleeding in patients with factor XI inhibitors has responded to increased fresh frozen plasma infusions, plasmapheresis, and bypassing products (prothrombin-complex concentrates and rVIIa).

Spontaneous factor XI inhibitors (autoantibodies) are more common; up to 26 cases were known in one report in 1984. Both IgG and IgM antibodies have been described. Most of the patients have underlying autoimmune disorders (rheumatoid arthritis, SLE, or drugs such as chlorpromazine) but rarely show significant hemorrhagic manifestations; most of the patients are diagnosed through evaluation of a prolonged APTT with a normal PT. Both allo- and autoantibodies to factor XI may be confused with an inhibitor to factor XI adsorption to glass surfaces (pseudo factor XI deficiency); specific assays for the other contact factors are frequently mildly abnormal. In the majority of cases, no specific therapy is necessary; however, immunosuppressive treatment of underlying SLE has been associated with disappearance of the inhibitor.

ACQUIRED INHIBITOR OF VON WILLEBRAND FACTOR

See Chap. 13 for a discussion of this inhibitor.

ACQUIRED FACTOR V INHIBITORS

Acquired antibodies in congenital factor V deficiency are exceedingly rare. In one patient, bleeding manifestations worsened and a time-dependent destruction of factor V activity was demonstrated using a factor V assay. Over 30 cases with spontaneous autoantibodies to factor V have occurred in patients who were previously normal although in the postoperative period; most were older adults except for a 3-year-old child after liver transplantation. Bleeding manifestations have been variable and perhaps related to the accessibility of the patient's platelet factor V to the acquired antibody. The duration of the antibody is relatively short (<10 weeks in most patients) and specific treatment is usually required for acute bleeding episodes. The immunoglobulin class of the antibody may be IgG, IgM, or IgA. The diagnosis is suspected when marked prolongation of the APTT and PT are seen in face of a normal thrombin time and negative tests for lupuslike anticoagulant. (In low titer inhibitor patients, the platelet neutralization test for lupus anticoagulant may be spuriously positive.) Confirmation is by factor V assay and demonstration of factor V inactivation in plasma mixing tests. Successful treatment of bleeding manifestations has been with platelet concentrates or the use of bypassing products.

Antithrombin Antibodies

Several recent reports suggest a link between patient exposure to bovine topical thrombin (previous surgeries) and the development of antithrombin antibodies. These patients present with no or occasional bleeding symptoms and a markedly prolonged TCT. In particular, the TCT is greatly prolonged when bovine thrombin is used as the reagent; less prolongation of the TCT is seen when human thrombin is used in the TCT. Some studies have indicated a cross-reactivity of the bovine antithrombin antibody with human thrombin. Avoidance of topical thrombin (bovine) as a hemostatic agent may prevent the occurrence of the antibodies although the ultimate clinical significance of the antibodies remains to be determined.

α_1-Antitrypsin Pittsburgh

A mutation in the α_1-antitrypsin molecule (358 Met→Arg) converts the protease to a thrombin and Xa inhibitor which does not require heparin for strong antithrombin activity. The nonimmune mutation designated α_1-AT Pittsburgh has been reported in two unrelated children; the first (age 10 years) reported had a lifelong history of severe and ultimately fatal soft tissue and postsurgical bleeding; the second patient (age 15 years) was asymptomatic but was noted to have abnormal presurgical screening tests. Both boys displayed marked prolongation of the APTT and thrombin time with moderate prolongation of the PT; 1:1 mixing with normal plasma showed no correction (inhibitory effect). A severe protein C deficiency was demonstrated in the second patient.

Table 21-2 contains information on other rare acquired inhibitor syndromes with antibody specificity for coagulation factors; inhibitors are also discussed in appropriate factor deficiency chapters.

BIBLIOGRAPHY

Aly AM et al: Histocompatibility antigen patterns in haemophilic patients with factor VIII antibodies. *Br J Haematol* 76:238, 1990.

Arai M et al: Molecular basis of factor VIII inhibition by human antibodies: Antibodies that bind to the factor VIII light chain prevent the interaction of 4-factor VIII with phospholipid. *J Clin Invest* 83:1978, 1989.

Bloom AL: The treatment of factor VIII inhibitors. In: Verstraete M, Vermylen J, Lijnen R, Arnout J (eds): *Thrombosis and Haemostasis*, Leuven, International Society for Thrombosis and Haemostasis and Leuven University Press, 1987, pp 447–471.

Brettler DB et al: The use of porcine factor VIII concentrate (Hyate:C) in the treatment of patients with inhibitor antibodies to factor VIII: A multicenter US experience. *Arch Intern Med* 149:1381, 1989.

Ehrenforth S et al: Incidence of development of factor VIII and factor IX inhibitors in haemophiliacs. *Lancet* 339:594, 1992.

Ewing NP, Kasper CK: In vitro detection of mild inhibitors to factor VIII in hemophilia. *Am J Clin Pathol*:77:749, 1982.

TABLE 21-2 Rare and Unusual Coagulation Factor Inhibitors

Inhibitor	Antibody Characteristics	Clinical Manifestations	Treatment
Factor VII autoantibody	IgG: progressive destruction of factor VII activity with incubation at 37°C.	Spontaneous occurrence in 2 older patients; mild to severe bleeding. PT prolonged; other tests normal	No response to IVIG: hemostasis with plasmapheresis and VII concentrate; disappearance with immunosuppression
Factor II autoantibody	IgG; nonprothrombin activity neutralizing; antibody binds to prothrombin fragment 1	Diffuse bleeding diatheses; PT and APTT abnormal; no evidence for lupus inhibitor Factor II level 0.06 U/mL; ↑ to 0.55 with 1:1 mix with normal plasma	Good response to corticosteroids; antibody disappeared in 1 wk

Autoimmune inhibitor of fibrin stabilization	Autoantibody (IgG1 and IgG3) against A and/or B chains of factor XIII	Severe bleeding in adults (1 child) Onset related to penicillin allergy and isoniazid usage. Only abnormal test is defective urea solubility of patient and 1:1 mix with normal plasma	Try immunosuppressive therapy
Heparin-like anticoagulant	Usually not an antibody; but is heparan sulfate proteoglycan: 1 case with immunoglobulin anticoagulant	Diffuse bleeding diathesis; laboratory tests show marked heparin effect; APTT and TT markedly prolonged; PT slightly prolonged; normal reptilase time. Underlying disorders include acute monoblastic leukemia (infant); multiple myeloma, systemic mastocytosis; neoplastic disease	Protamine sulfate

Goldsmith GH, Silverman P: Inhibitors of plasma thromboplastin antecedent (factor XI): Studies on mechanism of inhibition. *J Lab Clin Med* 106:279, 1985.

Green D, Lechner K: A survey of 215 non-hemophilic patients with inhibitors to factor VIII. *Thromb Haemost* 45:200, 1981.

Herbst KD et al: Syndrome of an acquired inhibitor of factor VIII responsive to cyclophosphamide and prednisone. *Ann Intern Med* 95:575,1981.

Horne MK III et al: A heparin-like anticoagulant as part of global abnormalities of plasma glycosaminoglycans in a patient with transitional cell carcinoma. *J Lab Clin Med* 118:250, 1991.

Kasper CK: Complications of hemophilia A treatment: Factor VIII inhibitors. *Ann NY Acad Sci* 614:97, 1991.

Kessler CM: An introduction to factor VIII inhibitors: The detection and quantitation. *Am J Med* 91:5A1s, 1991.

Lawson JH et al: Isolation and characterization of an acquired antithrombin antibody. *Blood* 76:2249, 1990.

Lippert LE et al: Relationship of major histocompatibility complex class II genes to inhibitor antibody formation in hemophilia A. *Thromb Haemost* 64:564, 1990.

McMillan C et al: The natural history of factor VIII:C inhibitors in patients with hemophilia A: A national coooperative study. II. Observations on the initial development of factor VIII:C inhibitors. *Blood* 71:344, 1988.

Nesheim ME et al: Isolation and study of an acquired inhibitor of human coagulation factor V. *J Clin Invest* 77:405, 1986.

Schnall SF et al: Acquired factor XI inhibitors in congenitally deficient patients. *Am J Hematol* 26:323, 1987.

Shapiro SS, Hultin M: Acquired inhibitors to the blood coagulation factors. *Semin Thromb Hemost* 1:336, 1975.

Bleeding Associated
with Vascular Disorders

A number of bleeding disorders are associated with abnormalities involving the blood vessels, usually without demonstrable defect in platelets or the coagulation system (exceptions will be noted). These vascular disorders, which are sometimes part of a systemic disease, include the spectrum of vasculitides (Henoch-Schönlein purpura, HSP), vascular malformations (hemangiomas, telangiectasias), collagen diseases (Ehlers-Danlos syndrome), and the purpuras (microvascular extravasation of blood into the skin). The hemorrhagic manifestations of these diseases are discussed below.

VASCULITIS

A major cutaneous manifestation of the spectrum of vasculitis (inflammation and necrosis of blood vessels) is raised purpuric lesions or palpable purpura which triggers the differential diagnosis of a possible bleeding tendency. Diseases which may have such skin lesions include hypersensitivity or leukocytoclastic vasculitis, polyarteritis nodosa, vasculitis associated with malignancy, Wegener's granulomatosis, livedo vasculitis, dysproteinemia including the cryoglobulinemias, rheumatoid arthritis, and systemic lupus erythematosus (SLE). In most instances, the diagnosis is related to the underlying disorder; however, an occasional patient may present with only the cutaneous lesions (skin biopsy is often indicated). With the exception of the petechial-purpuric vasculitic lesions of acute infection (meningococcemia, rickettsial diseases, etc.), which are easily recognized, the most common disorder associated with the differential diagnosis of palpable purpura is hypersensitivity angiitis, leukocytoclastic vasculitis, or anaphylactoid purpura (HSP) as it is usually called in children where it is most commonly seen.

Anaphylactoid purpura or HSP typically presents in a child (rarely in adults) as a nonthrombocytopenic raised rash occurring over the lower extremities and buttocks but occasionally involving other parts of the body. The rash is typical in appearance and does not require biopsy. The rash consists of urticarial wheals and ecchymoses, variable in size (petechiae to confluent spots) and raised to the touch ("palpable purpura"). The purpuric areas evolve from red to purple, to brown-rust colored and eventually fade; the rash can persist for weeks and recur in crops every few weeks or months. Angioedema of the scalp (20 percent) and extremities (48 percent of cases) may be striking in younger children and is associated with cockade (round papular) purpura on the face and arms as well as lower extremities (called infantile acute hemorrhagic edema).

Other typical manifestations include arthralgia-arthritis, abdominal pain (35 to 85 percent), and signs of nephritis, which may complicate the disease in 20 to 50 percent of cases within 3 months of onset; persistent glomerulonephritis occurs in about 1 percent of cases. Every system may be involved in unusual patients as shown in Table 22-1. Most laboratory tests are helpful only to eliminate other diagnoses or to follow a particular organ involvement; the diagnosis is based on the clinical manifestations and the typical rash. All hemostatic screening tests are normal except occasional thrombocytosis. About half the patients have elevated serum IgA levels. Interestingly, factor XIII levels are decreased (30 to 50 percent) in most patients and are approximately correlated with the activity of the disease. Although hemorrhage may complicate some of the local lesions (gastrointestinal, CNS, pulmonary), a

TABLE 22-1 Manifestations of Henoch-Schönlein Purpura (Anaphylactoid or Leukocytoclastic Purpura)

Organ	Manifestation
Skin	Palpable purpura, urticaria, petechiae, angioedema
Gastrointestinal tract	Colicky abdominal pain, bleeding, ileus, intussusception, pancreatitis, cholecystitis
Genitourinary	Nephritis, hematuria, nephrosis, scrotal edema, hemorrhage, orchitis
CNS	Apathy, headache, seizures, CNS bleeding (rare) peripheral neuropathy
Cardiac	Myocardial infarction
Musculoskeletal	Arthritis, arthralgia, muscle hematoma
Pulmonary	Hemorrhage, pleural effusion
Laboratory	Positive stool guaiac, hematuria, proteinuria, elevated blood urea nitrogen, and creatinine; elevated erythrocyte sedimentation rate, leukocytosis, thrombocytosis, occasionally elevated antistreptolysin O and decreased CH50, elevated IgA, decreased factor XIII

generalized bleeding tendency is not apparent, and surgery and biopsies may be performed without undue risk.

Henoch-Schönlein purpura is considered an immune complex disorder like other hypersensitivity vasculitides and has been associated with a plethora of underlying causes: infection (*Streptococcus*, hepatitis B, cytomegalovirus, Epstein-Barr virus), medications (penicillin, sulfa, phenytoin, iodides, cimetidine, allopurinol), chemicals (insecticides), systemic autoimmune diseases (SLE, rheumatoid arthritis, dermatomyositis), malignancy, and food products (dyes, preservatives). Treatment of HSP is mainly supportive; corticosteroids may slightly decrease the duration of gastrointestinal manifestations but do not appear to alter the course of nephritis. Infusions of factor XIII concentrate reportedly have benefited severe abdominal crises in HSP. The illness usually lasts 4 to 6 weeks in most cases, but recurrences are frequent, and in rare cases may occur months later; the overall prognosis is excellent with the exception of chronic glomerulonephritis in < 1 percent of patients.

ISOLATED PURPURAS

Patients who present with ecchymotic lesions appearing as small to large bruises and whose history reveals only easy bruising with few other bleeding manifestations may be considered for the diagnosis of one of the following causes of isolated purpura, so called because there is no systemic disease and all hemostatic screening tests are normal (see Chap. 5).

Psychogenic Purpura

Psychogenic purpura (Gardner-Diamond syndrome or autoerythrocyte sensitization syndrome) is a rare disorder characterized by occurrence of repeated crops of painful ecchymoses (which have an inflammatory component) in adult women with multiple systemic complaints and no generalized bleeding tendency. The purpuric lesion reportedly can be reproduced by intracutaneous injection of autologous blood and tends to occur mostly in individuals under emotional stress. A possibly related disorder is paroxysmal finger hematoma (see reference).

Factitious Purpura

Many well-documented examples of secretive self-inflicted injury producing purpuric and petechial lesions have been described. Mechanical maneuvers such as compression, or negative suction (mouth or cup or pinching) may produce lesions which are disturbing to patient or parents and in whom secondary gain is prominent. The patient usually responds to counseling after basic screening tests have proven negative.

Nonaccidental Trauma

A prominent feature of nonaccidental trauma (NAT) is ecchymoses; the pattern and physical characteristics of the lesions often suggest various types of trauma in both children and adults in whom physical abuse is suspected. The medical investigation of such cases should include a complete hemostatic screening battery (see Chap. 5) because the diagnosis of a mild bleeding disorder and NAT are not mutually exclusive; i.e., in a study of 50 children with suspected NAT (most with bruises), 8 (16 percent) showed abnormal screening tests leading to diagnoses of von Willebrand disease, platelet function disorders, and acquired factor VIII inhibitor. Tests done during the acute injury phase may be transiently abnormal also (mild disseminated intravascular coagulation [DIC] in head injury).

Purpura Simplex

Purpura simplex, "easy bruising," is a frequent complaint of adult women, some men, and active young children. If the ecchymoses are large (> 2 inches in diameter) or indurated and not easily explained by trauma, they should be considered abnormal and investigated (see Chap. 5). A recent report demonstrated increased metabolites of prostacyclin in blood oozing from incisions for bleeding time determinations in healthy children with easy bruising and suggested a role for increased endogenous prostacyclin production in their symptomatology.

Senile Purpura

Senile or atrophic purpura is seen in elderly individuals; the lesions are related to their skin and traction injury and are usually found on extensor surfaces of the extremities.

Hypercortisolism

Purpura may be seen in Cushing's syndrome and after long-term corticosteroid administration. The cause may be related to decreased collagen components in the skin.

Scurvy

Vitamin C is necessary in the final assembly of collagen when proline is converted to hydroproline, which stabilizes the helical structure of collagen. The bleeding tendency in scurvy is manifested by ecchymotic purpura, gingival bleeding, and subperiosteal hemorrhage despite usually normal hemostatic tests. Faulty diet is the usual cause and may also produce a megaloblastic anemia.

VASCULAR MALFORMATIONS

Hemangioma

Juvenile hemangioma or hemangioma of infancy is an angiomatoid malformation caused by abnormal proliferation of capillaries. These tumors grow rapidly in the first year of life and then slowly regress over the next 5 to 8 years or even sooner. More than 90 percent regress completely; however, a few persist (often giant cavernous type) into adult life. Most of the tumors are small and remain localized to the skin (strawberry nevus); a few grow rapidly to an alarming size or proliferate in multiple organs (liver, spleen, bone, lung) causing serious complications such as soft tissue destruction, endangerment of vital structures (eye, airway), congestive heart failure, and serious bleeding. The bleeding manifestations are due to intratumor hemorrhage (often producing significant anemia) and a generalized bleeding tendency due to acute and chronic DIC which occurs in a small percentage of cases. The consumption coagulopathy is usually characterized by thrombocytopenia, decreased fibrinogen, increased fibrinogen degradation products (FDP), and microangiopathic anemia and is called the Kasabach-Merritt syndrome.

Management consists of observation (serial photographs are helpful in following larger lesions) and possibly local compression of the lesion unless life-threatening complications appear (serious thrombocytopenia or DIC, limb or organ endangerment, congestive heart failure). Therapy with oral prednisone (3 to 4 mg/kg per day) is associated with regression in several weeks in about one third of the cases. Other modalities used with varying success include surgery, arterial embolization, low-dose radiation therapy, cyclophosphamide, and antifibrinolytic agents. The DIC may be controlled temporarily with intravenous heparin or the combination of aspirin and dipyridamole. Recent reports indicate that interferon-α2a induces early regressions of life-threatening corticosteroid-resistant cavernous hemangioma of infancy (tumors in 18 of 20 patients regressed by 50 percent or more after an average of 7.8 months of treatment; see Ezekowitz et al reference).

Hereditary Hemorrhagic Telangiectasia

Hereditary hemorrhagic telangiectasia (Osler-Weber-Rendu disease) is an autosomal dominant disorder with a frequency of about 1/50,000 and is manifested by lesions on the skin and mucous membranes varying from punctiform to spider-like to nodular, all o˚ which tend to bleed when traumatized. The lesions are found predominately under the tongue, perioral region, nasal mucosa, under nails, and on lips. Major clinical manifestations include bleeding mucosal and arteriovenous malformations, hypoxemia, cerebral embolism, and brain abscess due to pulmonary arteriovenous malformations, high output congestive heart failure, hepatovascular lesions, and symptoms related to CNS angiodysplasia. Although the disorder is rarely diagnosed in childhood, epistaxis is common and seems to worsen with age. Gastrointestinal bleeding may be chronic and produce iron deficiency anemia. Spider telangiectasias from liver disease must be differentiated (central prominent feeding vessel; head to nipple line). von Willebrand disease is sometimes an associated disorder and should be excluded; an occasional patient may show evidence of mild DIC with elevated FDP; hemostatic tests are otherwise normal.

COLLAGEN DISORDERS

The collagen diseases, also called heritable disorders of connective tissue, are those diseases in which the primary defect is due to a molecular alteration in collagen. These disorders, in which a mild bleeding tendency (easy bruising, hematoma formation, poor wound healing) is sometimes part of a distinctive phenotype, are due to defects in procollagen genes and abnormal collagen formation in the blood vessels and supporting tissues. Because the diagnosis may be first suspected during the evaluation of a possible bleeding diathesis, an awareness of the specific phenotypes is necessary.

Osteogenesis Imperfecta

Mutations in the collagen genes (located on chromosomes 17 and 7) produce a change in the structure of type 1 procollagen and the heterogeneous clinical syndrome of osteogenesis imperfecta. Brittle bones represent the main feature of the disorder; both autosomal and recessive forms of the disease are known, ranging in severity from death in utero to an occasional fracture and blue sclerae. Some of the patients bruise easily and show a mild platelet functional defect (abnormal aggregation pattern–failure to release) with slightly prolonged bleeding times.

Marfan's Syndrome

This disease is an autosomal dominant condition that produces multiple skeletal deformities (tall stature, long extremities and digits), ocular lens dislocations, and cardiovascular manifestations (aortic aneurysm). Connective tissues are often friable and surgical correction of the aortic defect has been associated with severe bleeding apparently on a vascular basis. A generalized bleeding tendency is not usually present.

Ehlers-Danlos Syndrome

The typical syndrome consists of easy bruising, friable tissues with paper thin scarring, hyperextensible joints, and loose skin. The bleeding manifestations are probably related to the underlying collagen defect (vessel or supporting tissue defect) but abnormalities in platelet aggregation (particularly to Ehlers-Danlos collagen) have been reported. Other hemostatic screening

TABLE 22-2 Clinical Variants of the Ehlers-Danlos Syndrome

Type	Name	Inheritance	Clinical Features
I	Gravis	AD	Hyperextensible skin; marked bleeding paper thin scars; hypermobile joints
II	Mitus	AD	Like I but less severe
III	Benign hypermobility	AD	Soft skin, marked large and small joint hypermobility, minimal bleeding
IV	Arterial, ecchymotic	AR or AD	Thin skin, visible veins, marked bleeding tendency, skin and joints less involved; arterial, bowel, uterine rupture
V	X-linked	XL	Like type II
VI	Ocular	AR	Ocular fragility and keratoconus; soft, velvety skin; hypermobile joints; scoliosis
VII	Arthrochalasis multiplex congenita	AD	Congenital hip dislocation; laxity of joints, bruising
VIII	Periodontal	AD	Periodontitis; skin like type II
IX	Cutis laxa (abnormal copper metabolism)	XL	Bladder diverticula and rupture; short arms, occipital horns; no bleeding
X	Fibronectin defect	AR	Like type II; mild bleeding

*AD, autosomal dominant; AR autosomal recessive; XL, X-linked

tests are normal. Multiple phenotypes are known (Table 22-2), the most clinically important of which is type IV (decreased synthesis or structure of type III collagen). Type IV is an often lethal disorder presenting in infancy (low birth weight, prematurity, congenital dislocation of hips, easy bruising, and a characteristic facies [large eyes, thin "pinched" nose and thin lips]). Hemostatic tests are usually normal. The patient may appear like a type 1 phenotype but often presents as an older child or young adult with ruptured hollow viscera (colon, rectal prolapse, gallbladder) or major artery rupture (femoral, iliac, renal, aorta) with disastrous results. Therefore, confirmation of the diagnosis by molecular analysis of the collagen genes should allow family counseling and genetic planning.

BIBLIOGRAPHY

Aylett SE et al: The Kasabach-Merritt syndrome: Treatment with intermittent pneumatic compression. *Arch Dis Child* 65:790, 1990.

Byers PH: Inherited disorders of collagen gene structure and expression. *Am J Med Genet* 34:72, 1989.

Ezekowitz RA et al: Interferon α2a therapy for life-threatening hemangiomas of infancy. *N Engl J Med* 326:1456, 1992.

Gibson LE: Cutaneous vasculitis: Approach to diagnosis and systemic associations. *Mayo Clin Proc* 65:221, 1990.

Hoffman R et al: *Hematology. Basic Principles and Practice*, New York, Churchill-Livingstone, 1991, color plates 96-18 to 96-25.

Hurvitz CH et al: Cyclophosphamide therapy in life-threatening vascular tumors. *J Pediatr* 109:360, 1986.

Kitchens CS: The anatomic basis of purpura. *Semin Hematol* 13:211, 1976.

Koerper MA et al: Use of aspirin and dipyridamole in children with platelet trapping syndromes. *J Pediatr* 102:311, 1983.

Lanzkowsky S et al: Henoch-Schoenlein purpura. *Pediatr Rev* 13:130, 1992.

O'Hare AE, Eden OB: Bleeding disorders and non-accidental injury. *Arch Dis Child* 59:860, 1984.

Pope FM et al: Clinical presentations of Ehlers Danlos syndrome type IV. *Arch Dis Child* 63:1016, 1988.

Ratnoff OD, Agle DP: Psychogenic purpura: A re-evaluation of the syndrome of autoerythrocyte sensitization. *Medicine* 47:475, 1968.

Shulkin BL et al: Kasabach-Merritt syndrome: Treatment with epsilon-aminocaproic acid and assessment by indium 111 platelet scintigraphy. *J Pediatr* 117:746, 1990.

Uden A: Collagen and bleeding diathesis in Ehlers-Danlos syndrome. *Scand J Haematol* 28:425, 1982.

Vitamin K Deficiency

Soon after the discovery of vitamin K by Henrik Dam in 1929, it was established that the generalized bleeding tendency, known as hemorrhagic disease of the newborn (HDN), was due to vitamin K deficiency. It is now known that vitamin K functions as an essential cofactor for the synthesis of the coagulation proteins, factors II, VII, IX, X, and protein C and protein S by promoting a unique posttranslational modification of specific glutamic acid residues to γ-carboxyglutamic acid (Gla), thus mediating calcium binding to negatively charged phospholipid surfaces. Other proteins dependent on vitamin K for completed synthesis include osteocalcin and protein Z (function unknown); Gla-containing proteins have been found in bone, cartilage, dentin, kidney, placenta, pancreas, spleen, lung, testes, and liver tissue.

STRUCTURE AND FUNCTION OF VITAMIN K

Vitamin K is 1,4-naphthoquinone with a methyl group at position 2 and a polyisoprenoid side chain at position 3. Vitamin K_1 or phylloquinone is made by green plants; vitamin K_2 includes a group of compounds made by bacteria and are called menaquinones (MK-n) with n being the number of isoprene units at position 3. The parent compound lacking the side chain is menadione (K_3), which has no vitamin K activity in vitro but can be alkylated to active MK-4 in animal tissues. Intestinal bacteria synthesize MK-10–13 forms resulting in < 50 percent of the total needed; in humans the major source comes from ingestion of phylloquinone. Table 23-1 indicates the major vitamin K analogues. The human dietary requirement of vitamin K is about 1 $\mu g/kg$ per day and is easily supplied by green and yellow leafy vegetables and other foods; human milk is low in vitamin K (~2 $\mu g/L$) as compared to cow's milk (4 to 18 $\mu g/L$). The role of endogenous vitamin K_2 as a significant source of vitamin K for man is poorly understood although menaquinone is the major form stored in the liver. Vitamin K is a lipid-soluble vitamin and is dependent on an intact intestinal fat absorption mechanism for optimal utilization of

TABLE 23-1   Vitamin K Analogues

Name	Source	Dosage Form
Phylloquinone (K_1)	Diet; green plants	AquaMEPHYTON Konakion
Menaquinones-n (K_2) (n = number of isoprene units)	Intestinal bacteria	Kaytwo (MK-4)
Menadione (K_3)	Parent compound	Synkayvite

oral forms of the vitamin. Vitamin K is poorly transported across the placenta; maternal fetal gradients of 18:1 and 30:1 have been reported.

The primary biologic function of vitamin K is to mediate the carboxylation of selected 9 to 12 glutamates located in the Gla domain at the NH_2 terminus of the protein to γ-carboxyglutamic acid residues used to bind calcium to phospholipid membranes, thus allowing formation of critical coagulation complexes ("factor Xase," "prothrombinase," and "protein Case"). Fig. 23-1 depicts the carboxylation step and the role of vitamin K. The carboxylation process is mediated by a vitamin K-dependent "carboxylase," reduced K, carbon dioxide and oxygen. Recent evidence suggests that vitamin K can work in a nonenzymatic reaction without evoking a specific "carboxylase" enzyme. The cycle is interrupted by warfarin-type compounds which block the epoxide reductase allowing accumulation of vitamin K epoxide to levels 50 times baseline.

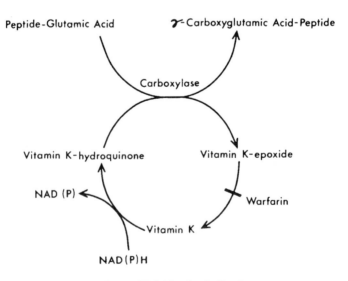

Figure 23-1 The vitamin K cycle.

Impairment in carboxylation that occurs in vitamin K deficiency or some types of liver dysfunction (cirrhosis, hepatocellular carcinoma) results in an accumulation of the clotting factor protein with absent or decreased γ-carboxylation sites and whose half-disappearance time in the circulation is approximately that of the native protein (60 h for noncarboxylated prothrombin). The non- or des-carboxylated protein is also called "protein induced in vitamin K absence" or PIVKA and can be used as a marker for vitamin K deficiency.

DIAGNOSIS OF VITAMIN K DEFICIENCY

Vitamin K deficiency results in:

- Decreased liver stores of phylloquinone
- Decreased plasma level of vitamin K_1
- Increased levels of K_1 epoxide (especially when due to warfarin effect), appearance of noncarboxylated proteins (PIVKA)
- Decreased levels of functioning vitamin K-dependent clotting factors
- Prolongation of the APTT, PT, and thrombotest

The progression of the deficiency state is in approximately the above order. The assays used to determine the deficiency state are listed (Table 23-2). Because *Echis carinatus* venom activates both normal and noncarboxylated prothrombin, a prolonged PT with a normal *Echis* clotting time indicates vitamin K deficiency. A bleeding tendency does not occur until the coagulation factor levels are < 30 to 35 percent and, therefore, the screening

TABLE 23-2 Assays Used to Determine Vitamin K Deficiency

	Assay Sensitivity
Prothrombin time	Abnormal time when factor levels < 50 percent of normal
Thrombotest	Abnormal time when factor levels < 50 percent of normal
Factors II, VII, IX, X	To < 0.01 U/mL
Noncarboxylated prothrombin (PIVKA)	
II-immunoelectrophorsis	1.0 μg/mL
II-ELISA	0.05–0.1 μg/mL
Vitamin K_1 assay	Adult mean = 0.5 ng/mL Cord blood = 0.2 ng/mL to ND
Urinary Gla assay	25–29 μmol/day

ND-nondetectable.

tests (PT, APTT) become abnormal. The more sensitive assays, plasma vitamin K level and noncarboxylated prothrombin (or protein C) assay as well as the urinary Gla assay (decreased Gla in vitamin K deficiency), are particularly useful in determination of subclinical deficiency states; however, in most clinical situations, the correction of the abnormal screening tests by vitamin K is the mainstay of diagnosis. Detectable amounts of non-carboxylated prothrombin (PIVKA-II) is indicative of vitamin K deficiency (currently being evaluated for monitoring of warfarin). With a few possible exceptions such as severe liver disease, hepatocellular carcinoma, and rare cases of multiple vitamin K-dependent coagulation factors, vitamin K deficiency is associated with increased noncarboxylated proteins. All of these exceptions may respond to large doses of vitamin K.

VITAMIN K DEFICIENCY IN INFANCY

Three syndromes of hemorrhagic disease may be seen in the newborn and young infant; these have been called early, classic, and late HDN and are described in Table 23-3. Of particular interest are early and late HDN, which raise controversial issues regarding management. Early HDN is most likely to occur in newborn infants whose mothers have been on anticonvulsant therapy (phenytoin, phenobarbital, valproic acid, carbamazepine). From 25 to 50 percent of these infants will show biochemical evidence (low vitamin K and increased noncarboxylated prothrombin levels) in cord blood, which can be eliminated by administering 10 mg vitamin K_1 orally daily 2 weeks before delivery.

Late HDN occurs mainly in exclusively breast-fed infants who have had no vitamin K or only oral vitamin K as neonatal prophylaxis. The prevalence varies from 5 to 20/100,000 births without neonatal prophylactic vitamin K. Late HDN is frequently associated with intracranial hemorrhage and neurologic residuals. Parenteral vitamin K at birth or multidose oral vitamin K prevents the syndrome.

Although the prevalence of late HDN can be reduced to 1 to 2 cases per 100,000, a single oral dose of vitamin K_1 or K_2 is not always effective for prevention, especially in infants with subclinical cholestatic liver disease. Current considerations for prophylaxis are further complicated by a recent British study indicating that intramuscular but not oral vitamin K at birth was associated with a 2.3 increased risk of childhood cancer (see Golding reference). Changing practices and various dosage forms of vitamin K have renewed old controversies.

Current guidelines for prevention of HDN are:

1. *Early HDN*: Mothers on anticonvulsants, antibiotics, or warfarin should receive 10 mg vitamin K_1 orally each day beginning 2 weeks before delivery.

TABLE 23-3 Vitamin K Deficiency Hemorrhagic Syndromes in Infancy

Syndrome	Age	Common Bleeding Sites	Cause	Prevention by Vitamin K Administration at Birth	Comments
Early HDN	0–24 h	Cephalhematoma, scalp monitor, intracranial, intrathoracic, intra-abdominal	Maternal drugs: warfarin, anticonvulsants, antituberulous chemotherapy, idiopathic	Not in all instances	Frequently life-threatening; daily oral vitamin K to mother for 2 wk before delivery
Classic HDN	1–7 d	Gastrointestinal, skin, nasal, circumcision	Idiopathic, maternal drugs	Yes, oral or IM	Incidence increased in breast-fed neonates and reduced by early formula feedings
Late HDN	1–6 mo	Intracranial, skin, gastrointestinal	Idiopathic	Probably yes	Common cause of intracranial hemorrhage in breast-fed infants aged 1–3 mo; may be aggravated by antibiotic administration
			Secondary: diarrhea, malabsorption (cystic fibrosis, a_1-antitrypsin deficiency, biliary atresia), hepatitis	No, need monthly IM injection	

*HDN, hemorrhagic disease of the newborn.

2. *Classic HDN*: Infants should receive 0.5 to 1 mg vitamin K_1 intramuscularly or 2 mg vitamin K_1 orally at birth.

3. *Late HDN*: Breast-fed infants should receive prophylaxis as for classic HDN at birth; repeat oral vitamin K during infancy when diarrhea for more than a few days occurs.

Multiple oral doses of K_1 or K_2 (birth, 1 week, 2 to 4 weeks) are necessary to approximate parenteral prophylaxis in breast-fed infants in preventing all late HDN. Repeat intramuscular dose monthly in infants with hepatitis or malabsorption syndromes. In the United States the standard neonatal prophylaxis with 0.5 to 1.0 mg vitamin K_1 oxide given parenterally (intramuscularly) prevents late HDN, but this recommendation may be altered in light of the potential risk of parenteral vitamin K plus the advent of new, better adsorbed oral preparations (mixed micellar vitamin K).

VITAMIN K DEFICIENCY IN OLDER CHILDREN AND ADULTS

Vitamin K deficiency with or without overt bleeding symptoms may occur at any age and should be suspected in any differential diagnosis of an acquired bleeding tendency. Malabsorption of fat-soluble vitamins (Table 23-4) may be subtle and a clue to a major disorder. Prolonged fasting (3 to 7 or more days) with or without antibiotic therapy may cause a symptomatic deficiency (i.e., elderly patients with poor oral intake or intravenous antibiotic therapy). Warfarin ingestion is an obvious and therapeutically important cause (see

TABLE 23-4 Associated Causes of Vitamin K Deficiency

Malabsorption
  a_1-Antitrypsin deficiency
  Abetalipoproteinemia
  Bile duct atresia
  Celiac disease
  Chronic diarrhea
  Cystic fibrosis
  Subclinical cholestasis
Fasting
Alcoholism
Drugs
  Coumarins: warfarin, herbal tea, long-acting rodenticides (brodifacoum)
  Maternal anticonvulsants
  Antibiotics (cephalosporins, NMTT chain)
  Vitamin E megadose
  Salicylates

*NMTT, N-Methyl-thiotetrazole.

Chap. 62); however, surreptitiously or accidental ingestion of short-acting warfarin or long-acting coumarin found in rodenticides (brodifacoum) should be considered in bleeding patients with prolonged PT and APTT (sometimes with a poor or no response to usual vitamin K doses). Antibiotics with a N-methyl-thiotetrazole side chain (β-lactam) and salicylates inhibit vitamin K epoxide reductase and elevate plasma K_1 epoxide levels.

The pattern of coagulation screening tests shows prolonged (often greatly) PT and APTT with normal thrombin time (ruling out heparin effect) and normal platelet count (unless disseminated intravascular coagulation is also present). The PT is often prolonged early and more severely. When this pattern is seen in a bleeding patient, vitamin K should be given parenterally (intramuscularly, subcutaneously, or *slowly* intravenously to avoid reactions) in the following dosage: infant or child 1 to 5 mg; older child 5 to 10 mg; and adult 10 to 20 mg. The usual response is cessation of bleeding and correction of PT in 4 to 8 h or less. Additional blood product replacement is rarely needed unless the patient is on warfarin and has significant bleeding at which time fresh frozen plasma should be used. Even though the PT and APTT have returned to normal, a diagnosis of vitamin K deficiency may be confirmed by elevated noncarboxylated prothrombin (which has a half-disappearance time of 60 h).

BIBLIOGRAPHY

Blanchard RA et al: Acquired vitamin K-dependent carboxylation deficiency in liver disease. *N Engl J Med* 305:242, 1981.

Bovill EG et al: Vitamin K_1 metabolism and the production of des-carboxy prothrombin and protein C in the term and premature neonate. *Blood* 81:77, 1993.

Dowd P et al: Mechanism of action of vitamin K. *J Am Chem Soc* 113:7734, 1991.

Golding J et al: Childhood cancer, intramuscular vitamin K, and pethidine given during labour. *Br Med J* 305:341, 1992.

Greer FR et al: Vitamin K status of lactating mothers, human milk, and breast-feeding infants. *Pediatrics* 88:751, 1991.

Hathaway WE: New insights on vitamin K. *Hematol Oncol Clin North Am* 1:367, 1987.

Hathaway WE et al: Comparison of oral and parenteral vitamin K prophylaxis for prevention of late hemorrhagic disease of the newborn. *J Pediatr* 119:461, 1991.

Hogan RP: Hemorrhagic diathesis caused by drinking an herbal tea. *JAMA* 249:2679, 1983.

Moslet U, Hansen ES: A review of vitamin K, epilepsy and pregnancy. *Acta Neurol Scand* 85:39, 1992.

Ono M et al: Measurement of immunoreactive prothrombin precursor and vitamin-K-dependent gamma-carboxylation in human hepatocellular carcinoma tissues: Decreased carboxylation of prothrombin precursor as a cause of des-gamma-carboxyprothrombin synthesis. *Tumor Biol* 11:319, 1990.

Ross GS et al: An acquired hemorrhagic disorder from long-acting rodenticide ingestion. *Arch Intern Med* 152:410, 1992.

Shearer MJ et al: Mechanism of cephalosporin-induced hypoprothrombinemia: Relation to cephalosporin side chain, vitamin K metabolism, and vitamin K status. *J Clin Pharmacol* 28:88, 1988.

Shearer MJ: Vitamin K and vitamin K-dependent proteins. *Br J Haematol* 75:156, 1990.

Solano C et al: Prediction of vitamin K response using the *Echis* time and *Echis*-prothrombin time ratio. *Thromb Haemost* 64:353, 1990.

Suttie JW et al: Vitamin K deficiency from dietary vitamin K restriction in humans. *Am J Clin Nutr* 47:475, 1988.

von Kries R et al: Vitamin K in infancy. *Eur J Pediatr* 147:106, 1988.

CHAPTER 24

Liver Diseases

Bleeding in patients with advanced liver disease is common and is usually due to local vascular lesions such as esophageal varices, or to failure of almost any facet of hemostasis; i.e., impaired clotting factor synthesis, platelet dysfunction, disseminated intravascular coagulation (DIC), or systemic fibrinolysis (Table 24-1). Surgery or trauma can precipitate sudden hemostatic failure in an otherwise stable patient. To conserve blood products, treatment directed at specific hemostatic abnormalities must often be combined with correction of vascular defects using techniques such as catheter-directed embolization of bleeding vessels, surgical alleviation of portal hypertension, or even emergent liver transplantation.

PATHOGENESIS

Liver failure can be acute (e.g., fulminant hepatitis, mushroom poisoning, hypoxia) or more chronic and progressive (e.g., alcoholic or viral cirrhosis,

TABLE 24-1 Hemostatic Defects in Liver Disease

Defect	Possible Mechanisms
Impaired coagulation	Decreased hepatic synthesis of clotting factors
	Vitamin K deficiency
Thrombocytopenia and platelet function defects	Hypersplenism
	Failure to clear platelet inhibitors
Disseminated intravascular coagulation	Procoagulants from liver cells
	Endotoxins in portal circulation
	Failure to clear activated clotting factors
	Reduced antithrombin III and protein C
	Elevated cytokines
Systemic fibrinolysis	Reduced a_2-antiplasmin
	Failure to clear fibrinolytic enzymes
	Release of tissue plasminogen activator during surgical stress

biliary atresia, primary biliary cirrhosis). Although the causes of liver disease are diverse, the coagulopathies associated with liver failure usually fall into one or more of the categories described below and in Tables 24-1 and 24-2.

Impaired Synthesis of Clotting Factors

When the synthetic function of the liver is suppressed by disease, the concentrations of clotting factors in the plasma often fall to levels that promote bleeding. Factor VII and factor V are sensitive indicators of hepatic protein synthesis and may be used as a guide to the severity of the liver disease. Abnormal forms of the vitamin K-dependent clotting factors such as des-γ-carboxyl prothrombin have been identified in patients with acute hepatitis and cirrhosis, although the concentrations of these abnormal clotting factors are sufficiently low that they do not contribute to bleeding. Malabsorption of fat-soluble vitamins from the bowel can lead to vitamin K deficiency.

Von Willebrand factor is not produced in the liver, but is synthesized by endothelial cells and megakaryocytes; it is markedly increased in patients with hepatic insufficiency. The reason for the elevation is not known, but it could reflect vascular stimulation or damage with release of von Willebrand factor into the blood. Although coagulation factor VIII is synthesized in the liver (liver transplantation brings factor VIII levels to normal in patients with hemophilia A), end-stage liver disease due to hepatitis, alcohol, or other cause does not produce a fall in plasma factor VIII activity. Indeed, the concentration of factor VIII rises in the blood parallel with, but somewhat behind, the increase of von Willebrand factor.

TABLE 24-2 Representative laboratory values in a patient with end-stage liver disease awaiting liver transplantation

	Patient	Normal Range
PT	22 s	11–13.5 s
APTT	56 s	25–35 s
TCT	42 s	< 30 s
Fibrinogen	42 mg/dL	175–350 mg/dL
Platelet count	82,000/μL	150,000–350,000/μL
Bleeding time	14 min	< 9.5 min
D-dimer	1.0 μg/mL	< 0.5 μg/mL
Euglobulin lysis time	20 min	> 60 min
Plasminogen	0.4 U/mL	0.7–1.3 U/mL
a_2-antiplasmin	0.2 U/mL	0.85–1.15 U/mL

Thrombocytopenia

A mild to moderate reduction in platelet count is common in chronic liver disease and is most often due to hypersplenism with sequestration of platelets within an enlarged spleen. Platelet survival is also reduced in cirrhosis, but the short survival is offset by increased platelet production in the bone marrow. The sites of platelet destruction are not known with certainty but could involve vascular damage in the liver or elsewhere.

Patients with alcoholic liver disease have additional reasons for thrombocytopenia. Alcohol can reduce platelet production by megakaryocytes and hasten platelet destruction. Folic acid deficiency may contribute to ineffective thrombopoiesis. Fulminant viral hepatitis, either in children or adults, is associated with more dramatic drops in platelet counts. Viral infections inhibit megakaryopoiesis or may lead to accelerated peripheral destruction of platelets that is mediated by immune complexes or acute vascular damage. Occult liver disease with borderline splenomegaly should be considered in the differential diagnosis of mild thrombocytopenia.

Platelet Function Defects

The bleeding time is often prolonged in patients with severe liver disease, but the cause of the platelet dysfunction is uncertain. Ex vivo platelet function tests have shown abnormalities in platelet adhesion and platelet aggregation in some patients, but the findings are by no means consistent. It is possible that circulating platelet inhibitors (e.g., fibrin degradation products) are not adequately cleared by the failing liver. Plasma levels of von Willebrand factor are increased in most patients with liver disease but little is known about the multimeric composition or function of the adhesive protein.

Disseminated Intravascular Coagulation

Most observers would agree that many patients with advanced liver disease show evidence of chronic low-grade DIC. Fibrinogen survival is reduced, and elevated levels of fibrin degradation products (D-dimer) and thrombin-antithrombin (TAT) complexes have been identified in the plasma. Infusions of heparin correct these abnormalities, which lends support to the concept that thrombin generation or activation of other clotting factors is involved. The cause of the DIC is not completely understood. Hypotheses include the release of procoagulants from degenerating or injured liver cells, low-grade endotoxemia of the portal circulation, failure of the liver to clear activated clotting factors, and decreases in antithrombin III (AT III) or protein C. In general however, the DIC is usually mild (in the absence of concurrent sepsis or malignancy).

Systemic Fibrinolysis

Many patients with severe liver disease have evidence of low-grade systemic fibrinolysis. The euglobulin lysis time (ELT) is short in up to 40 percent of patients awaiting liver transplantation, and one study identified elevated levels of plasmin-antiplasmin complexes in the circulation. Evidence that systemic fibrinolysis is not severe in stable patients is provided by the finding of elevated levels of fibrin, but not fibrinogen degradation products, in patients with advanced liver disease. Systemic fibrinolysis is most likely caused by reduced hepatic synthesis of a_2-antiplasmin (a_2-AP) and impaired clearance of circulating fibrinolytic enzymes by the diseased liver.

Even though the ELT is shortened in patients with chronic liver disease, it is unlikely that systemic fibrinolysis markedly increases the risk of hemorrhage in stable patients. However, major surgery (portal-systemic shunt procedures, orthopedic surgery) provokes the release of large amounts of plasminogen activator from injured tissues, which can temporarily overwhelm protective mechanisms impaired by liver disease and produce severe primary fibrinolysis and bleeding.

Abnormal Fibrinogen Function

Many patients with hepatic insufficiency synthesize an abnormal fibrinogen molecule that is enriched in sialic acid (similar to fetal fibrinogen). Although the dysfibrinogenemia may prolong the TCT, it is unlikely to be responsible for excessive bleeding. Abnormal fibrinogen and prothrombin (noncarboxylated prothrombin) are also synthesized by patients with primary hepatocellular carcinoma.

LABORATORY SCREENING TESTS

As indicated in Chapter 6, standard screening tests are used to assess possible hemostatic defects in hospitalized patients with liver disease who are actively bleeding or who require invasive diagnostic or therapeutic procedures. The tests help in the assessment of the severity of the hemostatic defects and provide baseline values for monitoring blood product replacement therapy. PT, APTT, fibrinogen, and platelet count are all that are necessary for patients with chronic liver disease who are otherwise stable and are not scheduled for surgery.

MANAGEMENT OF BLEEDING

General

Most of the bleeding in patients with advanced liver disease is caused by esophageal varices, peptic ulcer disease, or surgery. Hemostatic defects are often complex but can be divided into several components for purposes of diagnosis and therapy: coagulation defects, platelet function disorders, DIC, and systemic fibrinolysis.

Coagulation Defects

Vitamin K deficiency should be considered early in the management of patients with bleeding due to liver disease. Coagulation screening tests cannot distinguish impaired hepatic synthesis of clotting factors from lack of vitamin K, so that a therapeutic trial of vitamin K is usually indicated if the APTT or PT is prolonged. Doses of 5 to 10 mg should be administered orally or subcutaneously. Deep intramuscular injections should probably be avoided in patients with severe coagulopathies because of the possibility of hematoma formation.

Mild coagulation defects will be reflected in a slightly prolonged PT, with a normal APTT and fibrinogen concentration. Clotting factor replacement therapy is rarely necessary. If defects are more severe and the patient is bleeding (i.e., the PT and APTT are both moderately increased, but the fibrinogen is > 125 mg/dL), then the administration of fresh frozen plasma should be considered. Cryoprecipitate may be required if the coagulopathy is extremely severe and is associated with markedly low fibrinogen concentrations.

In a few patients with end-stage liver disease or acute hepatic failure (e.g., fulminant hepatitis B or herpes simplex hepatitis in an infant), the synthesis of clotting factors can be severely impaired and plasma exchange may be necessary to prepare patients for liver transplantation or to manage refractory bleeding in a patient who is likely to recover spontaneously. Prothrombin complex concentrates should not be used to replace coagulation factors II, VII, IX, and X because of the risks of thrombosis and viral hepatitis.

Platelet Function Defects

Platelet transfusions are indicated if a patient is actively bleeding and the platelet count is < 50,000 to 75,000/μL. The recovery of transfused platelets is impaired in the presence of splenomegaly, but hemostatically effective platelet counts can still be achieved with platelet transfusion in up to 50 percent of patients. The intravenous infusion of DDAVP in doses of $0.3\,\mu g/kg$ significantly but transiently shortens the bleeding time in over 60 percent of patients with liver disease. Although its therapeutic efficacy is unknown, DDAVP is worth a trial in patients with refractory hemorrhage and a prolonged bleeding time.

Disseminated Intravascular Coagulation

Although many patients with advanced liver disease have evidence of chronic low-level DIC, specific therapy is rarely required. Heparin administration is not indicated and is likely to make the bleeding worse. In the rare patient with fulminant liver failure, such as acute fatty liver of pregnancy or severe overwhelming viral hepatitis in children or adults, AT III concentrates may be useful.

Systemic Fibrinolysis

Patients with extremely short ELTs who continue to bleed despite optimal clotting factor and platelet replacement therapy may have clinically significant systemic fibrinolysis. Fibrinolysis is of particular concern during or following a major surgical procedure. Replacement of a_2-AP by the administration of fresh frozen plasma can be tried. If bleeding continues, then the use of antifibrinolytic agents such as ε-aminocaproic acid or tranexamic acid by intravenous infusion should be considered, although central abdominal or peripheral venous thrombosis is a concern.

SPECIAL PROBLEMS IN LIVER DISEASE

Liver Biopsy

Bleeding following liver biopsy is infrequent (e.g., 0.4 percent) although rates of hemorrhage are substantially increased in patients with malignant disease (up to 14 percent). The platelet count should preferably be $> 50,000/\mu L$ prior to liver biopsy. However, mild increases in the PT (e.g., 4 s) and PTT (9 s) are probably not a major contraindication to the procedure. The use of DDAVP should be considered in patients with a history of bleeding and a prolonged bleeding time.

Liver Transplantation

Bleeding can be extraordinarily severe during the course of orthotopic liver transplantation. Common reasons for bleeding include severe portal hypertension and previous right upper quadrant surgery. In addition, a brisk rise in plasma levels of tissue plasminogen activator (t-PA) commonly occurs during the anhepatic phase of the surgery and is associated with a reciprocal fall in fibrinogen (Fig. 24-1). A less well-characterized coagulopathy with a sudden prolongation of the APTT occurs immediately after reperfusion of the newly implanted liver. Management includes aggressive replacement of red blood cells and clotting factors and the occasional use of antifibrinolytic agents.

Peritoneal-Venous Shunts for Ascites

After the implantation of peritoneal-venous shunts, DIC is extremely common and is most likely due to the infusion of cellular or fluid phase procoagulants from the ascitic fluid into the venous circulation. In most instances, the coagulopathy is not sufficiently severe to require removal of the shunt. The DIC can be limited by drainage of the ascitic fluid prior to the placement of the shunt, by temporarily occluding the shunt, or simply by having the patient sit up which reduces the flow of ascitic fluid within the conduit.

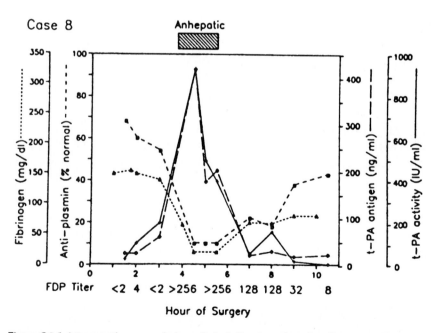

Figure 24-1 Intraoperative course during orthotopic liver transplantation. Note severe fibrinolysis as evidenced by rise in t-PA and fall in fibrinogen. (Used with permission from Dzik WH et al: Blood 71:1090, 1988.)

BIBLIOGRAPHY

Carr JM: Disseminated intravascular coagulation in cirrhosis. *Hepatology* 10:103, 1989.

Cattaneo M et al: Subcutaneous desmopressin (DDAVP) shortens the prolonged bleeding time in patients with liver cirrhosis. *Thromb Haemost* 64:358, 1990.

DiMichele DM, Hathaway WM: Use of DDAVP in inherited and acquired platelet dysfunction. *Am J Hematol* 33:39, 1990.

Dzik WH et al: Fibrinolysis during liver transplantation in humans: Role of tissue-type plasminogen activator. *Blood* 71:1090, 1988.

Gleysteen JJ et al: The cause of coagulopathy after peritoneovenous shunt for malignant ascites. *Arch Surg* 125:474, 1990.

Hussein MA et al: Platelet transfusions administered to patients with splenomegaly. *Transfusion* 30:508, 1990.

Langley PG et al: Thrombin-antithrombin III complex in fulminant hepatic failure: Evidence for disseminated intravascular coagulation and relationship to outcome. *Eur J Clin Invest* 20:627, 1990.

Leebeek FWG et al: A shift in balance between profibrinolytic and antifibrinolytic factors causes enhanced fibrinolysis in cirrhosis. *Gastroenterology* 101:1382, 1991.

Mannucci PM et al: Controlled trial of desmopressin in liver cirrhosis and other conditions associated with a prolonged bleeding time. *Blood* 67:1148, 1986.

McGill DB et al: A 21-year experience with major hemorrhage after percutaneous liver biopsy. *Gastroenterology* 99:1396, 1990.

McVay PA, Toy PTCY: Lack of increased bleeding after liver biopsy in patients with mild hemostatic abnormalities. *Am J Clin Pathol* 94:747, 1990.

Owen CA et al: Hemostatic evaluation of patients undergoing liver transplantation. *Mayo Clin Proc* 62:761, 1987.

Ritter DM et al: Evaluation of preoperative hematology-coagulation screening in liver transplantation. *Mayo Clin Proc* 64:216, 1989.

Stein SF, Harker LA: Kinetic and functional studies of platelets, fibrinogen, and plasminogen in patients with hepatic cirrhosis. *J Lab Clin Med* 99:217, 1982.

Violi F et al: Hyperfibrinolysis increases the risk of gastrointestinal hemorrhage in patients with advanced cirrhosis. *Hepatology* 15:672, 1992.

Disseminated

Intravascular

Coagulation

Disseminated intravascular coagulation (DIC) is a pathologic process in which a generalized activation of the hemostatic system occurs by one or more triggering pathways, causing widespread fibrin formation and subsequent lysis within the vascular system which may result in microthrombosis and consumption of platelets and clotting factors. The process, which results in the formation of thrombin and plasmin, may occur rapidly or slowly and with all degrees of magnitude; the result may be organ dysfunction, generalized hemorrhage, and hemolysis due to red blood cell fragmentation in the microvasculature. Other terms synonymous with DIC are consumption coagulopathy and defibrination syndrome. DIC may be acute (uncompensated) with decreased levels of hemostatic components or chronic (compensated) with normal or elevated levels of clotting factors. Several syndromes in which localized intravascular activation of coagulation occurs (hemolytic uremic syndrome-thrombotic thrombocytopenic purpura, vascular tumors, malignancies) or where the activation is related to toxins (toxic coagulopathy) are discussed in other parts of this book.

CAUSES

The major triggering mechanisms for DIC are (1) exposure or release of thromboplastin-like material containing tissue factor into the circulation; (2) endothelial cell damage; (3) endotoxin and activation of cytokines; (4) immune complexes and particulate matter (amniotic fluid, red blood cell stroma); (5) tissue injury; (6) direct infusion or release of activated clotting factors leading to thrombin (prothrombin complex concentrates [PCC]); (7)

release of proteolytic enzymes affecting the coagulation system (pancreas, granulocytes); (8) direct toxic or chemical effect on clotting factors (venoms, drugs); (9) massive thrombosis; and (10) severe hypoxia and acidosis. These trigger events are caused by a myriad of associated disorders as outlined in Table 25-1.

TABLE 25-1 Disorders Associated with Disseminated Intravascular Coagulation, Grouped According to Pathophysiologic Mechanism or Physiologic Status

Tissue damage (release/exposure of tissue factor) or other mediators
    Physical trauma (crushing and penetrating injuries, e.g., brain injury)
    Thermal injuries (burns, cold injury)
    Asphyxia-hypoxia
    Surgery
    Ischemia-infarction
    Rhabdomyolysis
    Fat embolism
    Hypovolemic-hemorrhagic shock
    Hyperthermia (heat stroke)
Malignancies (release of cancer procoagulants, tissue factor, tumor necrosis factor, cell proteases)
    Solid tumors
    Leukemias
Infections (endotoxin release, endothelial cell damage, platelet activation)
    Bacterial (*Meningococcus, Escherichia coli, Salmonella, Pseudomonas, Haemophilus, Pneumococcus,* hemolytic streptococci, *Staphylococcus*)
    Viral (dengue, Lassa, Ebola, Marburg, Hantaan, rubeola, herpes, etc.)
    Protozoan (malaria)
    Other (Rocky Mountain spotted fever, *Candida, Aspergillus, Clostridia, Mycobacterium tuberculosis*)
    Toxic shock syndrome
Vascular and circulatory disorders (abnormal endothelium, foreign surface coagulation, platelet activation)
    Giant hemangioma, vascular tumors
    Aortic aneurysm
    Vascular surgery
    Intracardiac tumor
    Cardiac bypass surgery
    Acute myocardial infarction
    Vasculitis
    Aortic balloon pump
    Malignant hypertension
    Pulmonary embolism
Immunologic disorders (complement activation, tissue factor release)
    Anaphylaxis
    Allergic reactions

(Continued on next page)

TABLE 25-1 Disorders Associated with Disseminated Intravascular Coagulation, Grouped According to Pathophysiologic Mechanism or Physiologic Status *(continued)*

Acute hemolytic transfusion reactions
Heparin-associated thrombocytopenia
Renal allograft reaction
Kawasaki disease
Drug (quinine, interleukin-1)
Direct enzyme activation
    Pancreatitis
    Snake, spider venoms
Other disorders
    Fulminant hepatic necrosis
    Reye's syndrome
    Cirrhosis
    Le Veen shunt reinfusion
    Adult respiratory distress syndrome
    Prothrombin-complex concentrate infusion
    Hemolytic uremic syndrome
    Inflammatory bowel diseases
    Sarcoidosis
    Amyloidosis
    Hemorrhagic shock and encephalopathy syndrome
    Homozygous protein C deficiency
    Homozygous protein S deficiency
Complications of pregnancy (tissue factor release, ischemia)
    Abruptio placentae
    Amniotic fluid embolism
    Eclampsia and preeclampsia
    Induced (saline) abortion
    Retained dead fetus or missed abortion
    Hydatidiform mole
    Placenta accreta
    Rupture of the uterus
    Chronic tubal pregnancy
    Degenerating fibromyoma
Neonatal DIC
    Infection
    Birth asphyxia
    Hyaline membrane disease
    Aspiration syndromes
    Apneic episodes
    Atelectasis, pneumonia
    Pulmonary hemorrhage
    Cold injury
    Polycythemia
    Abruptio placentae
    Small-for-gestational-age infant

TABLE 25-1 *(continued)*

Maternal hypertensive syndromes
Dead twin fetus
Chorangioma of placenta
Major vessel thrombosis
Purpura fulminans (protein C, protein S deficiency)
Necrotizing enterocolitis
Fetal neoplasms and leukemia
Brain injury (necrosis and hemorrhage)
Erythroblastosis fetalis
Hepatic disease
Hereditary fructose intolerance
Giant hemangiomas

In most instances the cause of the DIC is obvious; the more ill the patient, the worse the DIC. Only rarely does a patient present with clinical and laboratory signs of DIC without a known cause. Disorders such as dengue (or other hemorrhagic fever viruses), occult malignancies (mostly with chronic DIC), unrecognized pulmonary embolism, and infantile hemorrhagic shock and encephalopathy syndrome (encephalopathy, shock, diarrhea, acidosis, raised liver enzymes, decreased renal function, negative blood cultures) can present with DIC as the major manifestation sometimes without a recognizable cause.

The sick newborn infant is particularly prone to DIC because of a decrease in the usual defense mechanisms such as low protease inhibitors (low protein C, protein S, and antithrombin III [AT III]), low levels of fibrinectin, defective fibrinolysis, and an underdeveloped reticuloendothelial system. Pregnant women at term also present with a hypercoagulable state caused by an excess of procoagulants, and a mild activation of coagulation is observed during many normal births. Fetuses and pregnant women share the risk of exposure to thromboplastic material from abnormal or damaged placentas as well as birthing difficulties associated with hemorrhage and hypoxia. Thus, it is not unusual to observe the complication of DIC in the perinatal period (see Table 25-1). Infections and trauma (accidents, burns) are the major causes of DIC in the older child; mortality from head injury in children is four times greater in those with DIC. DIC in adults is frequently associated with infections and malignancies.

DIAGNOSIS

Clinical Manifestations

The clinical manifestations of DIC are frequently masked by the signs of the underlying disorder and laboratory evidence for the syndrome should be sought in any severely ill patient. The most common sign of DIC is bleeding, usually manifested as ecchymoses, petechiae, purpura, trauma-related oozing, and postsurgical hemorrhage. The bleeding diatheses are related to low levels of clotting factors (particularly fibrinogen, factor V, and prothrombin), increased levels of fibrinogen-fibrin degradation products (FDP), which act as an acquired anticoagulant prolonging the APTT and thrombin time and by interfering with platelet function, and thrombocytopenia. Other clinical manifestations relate to the microthrombosis which alters function in the kidneys (varying degrees of renal functional impairment), lungs (adult respiratory distress syndrome), and brain. Necrotic skin and bone and bone marrow lesions are common. Purpura fulminans, a lesion more apt to occur with meningococcemia, chickenpox, and Rocky Mountain spotted fever, is usually associated with severe DIC and low levels of protein C. A mild microangiopathic hemolytic anemia is frequently noted (up to 70 percent of cases of DIC).

Laboratory Manifestations

The laboratory tests which are most frequently abnormal in DIC are:

- Platelet count
- FDP level
- PT
- APTT
- Thrombin time
- Fibrinogen level

Depending on the triggering event, these tests may show varying degrees of abnormality. For instance, an infant after acute hypoxia may show normal platelets, a fibrinogen level of 50 mg/dL, and a mildly prolonged PT with elevated FDP while a young adult with meningococcemia may show a platelet count of 15,000/μL, mildly prolonged PT, and a borderline low fibrinogen level with elevated FDP; chronic DIC in adults with disseminated cancer may show only elevated FDP and a low fibrinogen level; the PT and APTT may be normal. In general, triggering events associated with "thromboplastin" exposure (cancer, hypoxia, brain injury) have greater decreases in fibrinogen, whereas infection is associated with lower platelet counts.

The diagnosis of DIC is made based on the clinical presentation (triggering event) plus laboratory evidence which shows abnormalities of elevated FDP plus reduction in platelets or low fibrinogen or prolonged PT. The APTT is less helpful (except in severe cases) because it is physiologically quite prolonged in the infant and prolongations may be masked by elevated factor VIII in adults.

In severe DIC, practically all coagulation factor assays are abnormal; more specifically proteases complexed with their inhibitors are elevated. Table 25-2 summarizes these assay results in DIC. In many instances, assays for individual coagulation factors such as AT III and protein C fail to add to diagnostic efficacy in evaluating consumptive coagulopathies; however, the use of the protease-inhibitor complex or activation peptide assays (thrombin-antithrombin, F1·2 fragment) has been helpful in clinical studies and holds promise for general clinical use. In our hands, the major benefit of factor assays has been in complicated and severe coagulopathies to guide replacement therapy (AT III, protein C, plasminogen), to offer

TABLE 25-2 Coagulation Assays Which May Be Abnormal in Disseminated Intravascular Coagulation

Assay	Normal Value for Adults	Representative Value(s) in DIC Patient*
A. Coagulation Factors		
Prothrombin	0.7–1.5 U/mL	0.2–0.6 U/mL
Factor V activity	0.6–1.5 U/mL	0.05–0.6 U/mL
Factor VIII:C	0.6–1.5 U/mL	0.8–6.0 U/mL
von Willebrand factor	0.6–1.5 U/mL	2.2–10 U/mL
Factor XII activity	0.7–1.3 U/mL	0.3–0.9 U/mL
Prekallikrein (PK) activity	0.75–1.25 U/mL	0.3–0.5 U/mL
C1-inhibitor	0.60–1.40 U/mL	0.64–2.3 U/mL
a_2-Macroglobulin	0.70–1.30 U/mL	0.60–1.20 U/mL
Antithrombin III	0.8–1.2 U/mL	0.25–0.7 U/mL
Protein C activity	0.7–1.3 U/mL	< 0.06–0.6 U/mL
Protein C inhibitor	0.65–1.3 U/mL	< 0.06–0.65 U/mL
Plasminogen	2.2–4.5 CTA U/mL	0.4–3.5 CTA U/mL
a_2-Antiplasmin	0.8–1.2 U/mL	0.2–1.2 U/mL
B. Activation Peptides or Fragments		
Fibrinopeptide A	0.9 ng/mL	13–346 ng/mL
Bβ 1–42 peptide	< 1.0 pmol/mL	5–10 pmol/mL
Bβ 15–42 peptide	< 1.0 pmol/mL	5–10 pmol/mL
F1·2 fragment	1.97 +/- 0.97 nM	18–56 nM
Factor X activation peptide	66 +/- 20 pmol/L	250–550 pmol/L
C. Enzyme-Inhibitor Complexes		
Thrombin-antithrombin	0.7–2.7 μg/L	3.3–145 μg/L
Plasmin-a_2-antiplasmin complex	0.0–0.5 mg/L	0.3–27

*Abnormal values are from patients with severe DIC.

prognostic help in severe liver disease (factor VII, see Chap. 24), to aid in confirmation of complicating vitamin K deficiency (noncarboxylated prothrombin, see Chap. 23), and to assess severity (AT III, protein C, factor V).

Pathologic Manifestations

Detailed necropsy studies of documented clinical DIC show pathologic evidence (disseminated microthrombi) in only 60 to 75 percent of patients. Fibrin deposition in small vessels may be altered by fibrinolysis and severe fibrinogen depletion.

FIBRINOGEN-FIBRIN DEGRADATION PRODUCTS

The *sine qua non* for the diagnosis of DIC is the presence of elevated levels of FDP. Over 95 percent of all reported instances of DIC have had elevated FDP; although FDP may be present in many inflammatory (systemic lupus erythematosis, renal disease, hemolytic uremic syndrome, necrotizing enterocolitis) and thrombotic (large vessel thrombosis) conditions without

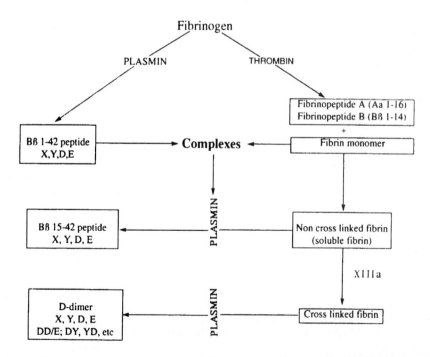

Figure 25-1 Action of thrombin and plasmin on fibrinogen and formation of fibrinogen-fibrin degradation products (FDP).

disseminated or consumption coagulopathy, it is difficult to make a diagnosis of DIC without elevation of FDP. As indicated in Fig. 25-1, the interaction of three key enzymes (thrombin, plasmin, XIIIa) on fibrinogen produces a series of circulating fragments and complexes called fibrinogen-fibrin degradation products or FDP. These products and the methods used to measure them are indicated in Table 25-3. Three types of tests have been used frequently to detect FDP in DIC.

1. The products formed early in the process are fibrin monomer and complexes of monomer with fibrinolytic fragments X, Y (later D, E) or soluble fibrin I; this material is detected by precipitation from plasma by

TABLE 25-3 Measurements of Fibrinogen-Fibrin Degradation Products

Product	Test (Reference)	Normal value	Specimen
FPA	RIA (1)	< 1.5 pmol/mL	Plasma
Bβ 1–42 peptide	ELISA (2)	< 1.0 pmol/mL	Plasma*
Bβ 15–42 peptide	ELISA (2)	0.4 pmol/mL	Plasma*
Monomer and "complexes" (soluble fibrin I)	(a) Ethanol precipitation	< 50 μg/mL	Plasma Plasma
	(b) Protamine precipitation	< 50 μg/mL	
Cross-linked fibrin complexes (soluble fibrin II)	SDS agarose gel electrophoresis	0.1 μg/mL	Plasma
D, E	Latex particles with D+E antibodies:		
	Thrombo-Wellcotest (3)	< 10 μg/mL	Serum
X, Y	Staphylococcal clumping test (4)	< 10 μg/mL	Serum
XYDE	Latex particles with antifibrinogen antibodies (Merskey) (5)	< 10 μg/mL	Serum
D-dimer	Monoclonal antibody latex agglutination (6)	< 200 ng/mL	Plasma
E	ELISA (monoclonal antibody to fragment E)	30–110 ng/mL	Plasma

*Ethanol treated
(1) Mallinckrodt, St. Louis, Missouri
(2) New York Blood Center, New York, New York
(3) Thrombo-Wellcotest, Wellcome Reagents Division, BW Company, Research Triangle Park, North Carolina
(4) Sigma Chemical Company, St. Louis, Missouri
(5) DADE FDP Detection Set, Dado Diagnostics, Aguada, Puerto Rico
(6) Dimertest Latex, American Diagnostica, Greenwich, Connecticut

ethanol or protamine sulfate; it is also the basis for cryofibrinogen. Although the "monomer" test is positive in DIC, it is not as sensitive as other tests.

2. A more sensitive test is the D-dimer determination, which can also be performed on plasma samples and detects cross-linked fibrin but not fibrinogen or the monomer complexes. Performed with a monoclonal antibody against the cross-linked D-dimer site, this procedure has great specificity for fibrin and is positive in DIC as well as in many patients with large vessel thrombosis.

3. A good correlation exists between the D-dimer test and the popular serum FDP or Thrombo-Wellcotest that measures D and E, which are present in both fibrin *and* fibrinogen degradation products. The Thrombo-Wellcotest is sensitive (measures down to 3 μg/mL) and should be drawn into a tube with fibrinolytic inhibitors to prevent an artifactual positive test (in vitro fibrinolysis).

Serum FDP procedures are also affected by heparin in the sample (incomplete clotting) causing a false positive test. Other measurements helpful in certain situations are agarose gel electrophoresis, which detects the cross-linked fibrin macromolecular complexes (soluble fibrin II) derived from extensive fibrin clots in vivo and the Bβ peptides, which offer a possible way to differentiate fibrinogenolysis (increased Bβ 1–42) from lysis of fibrin in the usual DIC patient (increased Bβ 15–42).

MANAGEMENT

Although the recognition of DIC is relatively straightforward, the management of the disorder has been controversial. More recent experience, anecdotal reports, and a few controlled studies have led to a general consensus of management, outlined in Fig. 25-2. The most important aspect of management is the recognition and removal or alleviation of the triggering event or underlying cause. When specific therapy and intensive support are successful, DIC is reversed and unless the consumption process has produced a bleeding tendency, no further treatment for the DIC is necessary. If an invasive procedure or surgery is planned, replacement therapy may be indicated. In this instance or if hemorrhage is ongoing or worsening, the main therapeutic endeavor should be replacement therapy as guided by the laboratory assessment, that is, administration of fresh frozen plasma, cryoprecipitates, and platelet concentrates to replace clotting factors, fibrinogen, and platelets to achieve hemostasis. In patients with shock and volume depletion, fresh frozen plasma should be used early for coagulation factor replacement as well as volume and oncotic effect. Additional therapy includes:

1. Heparin anticoagulation is sometimes indicated in acute leukemias (promyelocytic, monocytic) while induction is underway (see Chap. 34); in impending tissue destruction (skin necrosis in bacterial sepsis; in purpura

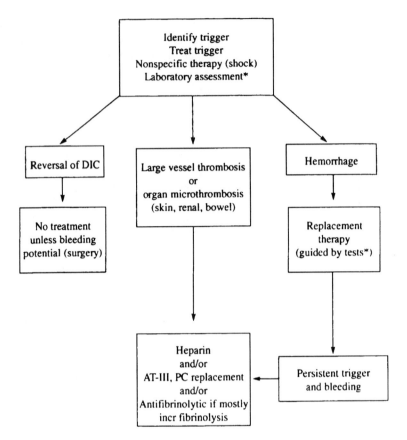

Figure 25-2 Guide to management of patient with diagnosis of acute DIC.

fulminans and in associated large vessel thrombotic disease. Consideration for heparin therapy should be given for giant hemangioma, necrotizing glomerulonephritis, and progressive necrotizing enterocolitis. The dose of heparin should be moderate; 5 to 10 U/kg per hour by continuous infusion as needed to interrupt the DIC (see Chaps. 30 and 34).

2. Specific factor concentrates may be helpful: AT III concentrate in intractable shock or fulminant hepatic necrosis; protein C concentrate in acquired purpura fulminans or severe neonatal DIC.

3. Although antifibrinolytic agents are usually contraindicated in DIC, in rare patients such as those with acute promyelocytic leukemia or prostatic cancer, systemic fibrinolysis can coexist. In these patients antifibrinolytic therapy may be warranted if the process has continued despite heparin.

These therapeutic considerations are appropriate for any age. However, fulminate DIC, especially if associated with liver disease (e.g., disseminated herpes simplex virus) in the newborn or young infant, is frequently amenable to exchange transfusion. Purpura fulminans in the neonate is usually associated with homozygous protein C (see Chap. 40) or protein S (see Chap. 41) deficiency.

BIBLIOGRAPHY

Bacon CJ, Hall SM: Haemorrhagic shock encephalopathy syndrome in the British Isles. *Arch Dis Child* 67:985, 1992.

Bauer KA: Laboratory workers of coagulation activation. *Arch Pathol Lab Med* 117:71, 1993.

Bick RL: Disseminated intravascular coagulation and related syndromes: A clinical review. *Semin Thromb Hemost* 14:299, 1988.

Cembrowski GS et al: Diagnostic efficacy of six plasma proteins in evaluating consumptive coagulopathies. Use of receiver operating characteristic curves to compare antithrombin III, plasminogen, a_2-plasmin inhibitor, fibronectin, prothrombin, and protein C. *Arch Intern Med* 146:1997, 1986.

Connaghan DG et al: Prevalence and clinical implications of heparin-associated false positive tests for serum fibrin(ogen) degradation products. *Am J Clin Pathol* 86:304, 1986.

Corrigan JJ Jr: *Hemorrhagic and Thrombotic Diseases in Childhood and Adolescence*, New York, Churchill Livingstone, 1985, pp 177–206.

Drewinko B et al: Comparative sensitivity of different methods to detect and quantify circulating fibrinogen/fibrin split products. *Am J Clin Pathol* 84:58, 1985.

Feinstein DI: Diagnosis and management of disseminated intravascular coagulation: The role of heparin therapy. *Blood* 60:284, 1982.

Marder VJ: What does the "Dimertest" test? *Circulation* 82:1514, 1990.

Marlar RA et al: Serial studies of protein C and its plasma inhibitor in patients with disseminated intravascular coagulation. *Blood* 66:59, 1985.

Miner ME et al: Disseminated intravascular coagulation fibrinolytic syndrome following head injury in children: Frequency and prognostic implications. *J Pediatr* 100:687, 1982.

Suvatte V: Dengue haemorrhagic fever. *Clin Haematol* 10:933, 1981.

Takada A et al: Prevention of severe bleeding by tranexamic acid in a patient with disseminated intravascular coagulation. *Thromb Res* 58:101, 1990.

Tallman MS, Kwaan HC: Reassessing the hemostatic disorder associated with acute promyelocytic leukemia. *Blood* 79:543, 1992.

Teitel JM et al: Studies of the prothrombin activation pathway utilizing radioimmunoassays for the F_2/F_{1+2} fragment and thrombin-antithrombin complex. *Blood* 59:1086, 1982.

Wilde JT et al: Association between necropsy evidence of disseminated intravascular coagulation and coagulation variables before death in patients in intensive care units. *J Clin Pathol* 41:138, 1988.

Systemic Fibrinolysis

Systemic (primary) fibrinolysis is a clinical disorder in which fibrinolytic enzymes circulate in an active form in the blood and attack clotting proteins as well as local hemostatic plugs within the vasculature. In contrast, fibrinolysis limited to the vicinity of a fibrin clot is termed *localized* or *secondary fibrinolysis*. Although systemic fibrinolysis is uncommon, bleeding may be extraordinarily severe. Prompt recognition of this syndrome is important because therapy with blood products or antifibrinolytic agents can often reduce bleeding.

PATHOPHYSIOLOGY

The fibrinolytic system functions to clear unneeded fibrin from vascular or extravascular sites and is normally highly regulated. Following vascular injury, the deposition of fibrin stimulates the release of tissue plasminogen activator (t-PA) from adjacent endothelial cells and perhaps other tissues in the neighborhood of the clot. Plasminogen activator binds to strands of fibrin and converts adsorbed plasminogen to plasmin, with lysis of the fibrin and formation of soluble fibrin degradation products (FDP). Under usual circumstances the fibrinolytic process remains strictly localized to the milieu of the fibrin clot by binding of the reactants to fibrin, immediate neutralization of any free plasmin by a_2-antiplasmin (a_2-AP), and inhibition of t-PA by plasminogen activator inhibitor (PAI). If fibrinolytic enzymes escape into the circulation in their active form, they are rapidly cleared by the liver before systemic fibrinolysis develops. Occasionally as a result of disease or the administration of thrombolytic agents, fibrinolysis becomes generalized, which leads to severe bleeding from sites of vascular injury. The fibrinolytic system is described in more detail in Chap. 1.

In general, systemic fibrinolysis occurs when excessive amounts of plasminogen activator accumulate in the blood, fibrinolytic inhibitors are deficient, or the liver is unable to clear plasminogen activator or plasmin (Table 26-1). Circulating fibrinolytic enzymes attack thrombi present anywhere within the vasculature, destroy fibrinogen and other clotting factors in the blood, and inhibit platelet function (Table 26-2).

TABLE 26-1 Mechanisms of Systemic Fibrinolysis

Mechanisms	Examples
Circulating plasminogen activators	Thrombolytic agents
	Malignancy, e.g., acute promyelocytic leukemia
	Cardiopulmonary bypass
Decreased inhibitors (a_2-antiplasmin; plasmin activator inhibitor-1)	Liver disease
	Amyloidosis
	Hereditary disorders
Reduced hepatic clearance of plasmin, plasminogen activators	Orthotopic liver transplantation
	End-stage liver disease with portal hypertension

LABORATORY TESTS

Table 26-3 lists the laboratory tests that are altered in patients with systemic fibrinolysis. The euglobulin lysis time (ELT) provides direct evidence of circulating plasmin or plasminogen activator, the standard hemostatic screening tests reflect clotting factor deficiencies and platelet dysfunction, and tests of FDP suggest proteolysis of fibrinogen or fibrin. The ELT is performed by creating a plasma-derived clot free of fibrinolytic inhibitors in a test tube and then observing it closely over the next 60 min for accelerated clot lysis. Because it is sensitive, a positive test (i.e., lysis in < 60 min) does not necessarily indicate that clinical bleeding is a result of systemic fibrinolysis. However, a negative test makes the diagnosis unlikely. Recently ELISA methods have been developed for circulating plasmin-a_2-antiplasmin complexes which are also useful in the identification of patients with excessive fibrinolysis.

The concentration of fibrinogen is an excellent guide to the severity of the fibrinolytic process, assuming other causes of hypofibrinogenemia have been excluded. Severe systemic fibrinolysis is frequently accompanied by a sub-

TABLE 26-2 Causes of Bleeding in Systemic Fibrinolysis

Cause	Mechanism
Lysis of hemostatic plugs	Circulating plasminogen activators or plasmin
Impaired fibrin formation	Plasmin-mediated proteolysis of fibrinogen, factors V and VIII
Platelet function defects	Inhibition of platelet aggregation (FDP) and adhesion ($\downarrow$ von Willebrand factor-glycoprotein Ib interactions)

TABLE 26-3 Clinical Laboratory Tests for Systemic Fibrinolysis

Process	Abnormal Tests
Circulating plasminogen activators or plasmin	Euglobulin lysis time
	t-Plasminogen activator activity
	Plasmin-antiplasmin complexes
Proteolysis of clotting factors by plasmin	PT
	PTT
	Fibrinogen
Platelet function defects	Bleeding time
Lysis of fibrin or fibrinogen	FDP
	TCT
Consumption of fibrinolytic reactants	Plasminogen
	a_2-antiplasmin
	Plasmin activator inhibitor-1

stantial fall in fibrinogen; for example, fibrinogen levels rapidly drop from 350 to 100 mg/dL or even lower following short-term thrombolytic therapy with streptokinase for acute coronary artery thrombosis.

Tests for FDP are often helpful in differentiating primary from secondary fibrinolysis. In general, high levels of D-dimer reflect secondary fibrinolysis, whereas less specific FDP assays (e.g., the Thrombo-Wellco test) identify the presence of either fibrinogen or fibrin degradation products. The combination of a normal D-dimer test along with a strikingly elevated assay that measures both fibrinogen and fibrin degradation products suggests recent systemic fibrinolysis, although a dysfibrinogenemia can produce similar results. Other tests are now available to help distinguish fibrin and fibrinogen degradation products including monoclonal antibody assays for the peptides Bβ 1–42, Bβ 15–42, and fragment E (see chap. 25).

CLINICAL DISORDERS

Bleeding due to brisk systemic fibrinolysis may be extraordinarily severe, particularly in patients undergoing surgery or other invasive procedures. Fig. 26-1 illustrates at least three reasons for hemorrhage:

1. Circulating fibrinolytic enzymes rapidly lyse any hemostatic plug in contact with the blood, so that virtually all vascular defects, large or small, begin to bleed.

2. Plasmin destroys fibrinogen, factor V, and factor VIII, producing a major impediment to fibrin formation.

3. Platelet function is seriously impaired due to aggregation defects in-

Massive Blood

Transfusion

Rapid and exceedingly severe blood loss is now commonplace with the advent of centralized trauma centers, organ transplantation, high-risk obstetrics, complex cardiovascular procedures, and aggressive cancer surgeries. *Massive transfusion* has been defined as the replacement of more than one blood volume (e.g., 10 U blood), in < 24 h. However, most major hemostatic defects occur when more than one blood volume is lost within 2 h. Hemostatic failure is common and results from dilution or consumption of clotting factors, disseminated intravascular coagulation (DIC), systemic fibrinolysis, or acquired platelet dysfunction. The overwhelming sense of urgency that surrounds these patients may be daunting, and optimal treatment demands a practical and simple but logical approach. Making the "right moves" can mean not only the difference between life and death but also allows conservation of valuable blood products.

PATHOPHYSIOLOGY

There are four major categories of hemostatic defects that must be promptly identified and treated in patients with severe bleeding.

Dilution/Consumption

The most common clinical problem is a dilutional coagulopathy resulting from the emergent support of vascular volume by replacement fluids that lack clotting factors or platelets (e.g., crystalloid solutions or packed red blood cells). Dilution is even more severe when packed red cells are administered that are prepared with Adsol®, a solution that adds approximately 100 mL normal saline to each unit of blood, and yields a final hematocrit of about 60 percent. Clotting factors and platelets are virtually absent in Adsol®-suspended red blood cells.

An indirect relationship exists between the number of units of blood given during a massive transfusion and the decrease in clotting factors and platelets (Fig. 27-1). The correlation between the two parameters is somewhat variable, possibly due to patient differences in the consumption of platelets and clotting factors at sites of tissue injury. Screening tests of hemostasis in patients with a dilutional coagulopathy typically show a prolongation of the PT and APTT, reduced concentrations of fibrinogen, and thrombocytopenia.

Disseminated Intravascular Coagulation

This defect frequently follows severe head injury with brain tissue trauma. Other causes of DIC associated with massive bleeding are placental abruption, severe hypotension with hypoxia and acidosis, bacterial sepsis, and

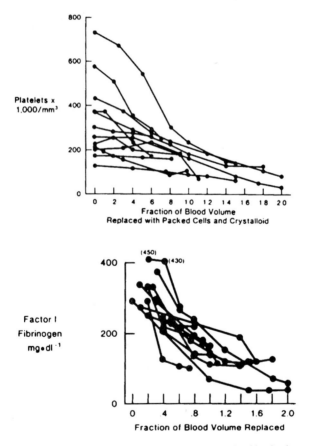

Figure 27-1 Decreases in platelet count and fibrinogen as increasing blood volumes are replaced with packed red cells and crystalloid solutions. Each patient is represented by a solid continuous line. (Used with permission from Murray DJ et al: Anesthesiology 69:839, 1988.)

malignancy. The sudden appearance of DIC following transfusion of red blood cells suggests a major hemolytic transfusion reaction. When DIC complicates the clinical course of patients with trauma or surgical bleeding, consumption of platelets and clotting factors is accelerated, and platelet function can be inhibited by circulating fibrin degradation products (FDP). Most patients with massive bleeding due to trauma usually have only minimal elevations of FDP. Markedly high levels suggest brain trauma or antecedent shock and acidosis.

Systemic Fibrinolysis

Massive hemorrhage, particularly from the gastrointestinal tract, is common in patients with advanced liver disease. These patients can develop systemic fibrinolysis with rapid lysis of thrombi at surgical sites and plasmin-induced destruction of circulating fibrinogen and other clotting factors. Systemic fibrinolysis that occurs during the anhepatic phase of liver transplantation is often associated with hemorrhage (see Chap. 24). The euglobulin lysis time (ELT) should be obtained in bleeding patients with liver disease (or thrombolytic therapy) or in patients who have persistent hemorrhage of unknown cause.

Platelet Dysfunction

Platelet dysfunction is one of the least well-characterized hemostatic defects in the massively bleeding/transfused patient but is a likely cause of hemorrhage. In addition to thrombocytopenia, platelet function can be impaired by high concentrations of fibrin or fibrinogen degradation products, the premature release of platelet granular contents within the circulation from intravascular platelet trauma ("exhausted" platelets), or dilution by transfused platelets that have been stored for several days before transfusion and require several hours to regain optimal function. Bleeding times are difficult to obtain in the emergency setting and are not likely to predict future bleeding. If other hemostatic defects have been corrected, but hemorrhage continues, platelet dysfunction should be suspected and treated with transfusion of platelets.

LABORATORY TESTS

A practical approach to the management of hemostatic failure in massively transfused patients is to obtain screening laboratory tests both for diagnosis and as a guide to blood product replacement therapy. An initial panel of tests should be obtained, followed by repeated testing at frequent intervals to monitor the impact of continued bleeding and blood product replacement (Table 27-1). The key to effective and efficient administration of blood

TABLE 27-1 Laboratory Tests in the Massively Bleeding Patient

INITIAL STUDIES

Test	Diagnostic Category
PT, APTT, fibrinogen, hematocrit	Dilution/consumption
Platelet count	Platelet function
FDP (e.g., D-dimer)	DIC
ELT	Systemic fibrinolysis

FOLLOW-UP TESTS

Test	Replacement Therapy
PT, APTT	Fresh frozen plasma
Fibrinogen	Cryoprecipitate
Platelet count	Platelet concentrates
Hematocrit	Packed red cells

products in the massively bleeding patient is the availability of frequent assessments of hemostasis. Blood must be transported immediately to the laboratory, the assays performed within 30 min, and the results rapidly returned to the emergency room, ICU, or operating suite. A flow sheet is essential to document and analyze results of the laboratory tests, major clinical events, and blood product use.

MANAGEMENT

Ideally, the management of patients with massive bleeding would involve replacement of lost blood with fresh whole blood that contains optimal amounts of platelets and clotting factors. However, fresh blood is rarely available because of limited supplies, rapid outdating, and the current emphasis on blood component therapy. In the past, the transfusion of a fixed ratio of plasma and platelets to units of red blood cells has been advocated. However, this strategy does not always correct all of the hemostatic defects and often wastes blood resources. A third method is to use screening laboratory tests of hemostasis (and hematocrit) to guide blood product replacement therapy (Table 27-2). Blood components used in the management of massively bleeding patients include packed red blood cells, fresh frozen plasma, cryoprecipitate, and platelet concentrates.

TABLE 27-2 Transfusion "Triggers" for Blood Product Replacement in Patients with Massive Bleeding

Hematocrit < 30%	→	Transfuse red blood cells
Platelet count < 75,000/μL	→	Transfuse platelets
Fibrinogen < 100 mg/dL	→	Transfuse cryoprecipitate (or fresh frozen plasma)
PT and/or APTT > 1.5 × control	→	Transfuse fresh frozen plasma

Red Blood Cells

The selection of red blood cells for transfusion follows standard blood banking practices. Compatible blood groups are outlined below:

Compatible Blood Groups

Patient	Red Cells	Plasma
O	O	Any
A	A (or O)	A(AB)
B	B (or O)	B(AB)
AB	Any	AB

In the majority of patients, blood group testing to provide type-specific red blood cells can be performed quickly (e.g., 10 min or less) so that the initial use of group O red blood cells is only necessary for short-term support. The full crossmatch takes 30 to 45 min. In emergencies, uncrossmatched group O Rh negative red blood cells should be administered. If necessary, group O Rh positive red blood cells can be given to older women and to males. When Rh sensitization is likely because of the transfusion of Rh positive red blood cells to an Rh negative recipient, Rh immune globulin is usually not effective because of the large quantity of red blood cells infused. However, Rh immune globulin should be considered when an Rh negative patient has received Rh negative red blood cells with Rh positive platelet concentrates.

Fresh Frozen Plasma

The preparation of fresh frozen plasma takes 15 to 30 min and its need should be anticipated so that time is allowed for the products to thaw. Each unit of fresh frozen plasma increases the concentration of each of the clotting factors by approximately 5 percent.

Cryoprecipitate

Cryoprecipitate is used to replace fibrinogen and factor VIII and can be given without regard to blood group. Approximately 10 to 15 min is required to thaw and pool the product. The infusion of 8 to 10 bags of cryoprecipitate will increase the fibrinogen concentration by 60 to 100 mg/dL in a 70-kg adult.

Platelet Concentrates

Platelet concentrates are usually available immediately although 10 to 15 min is required to pool the individual platelet packs. It is important to remember that 10 U random donor platelets contain approximately 500 mL plasma (300 mL for a platelet apheresis product). In the absence of marked dilution or consumption, 8 to 10 bags of platelets should raise the platelet count by approximately 80,000/μL in an adult.

The optimal "triggers" for the transfusion of blood components in the setting of massive bleeding are uncertain. However, studies in these patients have suggested that collapse of hemostasis, as judged by the appearance of generalized microvascular bleeding, commonly occurs when the platelet count falls below 50,000/μL, the concentration of fibrinogen is < 50 mg/dL, or the PT/APTT increases to more than 1.8 times control. In an otherwise stable patient, hematocrits as low as 18 to 20 percent are usually well tolerated. However, in a critically ill patient who is supported almost entirely by transfused blood, higher hematocrits are warranted. Criteria for the transfusion of blood products in massively bleeding patients are listed in Table 27-2. Controlled studies will be needed to determine if these values are appropriate as reflected by outcome measures such as salvage of life, expenditure of blood resources, and the transmission of viral disease.

In the most severe bleeding circumstances (and particularly in infants and small children), it is essential to give a mixture of blood products, so that one component does not become excessively diluted by administration of the others. Therefore, at regular intervals (e.g., every 30 to 60 min), appropriate proportions of red blood cells, fresh frozen plasma, cryoprecipitate, and platelets should be administered as indicated by the results of the laboratory tests; immediate correction of all the hemostatic defects may not be possible. For example, the infusion of large amounts of fresh frozen plasma for correction of a markedly prolonged APTT and low fibrinogen could cause the hematocrit to plummet if red blood cells are not administered at the same time.

Special Problems in Management

Uncorrectable APTT

One relatively frequent problem is the inability to correct a prolonged APTT in a patient who has a severe dilutional coagulopathy. The continued administration of fresh frozen plasma only seems to reduce the hematocrit because of dilution and fails to shorten the APTT. If marked systemic fibrinolysis can be excluded, a common cause of this often vexing problem is the administration of excessive volumes of crystalloid contained in the cell salvage blood (hematocrit of 45 to 50 percent), or the fluids that are being used by the anesthesiologist. The situation becomes even worse if urine output is low. Several approaches may be tried, including efforts to increase urine volume, reliance on packed red blood cells, and (if necessary) treatment of systemic fibrinolysis.

Long PT and Normal APTT

The PT is commonly minimally to moderately abnormal in patients with trauma, surgery, or sepsis (the mechanism is unknown). However, the APTT may be normal (or even short). In our experience, generalized bleeding tends to correlate with prolongation of the APTT rather than the PT. Therefore, large volumes of fresh frozen plasma should not be used only to correct a prolonged PT.

Citrate Toxicity–Hypocalcemia

Sudden falls in the concentration of ionized calcium are caused by very rapid infusions of citrated plasma. Hypocalcemia is more often observed during surgery in patients with liver insufficiency or during the anhepatic phase of liver transplantation. Most packed red blood cell products do not contain much citrate. However, if large amounts of plasma are being administered, frequent monitoring of the ionized calcium must be performed. Markedly low levels of ionized calcium can result in poor contractility and electrical instability of the heart.

Other Therapeutic Agents

In most instances, the administration of hemostatic agents other than blood products have not proven useful and may be dangerous. The use of DDAVP has not been prospectively studied in patients with massive trauma and bleeding. However, the stress involved in these situations would likely stimulate the release of von Willebrand factor. DDAVP can also lead to hyponatremia or alterations in blood pressure.

Clotting factor concentrates are not usually helpful. Prothrombin-complex concentrates (containing factors II, VII, IX, X) should not be administered because of their thrombogenic potential. Moreover, they cannot correct other clotting factor deficiencies, such as factor V and factor VIII. Because fresh frozen plasma is ordinarily needed for other indications, infusions of purified clotting factors such as factor VIII, factor IX, or antithrombin III are rarely warranted.

ε-Aminocaproic acid or tranexamic acid can be useful in patients with bleeding due to severe systemic fibrinolysis. Most often, the need for anti-fibrinolytic agents occurs during or following the anhepatic phase in patients undergoing liver transplantation. Even so, it is needed in only a minority of patients. Potential complications include vascular thrombosis and hypotension.

Use of Ancillary Equipment

A rapid infusion device that can quickly deliver large volumes of blood products via a large central intravenous line is extremely important. A blood warmer that is capable of a high infusion rate should also be available. The rapid infusion unit should contain a large reservoir into which blood products can be added. An intraoperative blood salvage device is useful in many cases of massive bleeding due to trauma or surgery. This equipment may not be appropriate in the presence of bowel injury or malignancy within the surgical field. However, salvage and reinfusion of red blood cells often substantially reduces packed red cell transfusions. The use of microaggregate blood filters may sometimes be helpful, although they can become obstructed and slow the infusion of blood. The issue as to whether routine microaggregate filtration of blood products reduces pulmonary vascular injury remains unresolved.

BIBLIOGRAPHY

Ciavarella D et al: Clotting factor levels and the risk of diffuse microvascular bleeding in the massively transfused patient. *Br J Haematol* 67:365, 1987.

Ciavarella D, Snyder E: Clinical use of blood transfusion devices. *Trans Med Rev* 2:95, 1988.

Counts RB et al: Hemostasis in massively transfused trauma patients. *Ann Surg* 190:91, 1979.

Dzik WH, Kirkley SA: Citrate toxicity during massive blood transfusion. *Trans Med Rev* 2:76, 1988.

Dzik WH: Massive transfusion. In: Churchill WH, Kurtz SR (eds): *Transfusion Medicine*, Cambridge, Mass., Blackwell Scientific, 1988, pp 211–229.

Goodnight SH et al: Defibrination following brain tissue destruction. *N Engl J Med* 290:1043, 1974.

Harrigan C et al: Serial changes in primary hemostasis after massive transfusion. *Surgery* 98:836, 1985.

Harrigan C et al: The effect of hemorrhagic shock on the clotting cascade in injured patients. *J Trauma* 29:1416, 1989.

Kruskall MS et al: Transfusion therapy in emergency medicine. *Ann Emerg Med* 17:327, 1988.

Leslie SD, Toy PTCY: Laboratory hemostatic abnormalities in massively transfused patients given red blood cells and crystalloid. *Am J Clin Pathol* 96:770, 1991.

Mannucci PM et al: Hemostasis testing during massive blood replacement. A study of 172 cases. *Vox Sang* 42:113, 1982.

Murray DJ et al: Coagulation changes during packed red cell replacement of major blood loss. *Anesthesiology* 69:839, 1988.

Nelson CC et al: Massive transfusion. *Lab Med* 22:94, 1991.

Phillips TF et al: Outcome of massive transfusion exceeding two blood volumes in trauma and emergency surgery. *J Trauma* 27:903, 1987.

Reed RL et al: Prophylactic platelet administration during massive transfusion. A prospective, randomized, double-blind clinical study. *Ann Surg* 203:40, 1986.

Hemostatic Defects

in Renal Disease

and Renal Failure

Hemorrhage was a serious and recurring problem for chronic renal failure patients before the routine use of dialysis. Bleeding rates have fallen sharply since then, but even with dialysis, superficial bleeding in the skin or from mucous membranes is not unusual. Severe hemorrhage is uncommon except perhaps as a consequence of major trauma or surgery. In contrast, patients with acute renal failure can have gastrointestinal bleeding which is usually related to anatomic lesions such as peptic ulcer disease or angiodysplasia of the bowel. Thrombosis and renal disease (e.g., nephrotic syndrome) is discussed in Chap. 45.

PATHOPHYSIOLOGY

Platelet function defects are seen in patients with uremia due to chronic renal failure (Table 28-1). The cause of the platelet dysfunction has been attributed to the accumulation of various "toxic" substances (e.g., guanidinosuccinic acid, phenols) in the plasma as a result of poor renal clearance. Clinical studies have suggested that some of these toxins are dialyzable, whereas others are not. More recently, it has been appreciated that a low erythrocyte or platelet mass contributes substantially to poor platelet function. Some of the evidence for impaired platelet vascular interactions in uremia is reviewed below.

Decreased Red Cell Mass
The severe anemia that accompanies uremia disrupts normal platelet vascular interactions. Several studies have shown that the prolongation of the bleeding time is inversely proportional to the hematocrit (Fig. 28-1). Correc-

TABLE 28-1 Possible Causes of Platelet Dysfunction in Uremia

Adhesion
    Elevated levels of plasma von Willebrand factor
    Abnormal plasma von Willebrand factor
    Reduction of platelet glycoprotein Ib
    Decreased adhesion via glycoprotein IIb/IIIa

Aggregation and secretion
    Elevated platelet cytosolic free calcium
    Decreased release of arachidonic acid from membrane
    Decreased conversion of arachidonic acid to thromboxane A_2
    Decreased storage pool contents and release

Procoagulant activity
    Decreased prothrombinase activity (platelet factor 3)

tion of the anemia (e.g., raising the hematocrit to approximately 30 percent) not only shortens the bleeding time but also reduces symptoms of bleeding.

Decreased Platelet Mass

Uremic patients have both mildly lowered platelet counts and decreased mean platelet volume (MPV) which results in a reduced platelet mass. The circulating platelet mass is inversely proportional to the bleeding time.

Reduced Platelet Adhesion

Experimental models that use high shear forces have suggested that platelet adhesion to vascular surfaces is impaired in patients with uremia. Some, but

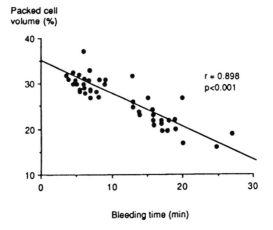

Figure 28-1 Correlation between bleeding time and hematocrit (packed cell volume) in patients treated with erythropoietin. (Reprinted with permission from Vignano G et al: Am J Kid Dis 18:44, 1991.)

not all, studies suggest that the high molecular weight multimers of von Willebrand factor are reduced and ristocetin-induced platelet aggregation is impaired. Moreover, glycoprotein Ib, the receptor for von Willebrand factor on the platelet surface, has recently been reported to be defective in uremic patients.

Defective Platelet Activation and Aggregation

Numerous platelet aggregation defects have been reported in uremic patients, but the defects have not been consistent. Decreased platelet synthesis of thromboxane A_2 and suboptimal exposure of the fibrinogen receptor (glycoprotein IIb/IIIa) on the surfaces of uremic platelets have been described.

Impairment of Platelet Function by Aspirin or Other Drugs

Aspirin decreases thromboxane synthesis in uremic platelets, but also produces a transient noncyclooxygenase-mediated inhibition of platelet function in uremia. This latter defect, when added to impaired thromboxane production, results in a greater than predicted aspirin-induced prolongation of the bleeding time.

Vascular Abnormalities in Uremia

Uremia augments production of endothelium-derived relaxing factor (EDRF) from blood vessels in experimental animal models. Other studies that used human venous tissue showed increased synthesis and release of prostacyclin (PGI_2) from the vasculature of uremic patients. Augmentation of EDRF and PGI_2 synthesis could lead to vasodilation and impaired platelet function in vivo.

Anticoagulant and Antiplatelet Effects of Heparin

The heparin required for dialysis in patients with chronic renal failure not only transiently inhibits coagulation, but also accentuates uremia-induced platelet function abnormalities.

LABORATORY FINDINGS

The bleeding time is frequently abnormal in patients with uremia and can be slightly, moderately, or often severely prolonged (i.e., > 30 min). Controversy exists as to whether the bleeding time has the ability to predict clinical bleeding in uremic subjects, particularly since the numbers of patients with significant hemorrhage are substantially fewer than those with long bleeding times. The platelet aggregation abnormalities are mild and variable and do not predict bleeding. Screening tests of coagulation (e.g., PT, APTT, TCT, fibrinogen) are generally normal, or may be slightly prolonged due to an improper anticoagulant plasma ratio as a result of severe anemia or the presence of ill-defined dialyzable inhibitors in the plasma. Bleeding due to systemic fibrinolysis has not been described in uremic patients.

Patients, particularly children, with the nephrotic syndrome may show abnormalities of the hemostatic screening tests even though they are not uremic. Prolongation of the APTT, due to low factor XII and sometimes factor IX, is not usually associated with a bleeding tendency. In addition, mild prolongations of the TCT are frequently seen and are probably due to a mild acquired dysfibrinogenemia associated with elevated fibrinogen levels. Low antithrombin-III (due to urinary loss) is sometimes associated with thrombosis (see Chap. 45).

MANAGEMENT

Since tests of hemostasis are frequently abnormal but severe hemorrhage is unusual in patients with chronic renal failure, therapy must focus on treatment or prevention of bleeding, rather than normalization of laboratory tests such as the bleeding time. An important first step is to review all medications so that aspirin or other drugs that interfere with platelet function can be stopped. Reduction or elimination of heparin for dialysis may be possible in patients who are at very high risk of bleeding (e.g., following surgery, CNS hemorrhage, hemorrhagic pericarditis).

Listed below are several strategies that can be used for control or prevention of bleeding in patients with chronic renal failure.

Increase Frequency of Dialysis

Accelerated schedules of dialysis tend to shorten bleeding times and reduce the severity of bleeding in some, but not all, patients with renal failure. This approach should be tried whenever possible. Peritoneal dialysis has been as effective as hemodialysis in restoring platelet function toward normal.

Improve Erythroid Mass

Correction of severe anemia produces long-term improvement of platelet function and may also allow other therapeutic measures to be more effective. Both red blood cell transfusions and parenteral erythropoietin are effective, but the latter is preferable because of the risks of chronic transfusion therapy. Hematocrits of 27 to 32 percent have been shown to optimize hemostasis (improved bleeding time, decreased bleeding), whereas higher hematocrits can lead to hypertension or thrombosis.

Improve Platelet Function with DDAVP

Short-term correction of the bleeding time and decreased symptoms of bleeding occur following infusions of DDAVP in 50 to 75 percent of uremic patients (Fig. 28-2). The action of DDAVP is rapid with effects on the

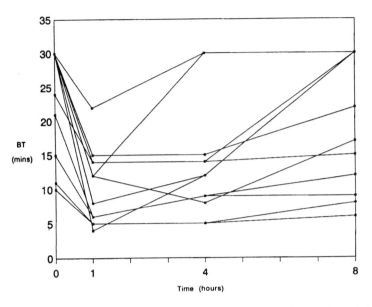

Figure 28-2 Bleeding times before and after DDAVP in uremic patients. (Data and permission obtained from Mannucci PM et al: N Engl J Med 308:8, 1983.)

bleeding time observed within minutes, which persists for at least 4 h. Shortening of the bleeding time correlates with a rise in the high molecular weight multimers of von Willebrand factor in the plasma. Although mild but transient flushing, headache, and abdominal cramps occur in up to 50 percent of treated patients following DDAVP, water retention and hyponatremia are rare because the diseased kidneys are unable to regulate water balance. Arterial thrombosis has been reported in elderly patients with atherosclerosis who were treated with DDAVP. Cryoprecipitate has also been used to treat bleeding in uremia, but variability of response, a lag in onset of action (1 to 12 h), and the risks of viral infection have made this approach less attractive.

Improve Platelet Vascular Interactions with Conjugated Estrogens

Large doses of conjugated estrogens (0.6 mg/kg per day for 5 days) can be given intravenously, subcutaneously, or orally, and have been reported to shorten the bleeding time and decrease bleeding in patients with chronic renal failure (Fig 28-3). Onset of action occurs in about 6 h and persists for 14 days. Maximal benefit is noted in 5 to 7 days. Since the duration of effect is substantially longer than that of DDAVP, estrogens have been used to prepare uremic patients for major surgical procedures.

An often difficult clinical problem is whether to attempt correction of the bleeding time with dialysis or DDAVP prior to percutaneous renal biopsy in

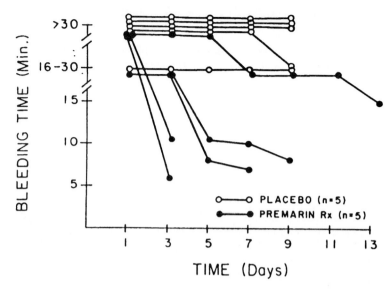

Figure 28-3 Patients with abnormal bleeding times and no clinical bleeding treated with conjugated estrogens or placebo. (Reprinted with permission from Shemin et al: Am J Med 89:436, 1990.)

patients with renal disease. Study of large series of subjects suggests that rates of hemorrhage are very low (< 1 percent) following biopsy in patients with near normal bleeding times. Whether the bleeding time can be used as a predictor of possible future hemorrhage is controversial. When patients with uremia are considered as a group, the prolonged bleeding time clearly suggests a disorder in platelet vascular interactions. However, it appears unlikely that the bleeding time reliably predicts future bleeding in individual patients. Until additional information is available, maneuvers to correct greatly prolonged bleeding times (> 30 min) with DDAVP or other modality prior to biopsy is probably warranted.

BIBLIOGRAPHY

Akizawa T et al: Effects of recombinant human erythropoietin and correction of anemia on platelet function in hemodialysis patients. *Nephron* 58:400, 1991.

Castillo R et al: Defective platelet adhesion on vessel subendothelium in uremic patients. *Blood* 68:337, 1986.

Di Minno G et al: Platelet dysfunction in uremia. Multifaceted defect partially corrected by dialysis. *Am J Med* 79:552, 1985.

Gaspari F et al: Aspirin prolongs bleeding time in uremia by a mechanism distinct from platelet cyclooxygenase inhibition. *J Clin Invest* 79:1788, 1987.

Gralnick HR et al: Plasma and platelet von Willebrand factor defects in uremia. *Am J Med* 85:806, 1988.

Kyrle PA et al: Evidence for an increased generation of prostacyclin in the microvasculature and an impairment of the platelet a-granule release in chronic renal failure. *Thromb Haemost* 60:205, 1988.

Livio M et al: Conjugated estrogens for the management of bleeding associated with renal failure. *N Engl J Med* 315:731, 1986.

Mannucci PM et al: Deamino-8-d-arginine vasopressin shortens the bleeding time in uremia. *N Engl J Med* 308:8, 1983.

Michalak E et al: The decreased circulating platelet mass and its relation to bleeding time in chronic renal failure. *Thromb Haemost* 65:11, 1991.

Remuzzi G: Bleeding in renal failure. *Lancet* 1:1205, 1988.

Remuzzi G et al: Role of endothelium-derived nitric oxide in the bleeding tendency of uremia. *J Clin Invest* 86:1768, 1990.

Sloand EM et al: Reduction of platelet glycoprotein Ib in uraemia. *Br J Haematol* 77:375, 1991.

Steiner RW et al: Bleeding time in uremia: A useful test to assess clinical bleeding. *Am J Hematol* 7:107, 1979.

Vignano G et al: Recombinant human erythropoietin to correct uremic bleeding. *Am J Kidney Dis* 18:44, 1991.

Zwaginga JJ et al: Defects in platelet adhesion and aggregate formation in uremic bleeding disorder can be attributed to factors in plasma. *Arteriosclerosis Thrombosis* 11:733, 1991.

Thrombotic

Thrombocytopenic

Purpura and the

Hemolytic Uremic

Syndrome

Thrombotic thrombocytopenic purpura (TTP) and the hemolytic uremic syndrome (HUS) are closely related disorders characterized by diffuse microvascular occlusion of the arterioles and capillaries producing ischemic dysfunction of multiple organs. The microthrombi are primarily composed of platelets and the disorders are presently considered to be due to endothelial cell damage and excessive platelet clumping. TTP is a syndrome (thrombocytopenia, microangiopathic hemolytic anemia, neurologic symptoms, renal disease, fever) which occurs mostly in adults (however, Moschowitz's original patient was a teenager) and may show acute (single episode), intermittent, or chronic-relapsing types.

Hemolytic uremic syndrome (thrombocytopenia, microangiopathic anemia, acute renal failure) occurs mostly in children and is of endemic-epidemic, sporadic, or familial types. Table 29-1 highlights the similarities and differences of the syndromes. Overlapping but clinically different syndromes due to vascular damage (thrombocytopenia, microangiopathic hemolysis, diffuse organ involvement) are some types of disseminated intravascular coagulation (DIC), preeclampsia-eclampsia (hemolysis, elevated liver enzymes, low platelet count) syndrome (see Chap. 31), malignant hypertension,

TABLE 29-1 Comparison of Major Features of Hemolytic Uremic Syndrome and Thrombotic Thrombocytopenic Purpura

Feature	HUS	TTP
Onset and course	Age usually < 3 y Males = females Prodrome (infection, bloody diarrhea) common Recurrence—rare	Peak incidence 3d decade Females > males Prodrome less common Recurrence—common
Diagnosis	*Triad* Acute renal failure Thrombocytopenia Microangiopathy (CNS involvement unusual) (Fever unusual)	*Pentad* CNS involvement Thrombocytopenia Microangiopathy Renal involvement Fever (Acute renal failure less common)
Etiologic factors	Most often infection (*E. coli, Shigella* gastroenteritis, pneumococcal, etc.) Rare familial and/or recurrent form Adult—postpartum, after mitomycin C, cyclosporin A	Not known in most cases Secondary causes: pregnancy, autoimmune disease, neoplastic, drugs (sulfa, oral contraceptives, iodine)
Treatment	Supportive Renal dialysis is mainstay Steroids—no help Heparin—for DIC if present	Steroids Plasma exchange Heparin—No Splenectomy
Prognosis	90% fully recover Rare death	Up to 90% gain remission with plasma exchange Mortality 9–15%

acute renal hemograft rejection, systemic lupus erythematosus (SLE), and severe vasculitis.

PATHOPHYSIOLOGY

The HUS syndromes may be divided into those with a prodromal diarrheal seasonal illness in children ("D+ " subtype, > 90 percent of cases) and those without the prodrome (often familial occurrence, children and adults, worse prognosis), which has been called "D–" subtype. The D+ group is known to be associated with infection with bacteria (*Escherichia coli* 0157; H7; *Shigella dysenteriae*, type 1) producing a renal endothelial cell cytotoxin (verocytotoxin, VT) which has been implicated in HUS. It is proposed that VT damages renal endothelial cells, thus releasing platelet clumping substances (ultralarge von Willebrand factor multimers or other substance) which form the microthrombi; indeed large molecular weight von Willebrand factor is decreased in many cases of HUS. Other microorganisms like pneumococci and endothelial-altering chemotherapeutic agents like mitomycin C or cyclosporin A may operate in a similar manner. In most susceptible individuals the kidney is the major target but other cells (brain, pancreas) may also be susceptible, or more likely, other organs are damaged by circulating microthrombi.

Likewise, TTP may follow the introduction of some platelet aggregating agent (a 37,000 Mr protein, a calcium-activated cysteine protease, a lysosomal cathepsin, autoantibody or ultralarge von Willebrand factor) into the circulation after endothelial cell damage or alteration (toxin, drug, virus, autoantibody). For example, if ultralarge von Willebrand factor multimers are released in excessive amounts or if they are processed defectively (lack of processing enzyme), TTP may occur. Plasma exchange, which is the current most successful therapy for an otherwise fatal disease, would be effective by removing the platelet clumping agent or replacing the ultralarge von Willebrand factor processing enzyme. In the chronic relapsing type of TTP, infusions of plasma alone may prevent recurrences.

Other mechanisms that may be operative in some cases of TTP-HUS include defective endothelial cell synthesis of prostacyclin which renders endothelial cells more susceptible to triggering events (decreased synthesis has been found in HUS, TTP, and during pregnancy), and platelet activation produced by thrombin or other aggregating agents associated with triggers of intravascular coagulation (limited DIC).

The red blood cell fragmentation (Fig. 29-1) and hemolytic anemia seen in both HUS and TTP are probably due to physical damage to red blood cells by the occlusive effect of the microangiopathy but the erythrocyte may also be made more susceptible to injury by a reduced antioxidant potential due to a relative deficiency of vitamin E. Reduced plasma levels of vitamin E and an apparent beneficial effect of supplementation has been observed in some children with HUS.

CLINICAL MANIFESTATIONS AND DIAGNOSIS

Hemolytic Uremic Syndrome

Almost all cases of childhood HUS ("D+" or endemic type) present acutely after a prodromal infectious illness which is frequently acute diarrhea or

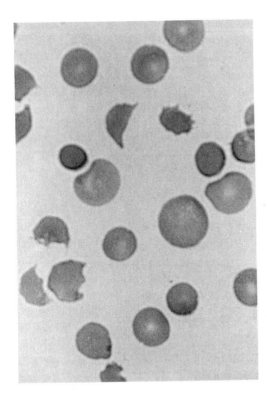

Figure 29-1 Oil power view of blood smear of patient with HUS. Note the fragmented red blood cells and microspherocytes. Identical findings are noted in TTP.

bloody diarrhea (colitis-like symptoms); other infections (*Mycoplasma*, viruses, microtatobiotes, *Pneumococcus*) have also been documented. Neuramidase from pneumococci exposes the Thomsen-Friedenreich receptor (T antigen) on red blood cells, platelets, and endothelium-producing IgM antibodies which agglutinate red blood cells and platelets; this mechanism has been associated with HUS (normal plasma contains anti-T agglutinins and could aggravate the anemia and thrombocytopenia). By the time the diagnosis is made and acute renal failure is established, an early complication may be excessive fluid administration and hyponatremic seizures.

Thrombocytopenia and anemia are usually present at the onset and last for 1 to 2 weeks and 2 to 4 weeks respectively; other laboratory tests include leukocytosis and derangements of blood urea nitrogen (BUN), creatine, and electrolytes for degree of renal failure. Abnormal coagulation tests include elevated fibrin degradation products (FDP) and raised levels of fibrinogen, factor VIII, and von Willebrand factor. The APTT, PT, and thrombin time are usually normal; an occasional patient has shown low antithrombin III (AT III) or protein C. A rare patient with a more complicated course will show evidence for DIC. Complications include CNS involvement (hyponatremic seizures, microthrombosis, cerebral infarction), pancreatic islet cell necrosis and diabetes, large bowel infarction, vitamin K deficiency, arterial thrombosis and extremity gangrene, and congestive heart failure. Risk factors for CNS involvement include female gender, prolonged use of antimotility agent, and an increased hemoglobin level.

A rare patient will present with HUS without a prodromal illness and with a tendency to recur. These patients are often older and family occurrence is known. This group is the sporadic or "D–" type in which an unknown genetic predisposition is present. We have followed a 9-year-old girl who has had four separate episodes of HUS since age 1 year; the episodes appeared to be triggered by urinary tract infections and often involved the CNS (seizures, disorientation). Coagulation studies including von Willebrand factor multimers were normal during remission. Adult HUS may occur sporadically in the postpartum period (occasionally in association with low AT III) and after chemotherapeutic agents (mitomycin C, cyclosporin A; see Chap. 30).

Thrombotic Thrombocytopenic Purpura

The pentad of neurologic symptoms and signs, hemolytic anemia, thrombocytopenia, renal disease, and fever are present in about 40 to 50 percent of the cases of adult TTP. About 75 percent of patients have hemolytic anemia, thrombocytopenia, and CNS changes. In addition, because of the rarity of the disorder and the confusion with similar diseases (autoimmune hemolytic anemia, Evan's syndrome, SLE, preeclampsia-eclampsia, postpartum renal failure, sepsis-endocarditis, vasculitis, and drug sensitivities), a firm diagnosis is difficult to make and is dependent on excluding the similar clinical disorders and on the presence of the characteristic red blood cell changes on the blood smear (fragmented cells, schistocytes, microspherocytes; see Fig. 29-1). Laboratory findings include anemia with elevated reticulocytes, thrombocytopenia, leukocytosis, bilirubinemia, and evidence of renal involvement. Although FDP are commonly present (about 60 to 70 percent of patients), most other coagulation tests are normal (APTT, PT, thrombin time, fibrinogen); von Willebrand factor and factor VIII are usually elevated. Lactic dehydrogenase is elevated (1200 to 1400 U/L) and is an indicator of disease activity. The direct antiglobin test is negative. Bone marrow and gingival biopsies are sometimes helpful by displaying the hyaline microthrombi in small vessels.

The clinical course of TTP is occasionally acute but usually differs from HUS in that the onset is more insidious (without a distinct prodromal illness); acute disease activity lasts longer (months rather than weeks) and has a characteristic tendency to recur. Without intensive treatment the mortality rate approaches 80 percent.

During pregnancy, the occurrence of TTP is often confused with severe preeclampsia-eclampsia. Consideration of the diagnostic pentad and exclusion of other causes of TTP-like disorders including HUS and renal failure and those that are drug related (mitomycin C, cyclosporine, ticlopidine) must be done before instituting therapy. With plasma exchange as a therapy, the prognosis for survival of both mother and fetus is good.

TREATMENT

Hemolytic Uremic Syndrome

Patients with HUS and acute renal failure are provided intensive supportive care (red blood cell transfusions if hemoglobin is < 7 g/dL; fluid and electrolyte balance, nutritional support, treatment of hypertension). Peritoneal dialysis or hemodialysis is instituted on clinical indications (usually a rising BUN or potassium, excessive fluid overload, hyponatremia) and continued until kidney recovery. About three fourths of patients will require dialysis. Thrombocytopenic bleeding is treated with platelet transfusions only if persistent wound bleeding or a vital site hematoma not responding to local measures occurs; most bleeding observed is mild skin purpura regardless of platelet count levels. No specific pharmacologic therapy (corticosteroids, antiplatelet agents, heparin) is used because most studies have not shown their superiority over no therapy. Heparin is used for thrombotic complications of intravascular catheters as needed. Most patients recover within 1 to 2 weeks but require long-term follow-up for renal status. A rare patient may develop serious extrarenal progressive organ involvement (brain, pancreas, colon); these patients should have early consideration of plasmapheresis with fresh frozen plasma replacement as a therapeutic trial.

Thrombocytic Thrombocytopenic Purpura

The approach to management of TTP is outlined in Fig. 29-2. Patients are monitored with hemoglobin, platelet count, reticulocyte count, BUN, creatinine, and lactate dehydrogenase as well as clinical signs. If the patient responds to steroids, the dose is dropped to 60 mg and then tapered slowly after the patient is in remission. If no response to steroids occurs in 48 h or if the patient shows general deterioration or has developed CNS signs, early plasmapheresis with fresh frozen plasma should be instituted. The average response time for daily plasma exchanges is 7 to 9 days. If the patient fails to improve or deteriorates further, cryoprecipitate-poor plasma should be substituted for fresh frozen plasma. If plasmapheresis is not immediately available, infusions of fresh frozen plasma may offer some benefit. Some patients, including two infants, with the chronic relapsing form of TTP have been

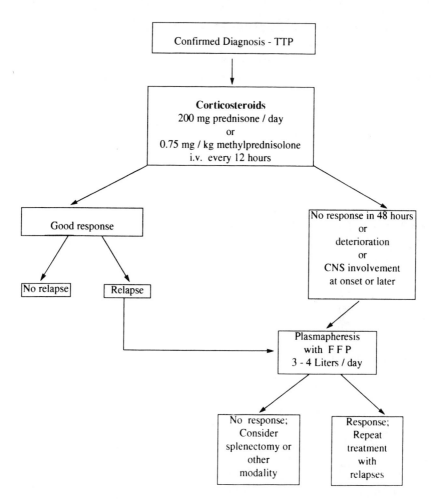

Figure 29-2 Schematic approach to management of TTP according to the reference of Bell and colleagues.

maintained in a relatively normal state with periodic (every few weeks) administration of fresh frozen plasma or cryoprecipitate-poor plasma.

PROGNOSIS

With strict attention to supportive care and renal dialysis, the prognosis for immediate survival is excellent in childhood ("D+") HUS. Long-term follow-up (5 to 21 years) in one group of children indicated considerable residual nephropathy (increased albumin secretion [31 percent]), reduced glomerular filtration (18 percent), and both (10 percent). Recent data demonstrates that the severity of the gastrointestinal prodrome (watery diarrhea versus bloody diarrhea or prolapse) reflects the severity of the process and resulting long-term outcome. Outcome will be variable in the less common types of HUS ("D-", drug induced, postpartum, and familial). Remarkable progress has been made in TTP, from a uniformly fatal disease to complete recovery in > 90 percent of patients in one recent series.

BIBLIOGRAPHY

Bell WR et al: Improved survival in thrombotic thrombocytopenic purpura-hemolytic uremic syndrome. Clinical experience in 108 patients. *N Engl J Med* 325:398, 1991.

Chintagumpala MM et al: Chronic relapsing thrombotic thrombocytopenic purpura in infants with large von Willebrand factor multimers during remission. *J Pediatr* 120:49, 1992.

Cimolai N et al: Risk factors for the central nervous system manifestations of gastroenteritis—associated hemolytic-uremic syndrome. *Pediat* 90:616, 1992.

Falanga A et al: A cathepsin-like cysteine proteinase proaggregating activity in thrombotic thrombocytopenic purpura. *Br J Haematol* 79:474, 1991.

Fitzpatrick MM et al: Long-term renal outcome of childhood haemolytic uraemic syndrome. *Br Med J* 303:489, 1991.

Lopez EL et al: Association between severity of gastrointestinal prodrome and long-term prognosis in classic hemolytic-uremic syndrome. *J Pediatr* 120:210, 1992.

Mattoo JK et al: Familial, recurrent hemolytic-uremic syndrome. *J Pediatr* 114:814, 1989.

Milford DV, Taylor CM: New insights into the haemolytic uraemic syndromes. *Arch Dis Child* 65:713, 1990.

Moake JL: TTP—Desperation, empiricism, progress. *N Engl J Med* 325:426, 1991.

Rarick MU et al: Thrombotic thrombocytopenic purpura in patients with human immunodeficiency virus infection: A report of three cases and review of the literature. *Am J Hematol* 40:103, 1992.

Ridolfi RL, Bell WR: Thrombotic thrombocytopenic purpura. Report of 25 cases and review of the literature. *Medicine* 60:413, 1981.

Rock GA et al: Comparison of plasma exchange with plasma infusion in the treatment of thrombotic thrombocytopenic purpura. Canadian Apheresis Study Group. *N Engl J Med* 325:393, 1991.

Ruggenenti P, Remuzzi G: Thrombotic thrombocytopenic purpura and related disorders. *Hematol Oncol Clin North Am* 4:219, 1990.

Tardy B et al: Intravenous prostacyclin in thrombotic thrombocytopenic purpura; case report and review of the literature. *J Intern Med* 230:279, 1991.

Thompson CE et al: Thrombotic microangiopathies in the 1980s: Clinical features, response to treatment, and the impact of the human immunodeficiency virus epidemic. *Blood* 80:1890, 1992.

Van Damme-Lombaerts R et al: Heparin plus dipyridamole in childhood hemolytic-uremic syndrome: A prospective, randomized study. *J Pediatr* 113:913, 1988.

Bleeding and Cancer

This chapter discusses hemorrhagic disorders that occur in patients with solid tumors, whereas bleeding that complicates the hematologic malignancies is covered later (Chaps. 33 and 34). The topic of thrombosis and malignancy is considered in Chap. 46. The most common hemostatic defect in cancer patients is thrombocytopenia, which usually develops late in the course of the illness. Less frequently, chronic disseminated intravascular coagulation (DIC) or disorders such as systemic fibrinolysis, circulating anticoagulants, or the synthesis of dysfunctional clotting factor molecules are seen.

THROMBOCYTOPENIA

Thrombocytopenia in patients with cancer is most often the result of suppression of marrow platelet production by malignancy, chemotherapy, or radiation treatments. Although immune thrombocytopenia (ITP) is classically associated with lymphoid neoplasms, patients with solid tumors also develop ITP. Immune-mediated thrombocytopenia can also be provoked by some of the drugs used in oncology practice, including vancomycin, penicillin, and heparin. The diagnosis and treatment of thrombocytopenia is reviewed in Chaps. 8, 29, and 52.

Some cancer patients have developed a severe microangiopathy accompanied by renal failure, anemia, and thrombocytopenia following chemotherapy strikingly reminiscent of the hemolytic uremic syndrome (HUS) (Table 30-1).

TABLE 30-1 Cancer-Associated Hemolytic Uremic Syndrome*

Adenocarcinoma in 89%
No evident malignancy at time of diagnosis in 35%
Mitomycin C therapy in 98%
Mortality—50% within 8 weeks
Consider therapy with staphylococcal protein A immunopheresis
Avoid transfusion of blood products

*From Lesesne JB et al: *J Clin Oncol* 7:781, 1989.

The drug that has been most commonly associated with this disorder is mitomycin C, but other agents have also been implicated, including cisplatin, bleomycin, and cyclosporin A. Cancer-related HUS is often fatal, but some benefit has been reported with staphylococcal protein A immunopheresis of the plasma.

DISSEMINATED INTRAVASCULAR COAGULATION

Pathogenesis

Many tumors can activate coagulation and fibrinolysis to facilitate the implantation of metastatic cells. The release of cells from the primary tumor can be augmented by the action of proteolytic or fibrinolytic enzymes on nearby blood vessels, and the growth and proliferation of disseminated tumor cells may be facilitated by the formation of a local fibrin meshwork.

Laboratory evidence of activation of coagulation (e.g., increased fibrinopeptide A) in both the early and late stages of cancer is exceedingly common. When the activation of clotting factors and platelets is mild or moderate, a propensity to thrombosis (e.g., venous, arterial, or involving a heart valve) may be found, but when stimulation of the clotting system is brisk and sustained, full-blown DIC can occur with severe hypofibrinogenemia and diffuse bleeding. Coagulation is instigated by tumor cell activation of factor VII, factor X, or prothrombin; platelets may also be activated and fibrinolysis can be inhibited as well. Of particular interest, cytokines such as interleukin-1 or tumor necrosis factor produced by tumor cells may stimulate nearby macrophages or endothelial cells to become prothrombotic via the synthesis and expression of cell surface tissue factor.

Hemorrhage as a result of DIC in patients with malignancy usually does not occur unless clotting factor depletion is severe; that is, fibrinogen concentrations of < 100 mg/dL, factor V or factor VIII of < 30 percent, or platelet counts < 50,000/μL. High concentrations of fibrin degradation products also impair platelet function. A rather wide spectrum of tumors are associated with DIC and bleeding. Common offenders include mucous-producing adenocarcinomas of the bowel or abdomen (e.g., pancreas, gastric, biliary tract), as well as neoplasms that originate in the lung. In childhood, activation of coagulation is most often found in patients with disseminated neuroblastoma and rarely occurs with other tumors.

The malignancy is often widely disseminated when severe hemostatic defects occur, and tumor cell emboli can be found in the microvasculature of the lung or other organs (Fig. 30-1). The intravascular collections of tumor cells can induce a severe microangiopathic hemolytic anemia with thrombocytopenia and circulating fragmented red blood cells.

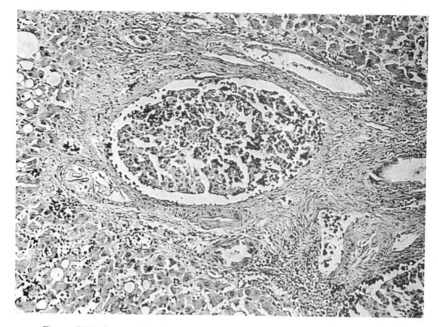

Figure 30-1 Tumor cell emboli in microvasculature of a patient with breast cancer.

Clinical Findings and Laboratory Tests

Most patients with malignancy do not have excessive bleeding and have normal screening tests of hemostasis. Hemorrhage, particularly after surgery or invasive diagnostic procedures, can be severe in patients who develop cancer-related DIC. Spontaneous bruising of the skin and bleeding from the mucous membranes or the gastrointestinal tract can occur.

Results of laboratory tests in cancer-related DIC are illustrated in Table 30-2. In addition, sensitive tests that reflect activation of coagulation or fibrinolysis such as circulating thrombin-antithrombin or plasmin-antiplasmin complexes are abnormal in 5 to 10 percent of patients. Fragmented red blood cells are prominent on the peripheral blood smear in patients with disseminated malignancy and DIC. The microangiopathic hemolytic anemia can produce marked elevations of lactic dehydrogenase and indirect hyperbilirubinemia as a result of the red blood cell destruction.

Management

Most patients with mild cancer-related DIC do not require specific therapy such as large volumes of blood products or therapeutic doses of anticoagulants. However, prophylactic antithrombotic measures should be strongly considered for surgical procedures because of the high likelihood of postoperative venous thromboembolism.

Effective chemotherapy or surgery is the best treatment for chronic DIC associated with cancer but unfortunately is often not possible. When antitumor treatment is effective, tumor cell lysis can expose the blood to even more procoagulant activity, which accelerates the consumption of clotting factors and platelets. In these circumstances, laboratory monitoring to include platelet counts, fibrinogen, and fibrin degradation products is warranted. Temporary anticoagulation with heparin may be necessary during periods of DIC as a consequence of early cycles of chemotherapy.

When cancer-related DIC is severe and associated with bleeding, correction of a prolonged PT and APTT with fresh frozen plasma, hypofibrinogenemia with cryoprecipitate, and thrombocytopenia with platelet concentrates may be required. Although in the past concerns were raised that the administration of blood products would "fuel the fire" and worsen the DIC, this phenomenon rarely occurs. However, if frequent blood product replacement therapy is needed to balance the accelerated consumption of clotting factors or platelets, then heparin may be needed to inhibit thrombin generation and reduce the intensity of the DIC.

When heparin is used, it should be given together with appropriate blood product replacement. Heparin should be infused at relatively low rates (e.g., 500 U/h) without a loading dose and increased as needed to maintain hemostatic levels of clotting factors and platelets. Unfortunately, unless effective cancer therapy is available, the prognosis in most of these patients is very poor.

SYSTEMIC FIBRINOLYSIS

Although many tumor cells produce and release fibrinolytic enzymes in culture, systemic fibrinolysis is unusual in cancer patients. Prostate cancer has been reported to be associated with primary fibrinolysis and bleeding, and

TABLE 30-2 Disseminated Intravascular Coagulation in Patients with Cancer

	Mild DIC	Severe DIC	Normal Range
PT	12.0	18	11–13.5 s
APTT	23	56	25–35 s
Fibrinogen	580	40	175–350 mg/dL
Platelets	650,000	56,000	175–325 $\times$ 10³/μL
D-dimer	4	32	< 0.5 μg/mL
ELT	> 60	> 60	> 60 min

Coagulation Factor Deficiencies

During normal pregnancy (see Chap. 3) fibrinogen, vWf, and factors II, VII, IX, X, VIII, and XII rise significantly by the third trimester while factors XI, XIII, and V remain the same or fall slightly. This physiologic change will have an effect on less severe congenital deficiencies but will not alter the severe defects. The experience with each hereditary disorder is briefly summarized.

Hemophilia A and B

Clinically significant factor VIII or IX deficiency is rare in women (see Chap. 14) except for the occasional carrier with extreme lyonization. Although factor VIII levels have risen appropriately in hemophilia A carriers, factor IX levels have risen only slightly in the few hemophilia B carriers with serial studies. Peripartum bleeding has occurred in factor IX carriers. Because the minimal hemostatic level for hemophilia A and B is about 0.20 to 0.30 U/mL, carriers should be monitored and if the level has not risen significantly, replacement therapy should be considered before delivery or for a cesarean section operation. For factor IX deficiency, use high purity factor IX concentrate (see Chap. 56).

Fibrinogen Abnormalities

Women with afibrinogenemia may have normal menses or severe menorrhagia and recurrent early abortions. A rare successful pregnancy and delivery was achieved with weekly fibrinogen infusions. Hypo- and dysfibrinogenemia are associated with recurrent abortion or abruptio placentae. Dysfibrinogenemic bleeding may even worsen as the synthesis of abnormal molecules increase during pregnancy. Bleeding episodes require the use of fibrinogen concentrate (cryoprecipitates, see Chap. 56). A woman weighing 60 kg would require 10 to 15 packs of cryoprecipitate to raise the normal fibrinogen level to above 100 mg/dL.

Other Deficiencies

First trimester spontaneous abortion has been reported in a patient with congenital dysprothrombinemia. Intrapartum and postpartum hemorrhage may be severe in patients with factor V deficiency; adequate hemostasis can be achieved by infusion of 15 mL/kg of fresh frozen plasma in the early puerperium. A patient with congenital factor X deficiency (level unknown) showed marked improvement of her bleeding tendency and PT during pregnancy. Severe menorrhagia occurs frequently in severe factor VII deficiency; however, only about one half of reported deliveries have had postpartum hemorrhage. Postpartum hemorrhage despite fresh frozen plasma in 2 patients was subsequently eliminated by use of a factor VII

concentrate. Homozygous factor XIII deficiency causes a severe hemorrhagic tendency but is readily treated with infusions of fresh frozen plasma
or concentrate. One patient had 12 previous pregnancies that were interrupted by severe bleeding and spontaneous abortions; because of regular
transfusions of plasma, the patient's 13th pregnancy was normal and no
bleeding occurred. Pregnancies in women with severe factor XII deficiency
and severe prekallikrein deficiency were uncomplicated and no excess
bleeding occurred. Some patients with severe factor XI deficiency do not
show any clinical bleeding tendency; one such patient known to us experienced a normal pregnancy and delivery without bleeding episodes. If
bleeding does occur, fresh frozen plasma or factor XI concentrate may be
needed (see Chap. 56).

ACQUIRED BLEEDING DISORDERS

Thrombocytopenia

The major causes of thrombocytopenia during pregnancy are listed in Table
31-2. The immune thrombocytopenias (ITP, pregnancy-associated thrombo-

TABLE 31-2 Causes of Thrombocytopenia in Pregnancy

Immune
   ITP
   SLE
   Evan's syndrome
   Thyrotoxicosis
   Lymphoproliferative diseases
   Pregnancy-associated thrombocytopenia
Infections
   Bacterial, viral, other
Drugs
   Alcohol, isoniazid, diphenylhydantoin, quinine, sulfonamides, heparin
Other
   TTP
   Preeclampsia/eclampsia, HELLP syndrome
   Chronic hepatitis
   Obstetrical complications with DIC
   Massive blood transfusions
   Bone marrow hypoplasia (toxic, idiopathic)
   Bone marrow malignant disease (cancer, leukemia)
   Megaloblastic anemias

*SLE, systemic lupus erythematosus; ITP, immune thrombocytopenic purpura; DIC, dissemin-
ated intravascular coagulation; HELLP, hemolysis, elevated liver enzymes, low platelet
counts; TTP, thrombocytic thrombocytopenic purpura.

cytopenia) are discussed in Chap. 9 and thrombocytic thrombocytopenic purpura (TTP) in Chap. 29. The differential diagnosis of low platelets and red blood cell fragmentation in the hypertensive pregnant woman in the third trimester may be particularly difficult and includes the following disorders: hypertensive disease of pregnancy (preeclampsia) with the severe form, the HELLP syndrome (hemolysis, elevated liver enzymes, low platelets), acute fatty liver of pregnancy (AFLP), TTP, hemolytic uremic syndrome, and abruptio placentae with disseminated intravascular coagulation (DIC). A precise diagnosis is important since therapy varies considerably with each disorder (Table 31-3).

A particularly difficult management problem is whether to use epidural anesthesia in patients with potential bleeding disorders, especially those with thrombocytopenia or prolonged bleeding time. Mild prolongation of the bleeding time is seen in patients with the above acquired disorders (microangiopathic thrombocytopenia) but no data are available to suggest the use of the bleeding time in management. In general, obstetric patients with

TABLE 31-3 Differential Diagnosis of Thrombocytopenia in "Preeclampsia"

Manifestation	HELLP	AFLP	Condition Abruption	TTP	HUS
Onset	Insidious	Acute	Acute	Insidious	Insidious
Thrombo-cytopenia	Severe	Mild, early	Mild to severe	Severe	Severe
Abnormal PTT, PT	When liver severely involved	Yes	20%of patients (DIC)	No	No
Elevated FDP	Yes	Yes	Yes	Yes	Yes
Jaundice	Rare	Yes	No	Rare	Rare
Increased liver enzymes	Yes	Yes	No	Occasional	No
Abdominal pain	Yes (epigastric)	Yes (epigastric)	Yes (uterine)	No	No
Renal failure	Rare	Rare	No	No	Yes
Neurologic involve-ment	Sometimes	Late	No	Yes	Rare

SOURCE: Adapted from Martin JN Jr, Stedman CM: *Obstet Gynecol Clin North Amer* 18:181, 1991.

*AFLP, acute fatty liver of pregnancy; HELLP, hemolysis, elevated liver enzymes, low platelets; DIC, disseminated intravascular coagulation; FDP, fibrin degradation products.

moderate thrombocytopenia do not display prolongation of the bleeding time. Coagulation factor-deficient patients are much more apt to bleed and deficiencies should be corrected if the procedure is performed. Epidural anesthesia is probably contraindicated in moderate and severe bleeding disorders.

Obstetric Causes of Disseminated Intravascular Coagulation

Hemorrhage produced or aggravated by DIC is associated with many of the major obstetric complications. Tissue factor-triggered DIC occurs in abruptio placentae, amniotic fluid emboli, saline-induced abortions, dead fetus, degenerating fibroma, hydatidiform mole, and placenta accreta. Other triggers include sepsis, massive hemorrhage, and shock. Diagnosis and management of DIC are discussed in Chap. 25. For details of the management of DIC associated with the specific obstetric complications see the Hathaway and Bonnar reference. Important principles (see Chap. 27) of patient management of women in coagulation failure (massive hemorrhage and shock) include:

1. Correction of circulating blood volume and tissue perfusion with appropriate volume replacement therapy. In patients who are believed to have a coagulation defect, fresh frozen plasma should be used for volume expansion so that replacement of clotting factors may be started early. The initial volume required for a significant effect on the coagulation status must be large and must be administered rapidly, that is, 600 to 2000 mL infused during a period of 1 to 2 h. Packed red blood cells should be given to maintain the hematocrit above 30 percent.

2. Vaginal delivery makes a less severe demand on the hemostatic mechanism than does delivery by cesarean section or by hysterotomy, both of which require the same degree of hemostatic competence as any other abdominal operation. When a coagulation defect exists, severe bleeding will occur at sites of surgical incisions and may not develop until after the operation. In the obstetric patient, extensive bleeding can occur into the abdomen from the cesarean section incision on the uterus. It is nearly always advisable in the absence of fetal distress to await spontaneous delivery, avoiding if possible all soft tissue damage to the vagina and perineum rather than embarking on operative interference. After delivery, the contracted and retracted myometrium will sharply diminish bleeding from the placental site.

3. The obstetric condition is responsible for the hemostatic defect, and spontaneous recovery will usually follow delivery of the patient, provided that the blood volume is maintained and hypovolemic shock is prevented. The treatment of the underlying obstetric complication is therefore an important part of the management of the bleeding tendency. In exceptional

circumstances when surgical intervention is deemed necessary, every effort should be made to correct the coagulation failure before and following operation.

Circulating Anticoagulants

A bleeding tendency similar to that which occurs in severe hemophilia A can occur secondary to development of an inhibitor to factor VIII (see Chap. 21).

Acute Fatty Liver of Pregnancy

Acute hepatic failure occurring at term and unrelated to preeclampsia, hepatitis, hepatotoxic agents, or HUS is termed *acute fatty liver of pregnancy*. These patients characteristically show biochemical evidence of liver disease (elevated bilirubins, enzymes, and low serum proteins) in association with a severe coagulopathy (low platelets, fibrinogen, and antithrombin III [AT III] with elevated fibrin degradation products). This coagulopathy of severe liver disease probably represents failure of both synthesis of clotting factor and activation of coagulation. At least two reports emphasized the extremely low AT III levels seen in AFLP patients and suggested a benefit from correction of the coagulopathy after administration of AT III concentrates.

BIBLIOGRAPHY

Bern MM: Acquired and congenital coagulation defects encountered during pregnancy and in the fetus. In: Bern MM, Frigoletto FD Jr (eds): *Hematologic Disorders in Maternal-Fetal Medicine*, New York, Wiley-Liss, 1990, pp 395–447.

Bjornsson S, Calder AA: Obstetric and gynaecological haemorrhage. In: Greer IA, Turpie GG, Forbes CD (eds): *Haemostasis and Thrombosis in Obstetrics and Gynaecology*, London, Chapman and Hall Medical, 1992, pp 45–76.

Cameron IT, Smith SK: Menorrhagia. In: Greer IA, Turpie GG, Forbes CD (eds): *Haemostasis and Thrombosis in Obstetrics and Gynaecology*, London, Chapman and Hall Medical, 1991, pp 77–93.

Giles AR, Hoogendoorn H, Benford K: Type IIB von Willebrand's disease presenting as thrombocytopenia during pregnancy. *Br J Haematol* 67:349, 1987.

Greer IA et al: Haemorrhagic problems in obstetrics and gynaecology in patients with congenital coagulopathies. *Br J Obstet Gynecol* 98:909, 1991.

Hathaway WE, Bonnar J: Hemorrhagic disorders during pregnancy. In: *Hemostatic Disorders of the Pregnant Women and Newborn Infant*, New York, Elsevier, 1987, pp 76–103.

Joseph G et al: Pregnancy in Henoch-Schonlein purpura. *Am J Obstet Gynecol* 157:911, 1987.

Martin JN Jr, Stedman CM: Imitators of preeclampsia and HELLP syndrome. *Obstet Gynecol Clin North Am* 18:181, 1991.

Peaceman AM, Cruikshank DP: Ehlers-Danlos syndrome and pregnancy: Association of type IV disease with maternal death. *Obstet Gynecol* 69:428, 1987.

Peaceman AM et al: Bernard-Soulier syndrome complicating pregnancy: A case report. *Obstet Gynecol* 73:457, 1989.

Robertson LE et al: Hereditary factor VII deficiency in pregnancy: Peripartum treatment with factor VII concentrate. *Am J Hematol* 40:38, 1992.

Vicente V et al: Normal pregnancy in a patient with a postpartum factor VIII inhibitor. *Am J Hematol* 24:107, 1987.

Bleeding Related

to Congenital

Heart Disease

and Cardiac Surgery

HEMOSTATIC DEFECTS DUE TO CONGENITAL HEART DISEASE

Severe congenital heart disease has been associated with a wide variety of hemostatic defects. As a consequence, excessive bleeding can become an important clinical problem when patients require cardiac or other major procedures. Fortunately, early surgical correction of the cardiac abnormalities is now the rule, so that bleeding symptoms are far less common than in the past. However, hemostatic defects may still occur in patients who are not candidates for corrective surgery or who must delay operation until a later date.

Pathogenesis

A wide spectrum of hemostatic abnormalities have been described in patients with congenital heart disease including defects in platelet function, coagulation, and fibrinolysis. In general, cyanotic patients with chronic hypoxia, polycythemia, and impaired blood flow have more prominent defects in hemostasis than those with acyanotic heart disease (e.g., ventricular septal defect).

Platelet Dysfunction

Mild to moderate thrombocytopenia (e.g., 90,000 to 100,000/μL) occurs in some patients with cyanotic congenital heart disease due to shortened platelet survival. Mild defects in platelet aggregation have also been reported and include reduced platelet aggregation with epinephrine and deaggregation when adenosine diphosphate is used as a stimulus. Bleeding times are occasionally prolonged (up to 8 percent of patients). The high molecular weight multimers of von Willebrand factor were lower than normal in a group of 12 patients with acyanotic congenital heart disease (Gill reference). Three of these subjects also had low levels of coagulation factor XII reminiscent of patients with a variant of von Willebrand disease (vWd—San Diego; see Chap. 12).

Coagulation

Many patients have been assumed to have a coagulopathy because the PT and PTT are frequently prolonged. However, some of these laboratory abnormalities (but not all) return to normal when the volume of anticoagulant is reduced in the collection tube to correct for the high hematocrit found in patients with cyanotic congenital heart disease. Some patients have reduced clotting factor synthesis due to chronic passive congestion of the liver. A few early reports suggested that low-grade disseminated intravascular coagulation (DIC) occurs, although more recent studies have not substantiated this observation.

Fibrinolysis

About 20 percent of patients have a short plasma euglobulin lysis time (ELT), but the origin and significance of this finding is uncertain. Clinically significant systemic fibrinolysis is unlikely because fibrinogen concentrations are not often reduced, and levels of fibrinogen degradation products are usually normal.

Laboratory Tests

Patients with congenital heart disease who have bleeding symptoms or who are candidates for major surgery should have screening tests of hemostasis (see Chap. 6). The volume of citrate anticoagulant in the collection tube must be adjusted to avoid spurious coagulation test results in patients with elevated hematocrits (see Chap. 2). Laboratory test results compiled from several large series of patients previously reported in the medical literature are listed in Table 32-1. However, at present the frequency of abnormal laboratory test

TABLE 32-1 Screening Laboratory Test Results Compiled from Several Reported Series of Patients with Cyanotic Congenital Heart Disease

Abnormal test results	Patients
Platelet count	42%
Bleeding time	8%
ELT	17%
PT	15%
APTT	8%
TT	6%

*From Colon-Otero G et al: *Mayo Clin Proc* 62:379, 1987.

results is likely to be lower because of early surgical repair of the cardiac lesions.

Clinical Manifestations

Most nonsurgical bleeding in patients with congenital heart disease is mild and limited to recurrent epistaxis and easy bruisability. Hemoptysis may occur and has been noted particularly in patients with pulmonary hypertension. Surgical bleeding is variable and unpredictable, although patients with severe hypoxia are at increased risk of hemorrhage. In rare patients, postoperative bleeding is exceedingly severe, and several hemorrhagic deaths have been reported. However, when surgery is successful, preoperative platelet function defects are almost always improved postoperatively, which suggests that the platelet abnormalities were acquired and related either to the cardiac lesion or to hypoxia and polycythemia.

Management

With modern medical and surgical management, most patients with congenital heart disease have minimal laboratory abnormalities or bleeding symptoms and do not require treatment. However, a few will have a history of severe bleeding or marked abnormalities in laboratory tests of hemostasis (mainly in association with severe cyanosis) and require correction of their coagulopathies prior to surgery. One therapeutic approach is to reduce the red blood cell mass by repeated isovolumetric phlebotomy to lower hematocrits to < 60 to 65 percent. The platelet count, bleeding time, and coagulation factor abnormalities will often improve. For adults, 500-mL phlebotomies with replacement of normal saline can be performed at daily intervals; smaller volumes (e.g., 50-mL increments) should be removed in children.

Desmopressin (DDAVP) has been administered prophylactically to increase plasma von Willebrand factor, shorten bleeding times, and reduce blood loss during and following cardiac surgery. However, the benefits remain uncertain. Patients with congenital heart disease have marked elevations in von Willebrand factor and factor VIII activity as a result of surgical stresses, and no further rise is seen after infusions of DDAVP. However, a therapeutic trial might be worthwhile in patients who have persistent postoperative bleeding. DDAVP should be used with caution in the nonsurgical setting because several patients with cyanotic congenital heart disease developed a sudden decrease in peripheral vascular resistance, hypotension, and death following its use.

Antifibrinolytic agents are commonly used in adult patients who undergo cardiac surgical procedures and cardiopulmonary bypass (see below), but they have not been used as extensively in patients with congenital heart disease. Potential problems include an increased risk of thromboembolism in cyanotic patients who have elevated hematocrits and sluggish blood flow.

HEMOSTATIC DEFECTS CAUSED BY CARDIAC SURGERY AND CARDIOPULMONARY BYPASS

Postoperative bleeding is often a major problem for patients who require cardiac surgery and cardiopulmonary bypass (CPB; Table 32-2). In many instances the bleeding is due to local vascular defects that require surgical repair. However, extracorporeal circulation regularly produces hemostatic abnormalities that can contribute to postoperative hemorrhage.

TABLE 32-2 Causes of Bleeding After Cardiopulmonary Bypass

Common (95–99%)
    Defective surgical hemostasis
    Acquired transient platelet dysfunction
Uncommon (1–5%)
    Other platelet dysfunction
    Thrombocytopenia
    Vitamin K deficiency
    DIC
    Inherited hemostatic defects
Doubtful Significance
    Systemic fibrinolysis
    Heparin
    Protamine excess

*Modified from Woodman RC et al: *Blood* 76:1680, 1990.

Pathogenesis

Platelet dysfunction is the most common hemostatic defect induced by CPB. Two problems have been described. First, platelets are activated in the oxygenator with the release of a-granule (but not dense granule) contents and exposure of specific a-granule proteins on the surface of the platelets (e.g., P-selectin). Activated mononuclear cells have recently been shown to bind to P-selectin with the formation of platelet-monocyte aggregates. Although not proven, these cellular aggregates could promote damage to the pulmonary microcirculation, a clinical problem that has been associated with the prolonged use of CPB.

A second platelet function defect is caused by physical damage to platelet membranes during extracorporeal circulation. Platelets transiently stick to the surfaces of the oxygenator, which damages membrane glycoproteins and results in decreased platelet adhesion and impaired binding of fibrinogen to platelet surfaces. Hypothermia magnifies the platelet function defects. Prolonged bleeding times and reduced quantities of thromboxane A_2 in blood issuing from bleeding time cuts have been documented.

Accelerated fibrinolysis occurs during CPB with marked increases in the concentration of tissue plasminogen activator (t-PA) and a moderate fall in a_2-antiplasmin (a_2-AP; Fig. 32-1). However, these abnormalities are short-lived and are not associated with clinically significant systemic fibrinolysis. Plasma fibrinogen falls only to the level expected by hemodilution and

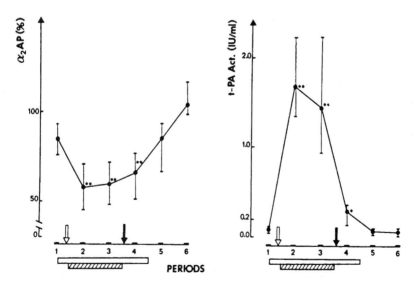

Figure 32-1 Median concentrations of a_2-AP and t-PA in 24 patients undergoing cardiopulmonary bypass in open heart surgery. (Used with permission from Gram J et al: Thromb Haemost 63:241, 1990.)

fibrinogen degradation products are not greatly elevated. In contrast, secondary fibrinolysis (presumably of thrombi formed in the surgical field) is brisk, as evidenced by a gradual increase in D-dimer concentrations throughout CPB and for several hours thereafter.

Clinical Manifestations

Excessive and persistent bleeding from chest tubes or wound sites is a common problem in the immediate postoperative period in cardiac surgery patients. The hourly volume of blood that issues from the chest tubes is an excellent indication of the magnitude of bleeding, which frequently exceeds several hundred milliliters per hour. Oozing of blood from venipuncture sites or other areas of trauma (catheters, nasotracheal or nasogastric tubes) suggests a systemic defect of hemostasis.

Laboratory Tests

Unfortunately, preoperative screening tests in cardiac surgery patients are seldom predictive of postoperative bleeding. However, the bleeding time can be of use when it is obtained immediately following the cessation of CPB. In one study, normothermic patients with prolonged bleeding times had significantly greater rates of postoperative bleeding.

Almost all laboratory tests of hemostasis are abnormal during and immediately following CPB because of hemodilution, the use of heparin, and platelet defects induced by the oxygenator. However, platelet counts are lower than predicted and plasma concentrations of the platelet-specific proteins such as β-thromboglobulin are increased, both of which suggests platelet activation. Thrombin-antithrombin complexes, D-dimer, and fibrinopeptide A are all elevated, but a_2-AP is decreased during CPB.

Laboratory tests should be obtained in cardiac surgery patients with postoperative bleeding and should include the PT, APTT, fibrinogen, bleeding time, and platelet count. In addition, D-dimer levels and the ELT may be of value (see Chap. 6). These tests are used to identify defects in coagulation, platelet function, and fibrinolysis, and as guides to clotting factor or platelet replacement therapy.

Management

Since thrombocytopenia and platelet function defects are so common, platelet concentrates are often given empirically to cardiac surgery patients who have postoperative bleeding. Several studies have documented normalization of platelet counts, bleeding times, and platelet aggregation tests along with cessation of bleeding following platelet transfusions. Hypothermia magnifies platelet dysfunction, so that rewarming the patient may also be of value. Coagulation abnormalities due to dilution or consumption of clotting factors must also be corrected (e.g., hypofibrinogenemia of < 100 mg/dL with cryoprecipitate and markedly prolonged PT and APTT with fresh frozen plasma; see Chap. 27).

Cardiac surgery teams have evaluated prophylactic infusions of DDAVP before or after CPB to improve platelet function and to decrease intraoperative or postoperative bleeding. Two early trials were encouraging, but subsequent studies have shown little benefit in terms of decreased blood loss or transfusion requirements in uncomplicated patients who received coronary artery bypass grafts. Levels of von Willebrand factor and factor VIII activity are almost invariably elevated by the stress of surgery so that additional benefit from DDAVP is unlikely. Most surgeons and cardiovascular anesthesiologists reserve DDAVP for complex and prolonged surgeries or for patients who develop uncontrolled bleeding.

Antifibrinolytic agents have also been used to decrease bleeding in cardiac surgery patients. Aprotinin (Trasylol), tranexamic acid (TA), and ε-aminocaproic acid (EACA) have been evaluated in clinical trials. In almost all of the studies, blood loss during and following surgery was decreased by 1/3 or more, red blood cell transfusions were reduced, and the number of patients who avoided transfusion significantly increased. Thromboembolism, a potential complication of antifibrinolytic therapy, was not observed. The antifibrinolytic agents not only inhibit fibrinolysis, but they also preserve platelet function, possibly by the prevention of platelet adhesion defects or by a reduction in circulating levels of fibrin degradation products.

The indications for antifibrinolytic agents in cardiac surgery patients continue to evolve. Most would agree that these drugs are useful when patients are at high risk for bleeding (e.g., reoperation, prolonged CPB, or uremia). Antifibrinolytic agents can also be used as adjunctive therapy in Jehovah's Witnesses when blood transfusion is not possible.

Other Hemostatic Problems Relative to Cardiac Surgery

Postoperative Coagulation Factor Inhibitors to Bovine Thrombin

Topical bovine thrombin is used frequently in cardiovascular surgery. Rare patients will produce antibodies either to bovine thrombin or to bovine factor V which is also present in most preparations of topical thrombin. These antibodies can cross-react in vivo with human thrombin or human factor V and cause bleeding. The diagnosis is suggested in postoperative patients with prolonged TCTs, particularly when bovine thrombin is used as the reagent for the thrombin time (see Chap. 21).

Protamine Toxicity

Some patients with diabetes mellitus who are treated with NPH insulin (which contains protamine) may develop IgG or IgE antiprotamine antibodies. When protamine sulfate is given to neutralize the heparin used for CPB, sensitized patients can suddenly develop pulmonary hypertension, hypoxia, and occasionally, overwhelming DIC. Since protamine contains arginine, one study suggested that arginine conversion to endothelium-derived relaxing factor is responsible for the systemic hypotension that has been observed in this syndrome. Reactions can be reduced if protamine is administered slowly and into the systemic rather than the venous circulation.

BIBLIOGRAPHY

Ansell J et al: Does desmopressin acetate prophylaxis reduce blood loss after valvular heart operations? A randomized, double-blind study. *J Thorac Cardiovasc Surg* 104:117, 1992.

Colon-Otero G et al: Preoperative evaluation of hemostasis in patients with congenital heart disease. *Mayo Clin Proc* 62:379, 1987.

Gill JC et al: Loss of the largest von Willebrand factor multimers from the plasma of patients with congenital cardiac defects. *Blood* 67:758, 1986.

Harder MP et al: Apotinin reduced intraoperative and postoperative blood loss in membrane oxygenator cardiopulmonary bypass. *Ann Thorac Surg* 51:936, 1991.

Horrow JC et al: Hemostatic effects of tranexamic acid and desmopressin during cardiac surgery. *Circulation* 84:2063, 1991.

Khuri SF et al: Hematologic changes during and after cardiopulmonary bypass and their relationship to the bleeding time and nonsurgical blood loss. *J Thorac Cardiovasc Surg* 104:94, 1992.

Manno CS et al: Comparison of the hemostatic effects of fresh whole blood, stored whole blood, and components after open heart surgery in children. *Blood* 77:930, 1991.

Perloff JK et al: Adults with cyanotic congenital heart disease: Hematologic management. *Ann Intern Med* 109:406, 1988.

Rinder CS et al: Cardiopulmonary bypass induces leukocyte-platelet adhesion. *Blood* 79:1201, 1992.

Valeri CR et al: Effect of skin temperature on platelet function in patients undergoing extracorporeal bypass. *J Thorac Cardiovasc Surg* 104:108, 1992.

van Oeveren W et al: Aprotinin protects platelets against the initial effect of cardiopulmonary bypass. *J Thorac Cardiovasc Surg* 99:788, 1990.

Weiss ME et al: Association of protamine IgE and IgG antibodies with life-threatening reactions to intravenous protamine. *N Engl J Med* 320:886, 1989.

Wenger RK et al: Loss of platelet fibrinogen receptors during clinical cardiopulmonary bypass. *J Thorac Cardiovasc Surg* 97:235, 1989.

Woodman RC, Harker LA: Bleeding complications associated with cardiopulmonary bypass. *Blood* 76:1680, 1990.

Zehnder JL, Leung LLK: Development of antibodies to thrombin and factor V with recurrent bleeding in a patient exposed to topical bovine thrombin. *Blood* 76:2011, 1990.

Lymphoproliferative

Disorders

In general, patients with lymphoproliferative disorders are troubled with excessive bleeding rather than arterial or venous thrombosis. Causes of hemorrhage are diverse although thrombocytopenia induced by marrow disease or chemotherapy is a common problem. A wide spectrum of platelet, coagulation, or fibrinolytic abnormalities have been described that often pose diagnostic and therapeutic dilemmas. This chapter covers acute and chronic lymphocytic leukemia, dysproteinemias including plasma cell myeloma and macroglobulinemia, and finally, the bleeding manifestations of systemic amyloidosis.

ACUTE LYMPHOCYTIC LEUKEMIA

Disseminated intravascular coagulation (DIC) can complicate acute lymphocytic leukemia (ALL) as well as acute promyelocytic or monocytic leukemia. This coagulopathy was recently identified in 12 percent of a large cohort of adults with ALL prior to treatment and was associated with a dramatic increase to 78 percent of patients following induction chemotherapy (Fig. 33-1). Bleeding ascribed to DIC was found in 9 of 153 patients in this series. Similar findings have been described in a group of patients with Philadelphia chromosome-positive ALL. Evidence of thrombin activation (based on screening tests of hemostasis including fibrin degradation products) has also been detected in a large proportion of children being treated for ALL, although overt DIC with bleeding was unusual (Table 33-1).

L-asparaginase is commonly used in the treatment of children and adults with ALL and can occasionally produce severe coagulation defects. L-asparaginase inhibits protein synthesis and, as a consequence, the formation of several clotting factors (or their inhibitors) by the liver. Bleeding may occur a few days after the completion of a course of therapy and is associated with prolongation of the PT and APTT and a fall in fibrinogen. Thrombosis occurs

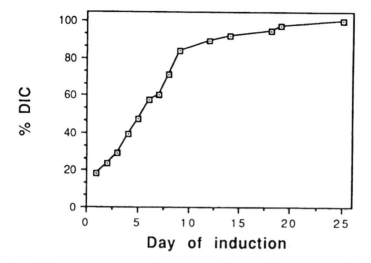

Figure 33-1 Cumulative occurrence of all DIC cases during remission induction of adult ALL patients. All cases of DIC occurring before day 1 of induction were plotted on day 1. (Used with permission from Sarris AH et al: Blood 79:1305, 1992.)

later, often after 2 to 3 weeks, and has been linked to decreased levels of protein C, antithrombin III (AT III), and protein S. Of note, both the bleeding and thromboembolic events show a predilection for the CNS, such as intracerebral hemorrhage and cerebral sinus vein thrombosis. The hemostatic complications of L-asparaginase are discussed in more detail in Chap. 35.

Therapy for the L-asparaginase-induced coagulopathies may include the administration of fresh frozen plasma in symptomatic patients. AT III concentrates have been used to elevate levels of AT III, but it is not known whether this approach will reduce rates of thrombosis.

TABLE 33-1 Hemostasis Laboratory Tests in 52 Children with Acute Leukemia

Test	Patients Abnormal
PT	27%
APTT	6%
TCT	17%
Fibrinogen	8%
D-dimer	38%
(activation of coagulation)	
Bβ 1–42	4%
(primary fibrinolysis)	

*From Abshire TC et al: *Cancer* 66:716, 1990.

CHRONIC LYMPHOCYTIC LEUKEMIA/LYMPHOMA

Patients with chronic lymphocytic leukemia (CLL), Hodgkin's disease, and non-Hodgkin's lymphoma occasionally become severely thrombocytopenic by an immune mechanism rather than due to marrow failure. Less commonly, acquired von Willebrand's disease or other coagulopathies have been described.

Immune Thrombocytopenic Purpura

Immune-mediated thrombocytopenic purpura (ITP) is relatively frequent in patients with CLL (perhaps 10 percent of patients at some point during their illness), and occurs in about 2 percent of patients with Hodgkin's disease. ITP is unusual but has been reported in sporadic patients with non-Hodgkin's lymphoma. When associated with Hodgkin's disease, thrombocytopenia is often associated with disease activity, but may also predate the diagnosis, or appear long after apparent complete remission. Although not proven, the immune dysregulation that so commonly occurs in the chronic lymphoproliferative disorders may permit the clinical expression of autoimmune phenomena such as ITP.

Standard therapy for ITP is usually successful and includes the use of corticosteroids, splenectomy, or immunosuppressive regimens. Aggressive treatment of the underlying lymphoproliferative disorder does not always correct the immune thrombocytopenia. A search for recurrent lymphoma is warranted when ITP develops in patients who have been previously treated for Hodgkin's disease.

Acquired von Willebrand Disease

In contrast to the hereditary disorder, acquired von Willebrand disease is uncommon but has been reported to occur in association with CLL, non-Hodgkin's lymphoma, and plasma cell myeloma. As expected, the bleeding time is prolonged, and the components of the von Willebrand factor-factor VIII macromolecular complex are decreased to 10 to 40 percent of normal. At least two mechanisms are responsible for the reductions in plasma von Willebrand factor. Some patients develop anti-von Willebrand factor antibodies, often IgG, that react with the high molecular weight components of von Willebrand factor. Another mechanism involves the adsorption of plasma von Willebrand factor onto the surfaces of neoplastic lymphoid cells. Bleeding varies from mild to severe. Therapeutic options include replacement of von Willebrand factor using large doses of cryoprecipitate or a von Willebrand factor concentrate, or stimulation of the vascular release of von Willebrand factor with DDAVP. Plasmapheresis or plasma exchange is sometimes necessary to remove a high titer anti-von Willebrand factor antibody. In several instances, splenectomy was performed to remove a large volume of malignant cells (presumably adsorbing von Willebrand factor) and was followed by remission of the von Willebrand disease (see Chap. 13).

HAIRY CELL LEUKEMIA

Thrombocytopenia is often a major clinical problem for patients with hairy cell leukemia and is usually due to a combination of marrow invasion by malignant cells and sequestration of platelets in an enlarged spleen. Platelet function defects, particularly a loss of platelet granules (as visualized by electron microscopy), and reduced platelet aggregation have also been noted. It has been suggested that the platelet release reaction occurs in the spleen where platelets are in contact with large numbers of malignant cells. Splenectomy reportedly normalizes platelet function and increases the platelet count.

PLASMA CELL MYELOMA AND MACROGLOBULINEMIA OF WALDENSTRÖM

Patients suffering from dysproteinemias such as plasma cell myeloma or macroglobulinemia often have abnormal laboratory tests of hemostasis although severe bleeding is relatively uncommon. Analyses of large numbers of patients have suggested that patients with IgA paraproteins, κ (rather than λ) light chains, high levels of serum proteins, or markedly increased serum viscosity are more likely to have overt bleeding. A wide array of hemostatic disorders have been described that involve both coagulation and platelet function (Table 33-2). Most of these defects are a consequence of elevated levels of monoclonal proteins. Therapy of these bleeding disorders involves treatment of the underlying disease to reduce or eliminate pathologic immunoglobulins and to reduce plasma viscosity. Intensive plasmapheresis may be necessary to temporarily control bleeding.

TABLE 33-2 Hemostatic Disorders in Patients with Dysproteinemia

Coagulation Defects	Platelet Abnormalities
Friable clot with increased fibrinolysis	Abnormal clot retraction
Inhibition of factor XIIIa receptor	Inhibition of glycoprotein IIIa
Inhibition of fibrin polymerization	Shortened platelet survival
Heparin-like anticoagulants	Inhibition of platelet adhesion

TABLE 33-3 Coagulation Studies in Five Patients with Circulating Heparin-like Anticoagulants

Patient	Pro- thrombin Time (17–19 s)	Activated Partial Thrombo- plastin Time (25–40 s)	Thrombin Time (20–23 s)	Reptilase Time (14–16 s)	Fibrin- ogen (190–365) (mg/dL)	Fibrin Split Products (< 6 l g/mL)
1	21	48	> 600	21	138	5
2	18	46	105	18	626	40
3	25	44	> 600	17	432	1
4	28	48	> 600	20	883	10
5	27	115	> 600	21	371	20

*Used with permission from Tefferi A et al: *Am J Med* 88:184, 1990.

Patients with plasma cell myeloma who develop circulating heparin-like anticoagulants pose challenging problems in management (Table 33-3). Most of these anticoagulants cause severe and unrelenting bleeding which is often fatal. Chemotherapy to reduce the malignant cell mass, intensive plasma- pheresis to remove the circulating anticoagulant, and intravenous protamine sulfate to neutralize the heparin-like glycosaminoglycan have all been tried, unfortunately with only modest success.

AMYLOIDOSIS

In one large series, about 10 percent of patients with systemic amyloidosis had severe bleeding. Easy bruisability is common and usually results from amyloid infiltration of blood vessels in the skin. However, systemic defects of hemostasis also occur.

Abnormalities of some laboratory tests, such as a prolonged TCT, are exceedingly frequent, but are not predictive of bleeding. However, more specific disorders have also been described that are associated with hem- orrhage. One of these is factor X deficiency which is due to adsorption of the clotting factor on amyloid fibrils. Circulating levels of factor X are sometimes as low as 2 to 4 percent of normal and are associated with recurrent hemorrhage. In a few instances, splenectomy was performed to remove a major site of amyloid deposition and was associated with a rise in circulating levels of factor X. However, long-term control of bleeding due to factor X deficiency usually requires a reduction in the amyloid burden with chemotherapy (e.g., melphalan and prednisone).

A second major hemostatic abnormality in amyloidosis is chronic systemic fibrinolysis which may also produce severe and recurrent bleeding. Primary fibrinolysis can be due to several different mechanisms including adsorption of a_2-antiplasmin (a_2-AP) on amyloid proteins, a process analogous to the loss of factor X. Elevated plasma levels of the plasminogen activators, t-PA and u-PA, and decreased concentrations of plasminogen activator inhibitor (PAI) have also been described. The mechanisms responsible for the increased plasminogen activators or depressed PAI are not known but could reflect vascular damage produced by amyloid proteins. Antifibrinolytic agents such as ε-aminocaproic acid or tranexamic acid are often useful for symptomatic control of bleeding.

Individual case reports have described other hemostatic defects in patients with amyloidosis. In one report, a patient developed a monoclonal IgA κ antibody that reacted strongly with factor VIII and was associated with severe bleeding. In another, a monoclonal Benz-Jones protein (i.e., an immunoglobulin light chain) bound tightly to fibrinogen produced a severe defect in fibrin polymerization; although the thrombin time was markedly prolonged, excessive bleeding did not occur.

Patients with systemic amyloidosis should have the usual screening tests of hemostasis, which should include a euglobulin lysis time and sometimes assays of plasminogen and a_2-AP. Conversely, if a patient with normal liver function is seen with a primary fibrinolytic syndrome, then a diagnosis of systemic amyloidosis should be considered.

The bleeding risk associated with liver biopsy in patients with amyloid has been reported to be about 3 percent as compared to 0.1 to 0.2 percent in patients with other forms of liver disease. Usually a diagnosis of amyloidosis can be made by biopsy of other sites such as rectal mucosa, skin, or bone marrow with less risk of bleeding.

BIBLIOGRAPHY

Abshire TC et al: The coagulopathy of childhood leukemia. Thrombin activation or primary fibrinolysis? *Cancer* 66:716, 1990.

Camoriano JK et al: Resolution of acquired factor X deficiency and amyloidosis with melphalan and prednisone therapy. *N Engl J Med* 316:1133, 1987.

Ey FS, Goodnight SH: Bleeding disorders in cancer. *Semin Oncol* 17:187, 1990.

Feinberg WM, Swenson MR: Cerebrovascular complications of L-asparaginase therapy. *Neurology* 38:127, 1988.

Gastineau DA et al: Inhibitor of the thrombin time in systemic amyloidosis: A common coagulation abnormality. *Blood* 77:2637, 1991.

Goodnight SH: Bleeding and thrombosis in hematologic neoplasia. In: Wiernik PH, Canellos GP, Kyle RA, Schiffer CA (eds): *Neoplastic Diseases of the Blood*, 2d ed., New York, Churchill-Livingstone, 1991, pp 967–982.

Hassidim K et al: Immune thrombocytopenic purpura in Hodgkin disease. *Am J Hematol* 6:149, 1979.

Homans AC et al: Effect of L-asparaginase administration on coagulation and platelet function in children with leukemia. *J Clin Oncol* 5:811, 1987.

Kaufman PA et al: Production of a novel anticoagulant by neoplastic plasma cells: Report of a case and review of the literature. *Am J Med* 86:612, 1989.

Rosove MH et al: Severe platelet dysfunction in hairy cell leukemia with improvement after splenectomy. *Blood* 55:903, 1980.

Sane DC et al: Elevated urokinase-type plasminogen activator level and bleeding in amyloidosis: Case report and literature review. *Am J Hematol* 31:53, 1989.

Sarris AH et al: High incidence of disseminated intravascular coagulation during remission induction of adult patients with acute lymphoblastic leukemia. *Blood* 79:1305, 1992.

Tefferi A et al: Circulating heparin-like anticoagulants: Report of five consecutive cases and a review. *Am J Med* 88:184, 1990.

Bleeding in the Myeloid Disorders— Acute Leukemia, Myelodysplasia, and Myeloproliferative Disease

This chapter focuses on bleeding in patients with three types of myeloid disorders—acute myeloid leukemia, myelodysplasia, and chronic myeloproliferative disease (MPD). Although all three diseases may be complicated by either hemorrhage or thrombosis, bleeding is most prominent in leukemia and myelodysplasia, whereas thrombosis predominates in MPD (see Chap. 44). In general, the primary hemostatic defect is severe thrombocytopenia in leukemia, whereas platelet function defects (PFD) are paramount in myelodysplasia, polycythemia rubra vera, myeloid metaplasia, and essential thrombocytosis. Acute promyelocytic leukemia (APL) produces a complex and often devastating coagulopathy consisting of disseminated intravascular coagulation (DIC) with or without systemic fibrinolysis.

ACUTE MYELOID LEUKEMIAS

A defibrination syndrome, often with severe bleeding, frequently complicates the clinical course of patients with APL, but also occurs in other categories of myeloid leukemia (approximately 5 percent) and acute mono-cytic leukemia (about 15 percent). Similar findings have been reported in childhood leukemia; a moderately severe coagulopathy is seen in about 15 percent of patients.

Pathogenesis

The coagulopathy in patients with myeloid leukemia, particularly APL, is often complex and consists of classic DIC, systemic fibrinolysis, or hemostatic and vascular defects produced by proteolytic enzymes such as leukocyte elastase (Fig. 34-1).

Disseminated Intravascular Coagulation

The malignant progranulocytes in patients with APL contain tissue factor which promotes the formation of thrombin via the extrinsic pathway. One report has suggested that leukemic cells activate factor X directly via a cysteine protease which is analogous to the procoagulant activity described in various solid tumors. Finally, it has been suggested that the malignant cells

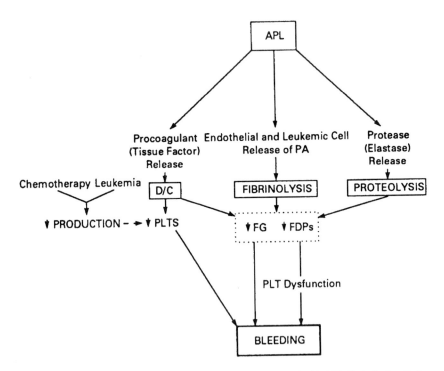

Figure 34-1 Pathogenesis of the complex coagulopathy associated with APL. Fg indicates fibrino-gen; PLTS indicates platelets. (Used with permission from Tallman MS, Kwaan HC: Blood 79:543, 1992.)

can produce large amounts of a cytokine, interleukin-1, which stimulates the synthesis and expression of tissue factor by other cells such as endothelium or monocytes within the vasculature. DIC often becomes dramatically worse following cytoreductive chemotherapy. The process is most likely due to the lysis of leukemic cells and release of preformed tissue factor or other pro-coagulants into the circulation. In contrast, retinoic acid has been reported to promote differentiation of the promyelocytes to more mature forms with subsequent lessening or even resolution of the DIC.

Primary Fibrinolysis

The leukemic cells from some patients with APL synthesize and secrete plasminogen activators which, if severe, can produce systemic fibrinolysis. Approximately 20 percent of patients have an accelerated euglobulin lysis time (ELT) and a_2-antiplasmin (a_2-AP) levels of < 30 percent. The primary fibrinolytic state is associated with DIC in some patients but not in others.

Defibrination Caused by Other Circulating Proteases

Several studies have recently suggested that proteases other than thrombin or plasmin are produced by myeloid cells in patients with acute leukemia. One proteolytic enzyme, elastase, has been identified in leukemia cell cultures. Elastase has a broad spectrum of proteolytic activity and degrades fibrinogen to large and small fibrinogen degradation products (FDP). It is not yet clear whether these proteases are responsible for bleeding in patients with acute leukemia.

Platelet Dysfunction

Although overshadowed by thrombocytopenia, patients with acute leukemia also have intrinsic PFD which may contribute to bleeding. Chemotherapeutic agents, antibiotics, or circulating FDP also contribute to platelet dysfunction and failure of hemostatic plug formation.

Clinical Findings/Laboratory Tests

Bleeding occurs in diverse sites in patients with acute leukemia including the skin, mucous membranes, and gastrointestinal tract. However, CNS hemorrhage is particularly common (and often fatal) in patients with APL. Risk factors for this complication include age over 50 years, large numbers of circulating blasts or promyelocytes, severe anemia, and marked thrombocytopenia especially in patients who are refractory to platelet transfusions. The risk of CNS bleeding is < 5 percent in patients without any of the above conditions, but increases to > 50 percent in those who have > two risk factors.

When first seen, patients with all forms of myeloid leukemia (not just APL) should have a baseline set of laboratory tests (Table 34-1). In patients with severe coagulopathies, the battery of tests should be repeated at least

TABLE 34-1 Baseline Laboratory Tests in Patients with Acute Leukemia

Tests	Uses
PT, APTT, fibrinogen	Reflect severity of the coagulopathy
Platelet count	Bleeding time is not usually necessary
D-dimer	Measure of secondary fibrinolysis
Euglobulin lysis time	Measure of systemic fibrinolysis
a_2-Antiplasmin	Reflects the intensity of fibrinolysis

daily and particularly just before and following major therapeutic interventions (e.g., chemotherapy, blood product replacement, or heparin) or when the clinical situation changes abruptly (e.g., with sepsis).

If only mild DIC is present, fibrinogen concentrations are usually normal, FDP are only minimally elevated, and the APTT is often short (e.g., < 25 s). In contrast, if the DIC is severe, fibrinogen concentration frequently falls to < 50 mg/dL, levels of D-dimer may be extraordinarily high, and the PT and APTT are markedly prolonged. When primary fibrinolysis occurs, with or without DIC, the ELT will be shortened to < 1 h, and a_2-AP levels reduced to < 30 percent of normal. It should be noted that a_2-AP will also be low in patients with brisk secondary fibrinolysis as a result of DIC. Although markedly low levels of antithrombin III and protein C would be expected in patients with severe DIC, circulating levels of these natural anticoagulants are often normal or only mildly reduced. The relative normality of these factors suggests that DIC is only one part of a much more complex coagulopathy.

Management

A consensus on the best strategy for managing acute myeloid leukemia patients with DIC or other defibrination syndromes has not yet been reached. However, most would agree that optimal blood product replacement is a cornerstone of therapy. For patients who are not actively bleeding, management should include:

1. Administering cryoprecipitate if fibrinogen concentrations fall to < 100 mg/dL.
2. Giving platelet concentrates if the platelet count is < 20,000/μL.
3. Infusing fresh frozen plasma if the APTT is prolonged to > 1.5 times control.

Replacement therapy for patients who are bleeding should be more vigorous, with goals of keeping the fibrinogen > 125 mg/dL, platelets >

50,000/μL, and the APTT more nearly normal. However, if the DIC is quite brisk, correcting clotting factor and platelet defects by administering blood products without producing massive fluid overload is nearly impossible. When rapid destruction of fibrinogen and platelets is present, intravenous heparin should be used to slow the pace of the consumption coagulopathy and allow more optimal correction of hemostatic defects. Because prospective randomized clinical trials have not yet been conducted in sufficiently large numbers of patients, it is not known whether heparin should be given prophylactically to all patients with DIC in APL.

Heparin should be administered by continuous intravenous infusion beginning with a dose of approximately 500 U/h (e.g., 7 U/kg body weight) with a goal of using the lowest dose possible to control DIC and allow effective blood product replacement. When DIC is severe, monitoring heparin therapy is often a problem, particularly if the APTT is markedly prolonged. As an alternative, an anti-X_a inhibition assay (heparin assay) could be used, although optimal heparin levels for treatment of DIC have not been determined. However, giving sufficient heparin to maintain the plasma anti-X_a activity from 0.1 to 0.3 U/mL is a reasonable starting point, although higher levels may be ultimately required to reduce levels of FDP and normalize fibrinogen concentrations without administering cryoprecipitate.

In a few patients, bleeding may persist despite optimal heparin therapy and clotting factor replacement. If the ELT is short and a_2-AP levels are markedly reduced (e.g., < 30 percent), then consideration should be given to the use of an antifibrinolytic agent such as ε-aminocaproic acid (EACA) or tranexamic acid (TA) in conjunction with heparin and blood products. Although intriguing, it is not known whether aprotinin, an antifibrinolytic agent with a wider spectrum of antiproteolytic activity, might be more effective than EACA and TA (see Chap. 60).

CHRONIC MYELOID DISORDERS: MYELODYSPLASIA AND MYELOPROLIFERATIVE DISEASE

Myelodysplasia (Preleukemia)

Bleeding in patients with myelodysplasia is almost always due to a platelet defect, either chronic thrombocytopenia or intrinsic platelet dysfunction. Platelets often appear abnormal on light and electron microscopy, with variations in shape, size, and granulation. A wide spectrum of PFD have been described including abnormalities in platelet aggregation, the release reaction, and thromboxane synthesis. Some patients, including one child with a major defect in glycoprotein Ib, have defective platelet adhesion. Thrombocytopenia or platelet dysfunction occasionally precedes diagnostic changes in myeloid cells and can provide a clue to the correct diagnosis.

Patients with myelodysplasia who have PFD and bleeding may require transfusion of platelets. DDAVP is sometimes useful, although advanced atherosclerosis could increase the risks of thrombosis in older patients. Antifibrinolytic therapy with EACA or TA can be used to suppress local fibrinolysis in subjects with refractory oral, nasopharyngeal, or gastrointestinal bleeding.

Chronic Myeloproliferative Disease (Essential Thrombocythemia, Polycythemia Rubra Vera, Myelofibrosis with Myeloid Metaplasia)

Patients with MPD have an increased risk of bleeding due to platelet function defects despite thrombocytosis, or they may develop venous or arterial thrombosis (see Chap. 44). Excessive bleeding has been reported in approximately 15 percent of patients with MPD, most often in patients with myelofibrosis with myeloid metaplasia and essential thrombocythemia. Bleeding is uncommon in patients with chronic granulocytic leukemia during the chronic phase of the disease.

Distorted platelet morphology is commonly observed both on light and electron microscopy. Platelets often appear large with strange shapes and bizarre granulation (Fig. 34-2). An array of PFD have been reported, as listed

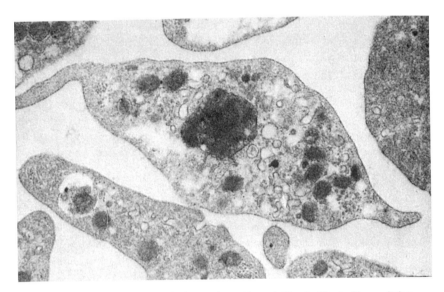

Figure 34-2 Giant-size fused granules in a patient with myelofibrosis. (Used with permission from Ramen BKS et al: Am J Clin Pathol 91:647, 1989.)

TABLE 34-2   Platelet Function Defects Reported in Patients with Myeloproliferative Disease

---

Aggregation defects: epinephrine, adenosine diphosphate, collagen
Acquired storage pool disease
Membrane defects
  • Glycoprotein IIb/IIIa
  • Increased Fc receptor
  • Decreased prostaglandin D_2 receptor
  • Decreased thromboxane A_2 receptor
  • Decreased a-adrenergic receptors
Prostanoid abnormalities
  • Decreased thromboxane A_2
  • Decreased lipoxygenase
Acquired von Willebrand disease

---

in Table 34-2. Notably, the platelet count, PFD, and the bleeding time often do not correlate with excessive bleeding.

The management of bleeding in patients with uncontrolled MPD and thrombocytosis may require acute lowering of the platelet count by platelet apheresis followed by chronic suppression of megakaryocytopoiesis with hydroxyurea or other suppressive agent. If bleeding persists, transfusion of platelets may be necessary. In the rare patient with acquired von Willebrand disease (see Chap. 13), cryoprecipitate or DDAVP can be useful. Fibrinolytic inhibitors should be used with caution in patients with MPD for fear of producing or potentiating thrombosis.

BIBLIOGRAPHY

Avvisati G et al: Tranexamic acid for control of haemorrhage in acute promyelocytic leukaemia. *Lancet* July 15:122, 1989.

Bennett B et al: The bleeding disorder in acute promyelocytic leukaemia: Fibrinolysis due to u-PA rather than defibrination. *Br J Haematol* 71:511, 1989.

Berndt MC et al: An acquired Bernard-Soulier-like platelet defect associated with juvenile myelodysplastic syndrome. *Br J Haematol* 68:97, 1988.

Budde U et al: Acquired von Willebrand's disease in the myeloproliferative syndrome. *Blood* 64:981, 1984.

Ey FS, Goodnight SH: Bleeding disorders in cancer. *Semin Oncol* 17:187, 1990.

Feinstein DI: Treatment of disseminated intravascular coagulation. *Semin Thromb Hemost* 14:351, 1988.

Fenaux P et al: Clinical course of essential thrombocythemia in 147 cases. *Cancer* 66:549, 1990.

Goodnight SH: Bleeding and thrombosis in hematologic neoplasia. In: Wiernik PH, Canellos GP, Kyle RA, Schiffer CA (eds): *Neoplastic Diseases of the Blood*, 2d ed., New York, Churchill Livingstone, 1991, pp 967–982.

Ramen BKS et al: Platelet function and structure in myeloproliferative disease, myelodysplastic syndrome, and secondary thrombocytosis. *Am J Clin Pathol* 91:647, 1989.

Schafer AI: Bleeding and thrombosis in the myeloproliferative disorders. *Blood* 64:1, 1984.

Schwartz BS et al: Epsilon-aminocaproic acid in the treatment of patients with acute promyelocytic leukemia and acquired alpha-2-plasmin inhibitor deficiency. *Ann Intern Med* 105:873, 1986.

Tobelem G et al: Acute monoblastic leukemia: A clinical and biologic study of 74 cases. *Blood* 55:71, 1980.

Ventura GJ et al: Analysis of risk factors for fatal hemorrhage during induction therapy of patients with acute promyelocytic leukemia. *Hemat Pathol* 3:23, 1989.

Wijermans PW et al: Combined procoagulant activity and proteolytic activity of acute promyelocytic leukemic cells: Reversal of the bleeding disorder by cell differentiation. *Blood* 73:800, 1989.

Toxic Coagulopathies

Several exogenous agents are sometimes associated with profound derangements in the hemostatic system leading to bleeding, thrombosis, or the potential for both. The "toxic coagulopathies," some of which are discussed elsewhere in this book, are caused by direct or sometimes secondary effects on the coagulation system by chemicals, venoms, physical agents, poisons, pharmacologic substances, or biologic mediators. The mechanism for the abnormality is frequently disseminated intravascular coagulation (DIC) or a DIC-like syndrome, direct activation and destruction of clotting factors, or inhibition of their synthesis. These coagulopathies will be discussed under the responsible exogenous causative agent.

VENOMS

Snake venoms produce a hemorrhagic syndrome by activation of the hemostatic system in several different ways. Some venoms are serine proteases which cleave either fibrinopeptide A or B (FPA, FPB) or both from fibrinogen, thus initiating coagulation and secondary fibrinolysis. Other venoms destroy fibrinogen directly by degrading the α-chain of fibrinogen first and then the β-chain (zinc-containing metalloendoproteinases) or degrade the β-chain directly by serine proteolytic activity (β-chain fibrinogenases). Other venoms cleave prothrombin or factor X into active enzymes or aggregate platelets directly. The laboratory and clinical uses of various venoms are well known and have been mentioned throughout this book; for example, the Stypven test using Russell viper venom (RVV) to cleave factor VII and the defibrination property of Ancrod used in anticoagulation therapy.

The resulting defibrination syndromes or DIC-like disorder may be mild to severe depending on the degree of envenomation. Examples of the clinical syndromes are shown in Table 35-1. The mainstay of treatment is the proper use of specific antivenin with replacement therapy for correction of the coagulopathy when necessary to halt hemorrhage.

A particularly severe bleeding diathesis noted in Venezuela and Brazil is associated with caterpillar stings or skin contact a few days after exposure;

TABLE 35-1 Coagulopathies Produced by Various Snake Venoms

Venom	Mechanism	Syndrome
Crotalus adamanteus (Eastern diamondback rattlesnake)	Cleavage of FPA with incr soluble fibrin and secondary fibrinolysis	Mild oozing; Fib, plasm decr; incr FDP; normal factors II, AT III; markedly incr TCT; mildly decr platelets; Peak changes at 24–36 h
Crotalus atrox (Western diamondback rattlesnake)	Fibrinogenase for Aα-chain	Incr APTT, PT; Decr Fib; Mild thrombocytopenia; Peak changes at 24 h
Vipera russeli (Russell's viper)	Activation of factor X: defibrination, secondary fibrinolysis	Local bleeding: Fib, factor X and V decr; FDP incr; mild decr platelets, AT-III, protein C; marked incr APTT, PT, TCT; Peak changes few hours after bite
Echis carinatus (Saw-scaled viper)	Activates prothrombin	Generalized hemorrhage; Severely decr Fib, protein C; Mod thrombocytopenia; Incr APTT, PT, FDP; Peak changes at 48 h
Bothrops jararaca (Viperine)	Thrombin-like; factor X activation; platelet aggregating	Severe bleeding; Mod severe thrombocytopenia; defibrination, high von Willebrand factor, TAT complexes, D-dimer incr; Peak changes at 2–3 h

*AT III, antithrombin III; incr, increase; decr, decrease; Nl, normal; Fib, fibrinogen; plasm, plasminogen; FPA, fibrinopeptide A; FDP, fibrin/fibrinogen degradation products; mod, moderate.

the contact is with *Lonoma achelous* caterpillars (saliva and hemolymph). The coagulopathy is characterized by hypofibrinogenemia in association with low levels of factor XIII and V. Fibrin degradation products (FDP, D-dimer) are increased and plasminogen is decreased. Screening tests (APTT, PT, TCT) are markedly prolonged. The fibrinolytic state has responded well to aprotinin and the judicious use of fresh frozen plasma. The bite of the brown recluse spider has been associated with DIC.

PHARMACOLOGIC AND BIOLOGIC AGENTS

Changes in the hemostatic system are well known side effects of several drugs and chemical compounds. Many of these changes are related to hepatic toxicity (acetaminophen, valproic acid, chlorinated hydrocarbons) or plate-let-vascular changes (salicylates, antibiotics) and have been mentioned else-where. Certain substances are less well known to produce alterations in the hemostatic system; a few of these are listed in Table 35-2. The thrombotic potential of contrast media used for angiographic procedures is now recog-nized and is related to increased thrombin generation associated with the nonionic media (iopamidol, iohexol, etc.) but not with ioxaglate or diatrizo-ate. These potentially thrombogenic media should be used with caution, if at all, in individuals at high risk of thrombosis (hereditary thrombotic defects, newborn infants, inflammatory states, hyperviscosity syndromes, and malig-nancies).

High-dose interleukin-2 (IL-2) immunotherapy is regularly associated with in vivo activation of the coagulation system (systemic fibrinolysis and mild DIC) even though IL-2 has no direct effect on coagulation factors in vitro; the clinical effect (including shock and edema) may be related to activation of the contact system (see Chap. 17). The use of hematin in the treatment of patients with acute porphyria is sometimes associated with bleeding or superficial thrombophlebitis. Extensive studies have shown the

TABLE 35-2 Biologic and Pharmacologic Substances Associated with Coagulopathy

Substance	Mechanism	Syndrome
Nonionic low osmolality contrast media (iopamidol, iohexol, ioversol)	Increased thrombin generation, TAT, FPA with hypercoagulability	Formation of thrombi in catheters; thrombotic complications of angiographic procedures
Interleukin-2	IL-2 damage of endothelial cells (other cytokines)	Hypotension, RDS, edema, decr platelets, incr D-dimer; slight decr II, VII, and contact factors; (DIC)
Hematin	Hematin degradation products activates platelets and alters clotting factors	Occasional bleeding and thrombophlebitis; decr platelets, fibrinogen, V, VIII; Incr FDP
L-Asparaginase	Decr levels of fibrinogen, antithrombin III, plasminogen, protein C; abnormal von Willebrand factor multimers	Thrombotic complications of ALL induction therapy; rare ICH

*FPA, fibrinopeptide A; RDS, respiratory distress syndrome; decr, decreased; incr, increased; FDP, fibrin/fibrinogen degradation products; ALL, acute lymphatic leukemia; ICH, intracran-ial hemorrhage; DIC, disseminated intravascular coagulation.

effects of hematin to be platelet activation, thrombocytopenia, decreased fibrinogen, factor V, and intrinsic fibrinolysis with factor XII activation. These changes, due to degradation products of hematin, can be mostly eliminated by the use of a more stable product now available, hematin-sorbitol (Panhematin).

Since the early 1980s a syndrome of thrombosis and occasionally hemorrhage complicating L-asparaginase therapy during the induction phase of acute lymphatic leukemia has been known (prevalence of 1 to 2 percent). The administration of L-asparaginase causes a gradual reduction due to decreased synthesis (over 3 to 4 days) in levels of several clotting factors (fibrinogen, plasminogen, protein C, protein S, antithrombin III [AT III], and factors IX and I), which persists for the 2 to 3 weeks of the therapy. However, these abnormalities are inconsistent and do not correlate with the onset of the thrombotic complications (deep vein thrombosis, indwelling catheter related, cerebral venous thrombosis). The thromboses frequently occur at the second to third week of therapy when the platelets are recovering: an alteration in ultralarge von Willebrand factor multimers has been demonstrated in a few patients and suggested as a contributing factor to platelet clumping (platelet aggregation is increased). At present, until the patient at risk can be identified, close observation and weekly monitoring of levels of clotting factors (fibrinogen, AT III, plasminogen) is preferred to prophylactic treatment with fresh frozen plasma. Acute thrombosis is managed in a routine manner with heparin until resolution of the thrombosis and normalization of clotting factors.

COAGULOPATHY OF IRON POISONING

A hemostatic defect is one of many serious complications seen in acute iron poisoning in man. The disorder has occurred in infants and children from accidental ingestion and in adolescents and adults from suicide attempts. A biphasic coagulopathy has been described. The first phase occurs within 24 h of ingestion of the iron and is manifested by marked prolongation of the basic screening tests (APTT, PT, TCT) with sparse evidence for DIC (normal fibrinogen, low FDP, normal platelet count). Studies in animals and in vitro plasma-iron mixing studies indicate that early changes (phase one) are serum iron concentration dependent and are due to a reversible functional impairment of serine proteases (thrombin, Xa, kallikrein) by ferrous sulfate. After 24 h a severe hepatotoxic coagulopathy may ensue (phase two) with evidence of marked transaminase elevation and a fall in liver-produced clotting factors (factors V, VII, X, IX, and later fibrinogen); factor VIII-von Willebrand factor level is raised. If chelation (desferoxamine) is successful early, the hepatotoxic phase may be avoided. Otherwise, therapy for bleeding manifestations follow those outlined for acute liver failure (see Chap. 24).

BIBLIOGRAPHY

Arocha-Pinango CL et al: Six new cases of a caterpillar-induced bleeding syndrome. *Thromb Hemost* 67:402, 1992.

Casalini E: Role of low-osmolality contrast media in thromboembolic complications: Scanning electron microscopy study. *Radiology* 183:741, 1992.

Fareed J et al: Thrombogenic potential of nonionic contrast media? *Radiology* 174:321, 1990.

Fleischmann JD et al: Fibrinolysis, thrombocytopenia, and coagulation abnormalitiies complicating high-dose interleukin-2 immunotherapy. *J Lab Clin Med* 117:76, 1991.

Green D, Tsao CH: Hematin: Effects on hemostasis. *J Lab Clin Med* 115:144, 1990.

Kamiguti AS et al: The role of venom haemorrhagin in spontaneous bleeding in *Bothrops jararaca* envenoming. *Thromb Haemost* 67:484, 1992.

Kitchens CS, Van Mierop LHS: Mechanism of defibrination in humans after envenomation by the Eastern Diamondback rattlesnake. *Am J Hematol* 14:345, 1983.

Kucuk O et al: Thromboembolic complications associated with L-asparaginase therapy. Etiologic role of low antithrombin III and plasminogen levels and therapeutic correction by fresh frozen plasma. *Cancer* 55:702, 1985.

Ouyang C et al: Characterization of snake venom components acting on blood coagulation and platelet function. *Toxicon* 30:945, 1992.

Priest JR et al: A syndrome of thrombosis and hemorrhage complicating L-asparaginase therapy for childhood acute lymphoblastic leukemia. *J Pediatr* 100:984, 1982.

Pui CH et al: Sequential changes in platelet function and coagulation in leukemic children treated with L-asparaginase, prednisone, and vincristine. *J Clin Oncol* 1:380, 1983.

Pui CH et al: Involvement of von Willebrand factor in thrombosis following asparaginase-prednisone-vincristine therapy for leukemia: *Am J Hematol* 25:291, 1987.

Rosenmund A et al: Blood coagulation and acute iron toxicity: Reversible iron-induced inactivation of serine proteases in vitro. *J Lab Clin Med* 103:524, 1984.

Smeets REH et al: Severe coagulopoathy after a bite from a 'harmless' snake (*Rhabdophis subminiatus*). *J Int Med* 230:351, 1991.

Than T et al: Evolution of coagulation abnormalities following Russell's viper bite in Burma: *Br J Haematol* 65:193, 1987.

Thrombotic

Disorders

The Infant and Child
with Thrombosis

Thrombotic disorders (deep vein thrombosis, DVT; venous thromboembolic disease; arterial thrombosis) are important causes of morbidity in infants and children. Although the overall prevalence and predisposing conditions are different from those in adults, the principles of diagnosis and therapy, with a few exceptions, are similar in the pediatric age group. This chapter emphasizes the differences and presents management guidelines.

Developmental influences are significant in the infant and child. The neonate and young infant are particularly prone to thrombosis; the older infant and child rarely display thrombotic disease except as a complication of another disorder; the adolescent behaves more like the adult and may present with "spontaneous" thrombosis or often related to other events like trauma, oral contraceptive agent (OCA) therapy, or pregnancy. Many of the treatment recommendations are based on extrapolations of well-studied disorders in adults; a great need for clinical research of pediatric thrombotic disease remains.

NEONATAL THROMBOTIC DISEASE

Thrombosis in the neonate is characterized by an increased incidence in premature and other high-risk infants, a predilection for major vessels, and frequent involvement of the arterial circulation related to indwelling catheters (umbilical artery catheter [UAC]). At least 1 percent of all UACs show clinical evidence of associated thrombosis while most of the catheters are associated with clinically "silent" large thromboses. Spontaneous thromboses do occur and most frequently involve the inferior vena cava and renal veins, the aortic, renal and femoral arteries as well as the middle cerebral artery.

The fetus and newborn are more susceptible to thrombosis because their blood exhibits a deficiency of thrombin inhibition and relatively deficient fibrinolysis. The infant shows low levels of antithrombin III (AT III) and protein C (sick infants frequently have protein C levels < 0.1 U/mL) as well as prolonged euglobulin lysis times probably related to low and altered plasminogen with near normal levels of a_2-antiplasmin (a_2-AP) and plasminogen activator inhibitor (PAI). The infant is protected from thrombosis by physiologic depression of factors II, VII, IX, and X but the balance favors thrombin formation over inhibition especially in the sick infant. Predisposing conditions associated with increased thrombosis include maternal diabetes mellitus, hypoxia, polycythemia, infection, and other causes of disseminated intravascular coagulation (DIC), and, of course, the indwelling catheter.

The diagnosis of neonatal thrombosis is based on clinical observations, contrast angiography, or imaging techniques (ultrasound, magnetic resonance imaging, color Doppler sonography). Angiography is contraindicated in infants with renal failure or gut ischemia. Subtle evidence for DIC is common in the sick newborn so that more sensitive laboratory markers of coagulation activation (D-dimer, TAT, etc.) have not been helpful thus far. The most common large vessel thromboses are renal vein thrombosis (RVT) and aortic thrombosis. RVT often presents in a term or large preterm infant with hematuria and a flank mass; anemia, thrombocytopenia, and mild DIC may also be present. Response to heparinization is usually good, although the optimal mode of therapy has not been established.

Aortic thrombosis often presents in preterm asphyxiated infants with a UAC in place. Associated symptoms include pallor of lower extremities, poor femoral pulses, hypertension, persistent pulmonary hypertension, and evidence for DIC (low platelets, fibrinogen, elevated fibrin-fibrinogen degradation products). Optimal treatment is controversial but successful therapy has included thrombectomy, heparinization, and use of fibrinolytic agents. Our approach would be the use of heparinization and thrombectomy if surgically feasible. Fibrinolytic therapy and low-dose heparin plus infusions of fresh frozen plasma (to replace plasminogen) are used for infants who are not surgical candidates.

Treatment of Neonatal Thrombosis

Heparin Anticoagulation

Although there are almost no controlled trials of heparinization for neonatal thrombotic lesions, the administration of heparin has been associated with resolution of the vascular occlusion in most instances. Neonatologists and others caring for sick infants are sometimes reluctant to use heparin in clinical situations where it is used in adults because of the difficulty in monitoring the effect and fear of aggravating intracranial hemorrhage (ICH). Guidelines based on our experience with heparin are shown in Table 36-1.

TABLE 36-1 **Pharmacologic Therapy of Neonatal Thrombosis**

A. Heparin infusion dosage
  1. Heparin sodium 50 U/kg by IV bolus followed by a continuous IV infusion of heparin in doses of:

Preterm (28 wk):	15 U/kg per h
Preterm (28-36 wk)	20 U/kg per h
Full term	25 U/kg per h

  2. Monitor effect with micro whole blood clotting time, plasma heparin assay (0.3–0.5 U/mL) or APTT.
  3. Continue infusion (proper dose infusing smoothly); adjust by amounts of 5 U/kg: some infants will require up to 50 U/kg to keep adequate level early in treatment.
  4. Continue treatment until infant is stable and thrombus is mostly resolved; i.e., 48–72 h for catheter toes and up to 14 days for renal vein thrombosis with vena caval involvement.
B. Warfarin is usually not used in the neonate.
C. Fibrinolytic therapy

Urokinase 4400 U/kg/h by continuous infusion; the dose may be doubled (8800) or tripled if no lysis can be documented and if plasminogen and fibrinogen have not decreased below half the initial level. Fresh frozen plasma may be given as source of plasminogen; low-dose heparin (5–10 U/kg/h) is usually maintained. Contraindications for use of urokinase include intracranial hemorrhage or recent surgical wound in area difficult to control bleeding.

Newborns show a relative resistance to heparin; however, heparinization can be achieved despite low AT III levels. The half-life of heparin is 35 min after intravenous doses of 50 to 100 U/kg as compared with 65 min in adults. The APTT is less satisfactory for monitoring because it is already considerably prolonged in sick preterm infants. Until a better test has been shown effective, a micro whole blood clotting time or the direct assay of heparin (heparin level) can be used. In a recent controlled study of therapeutic heparin to prevent catheter-related thrombosis in sick newborns, less bleeding (particularly intraventricular hemorrhage) occurred in the heparinized group than in the controls.

Thrombolytic Therapy

Fibrinolytic therapy (see Table 36-1) is reserved for recent thrombotic lesions which are not responding to heparinization (i.e., such as aortic thrombosis) or have occurred in vital areas (intracardiac thrombosis). As noted above, the newborn infant has a decreased fibrinolytic response but is able to resolve most clots during heparin therapy alone. The infant is also relatively resistant to fibrinolytic agents and may require much larger doses of urokinase (than used in adults) to maintain a lytic state. Supplementation of plasminogen (fresh frozen plasma) during fibrinolytic therapy may be helpful. Even less neonatal experience with the use of recombinant tissue plasminogen activator (t-PA) is available. Although t-PA is effective in newborn infants and children, bleeding complications do occur (see Levy reference).

Catheter-related Thrombotic Disease

As indicated previously, the association of umbilical vessel catheters with major vessel thrombosis is almost universal. Although many serious late thrombotic complications have been reported, including renal hypertension, aortic thromboatheromata, false aortic aneurysm, paraplegia, endocarditis, and organ infarction and death, it is a wonder that these severe sequelae do not occur more often. Attempts to prevent thrombotic lesions by heparin "flush" or continuous infusions of low-dose (1 to 2 U/mL) heparin have not been successful. Preliminary studies suggest that only "therapeutic" heparinization with demonstrated systemic heparin effect will prevent catheter-related thromboses. Our impression is that symptomatic thrombosis can be kept at a minimum if repeated attempts at catheter placement are avoided and the catheter is removed at first sign of decreased pulses, "vasospasm," extremity color changes or decreased perfusion, or darkening of the toes ("catheter toes"). If these signs persist despite catheter removal, assume that a thrombus is present or document with ultrasound examination and treat appropriately with anticoagulation. Other vascular complications may be related to the type of infusate; peripheral gangrene has followed infusion of dopamine.

CHILDHOOD THROMBOTIC DISEASE

By 6 months of age the infant coagulation system approximates that of the adult, and the deficiencies noted above are no longer present except for protein C which does not reach the normal adult range until 6 years of age. Nevertheless, the occurrence of thrombotic disease in the child is almost completely limited to complications of other serious illnesses (Table 36-2). A spontaneous thrombosis in an otherwise healthy child is suggestive of an hereditary deficiency.

During adolescence, additional risk factors such as athletic-related muscle and joint injury, use of OCA, pregnancy, and smoking add to the predisposition for thrombosis. These risk factors are associated with clinical onset of hereditary thrombotic disorders in many instances (such as AT III, protein C, and protein S deficiency). The diagnosis and initial management of thrombotic disease in children and adolescents is essentially the same as for adults

TABLE 36-2 Disorders Associated with
Deep Venous Thrombosis in Children

Congenital heart diseasee
After major surgery
Dehydration
Infection
Malnutrition
Lupus anticoagulant
Liver disease
Nephrotic syndrome
Inflammatory bowel syndrome
Chronic renal disease
Sickle cell disease
Thalassemia
After prothrombin-complex concentration
L-Asparaginase therapy
Stroke

(see Chap. 37). Heparinization with continuous infusion, a bolus of 50 U/kg followed by 15 U/kg per hour to keep the APTT 1.5 to 2 times the control, is followed by the initiation of warfarin therapy on day 1 or 2 of treatment. Warfarin is given in a dose of 0.4–0.6 mg/kg for 2 days (total maximal daily dose 10 mg) and then reduced to one fourth to one fifth of the loading dose. When the PT is holding at the desired INR (usually 2 to 3) for 24 to 48 h, the heparin is stopped. Children with severe DVT of the lower extremities and those patients with arterial or pulmonary artery lesions are candidates for a short course of fibrinolytic therapy to prevent venous valvular damage.

PERFORMANCE OF COAGULATION TESTING FOR HEREDITARY DEFECTS

Thromboses due to hereditary deficiencies of coagulation proteins rarely occur in the infant and child. The late second and third decades are the usual time for diagnosis. Nevertheless heterozygotes for AT III, protein C, protein S, plasminogen defects, and dysfibrinogenemias have been occasionally recognized at all ages including the newborn infant. The diagnostic level for the adult heterozygote frequently overlaps with the physiologic range of that factor in the newborn period and, therefore, it is difficult to make a firm association between the level and thrombotic tendency. Known heterozygotes in the newborn period have levels in or only slightly lower than normal newborn range. Family studies (an affected parent) and follow-up tests are usually necessary to confirm the diagnosis. In older children the suspected factor level may be associated with the acute thrombotic event (AT III and protein C may be low due to factor consumption with a large thrombosis). Because of these difficulties, the scheme in Fig. 36-1 may be helpful and is reserved for those infants and children in whom a clearly associated cause of the thrombosis is not apparent or in whom a positive family history is present. In the absence of a known cause, all infants and children with spontaneous or induced thromboembolism should be suspected of having a hereditary clotting defect (especially those with stroke, DVT, and pulmonary embolism).

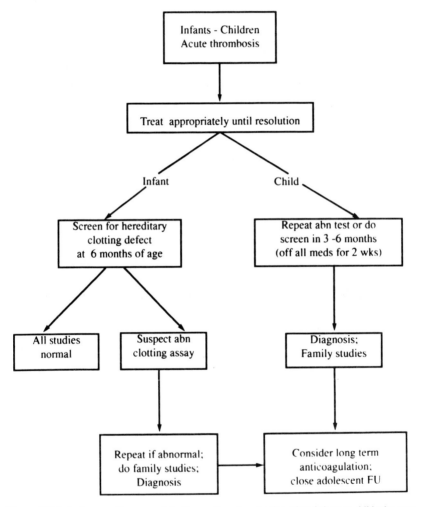

Figure 36-1 A diagramatic approach to the continued evaluation of an infant or child who presents with acute thrombosis. If the patient has abnormal (abn) results on testing for hereditary defects (AT III, protein C, protein S, dysfibrinogen screen, plasminogen), a scheme for retesting is suggested. Meds, anticoagulant medication such as warfarin.

PURPURA FULMINANS

Purpura fulminans is the sudden onset of massive microthrombosis and bleeding in the skin associated with skin necrosis and ischemia, systemic DIC, and anemia. It usually occurs in children but can also be seen in adults. The associated causes for the often rapidly progressing lesion are infection (varicella, gram-negative sepsis, group B streptococcal disease, meningococcemia; often with low protein C or S levels), homozygous protein C or protein S deficiency in the newborn infant or warfarin-induced skin necrosis in protein C and protein S-deficient heterozygotes, cancer, cholestasis, heparin-associated thrombocytopenia (HAT, see Chap. 46), or without known cause. Treatment of this disorder should include assessment of protein C and protein S levels, replacement of the appropriate factors (fresh frozen plasma or concentrate) as well as heparinization (except in HAT) especially if DIC or large vessel thrombosis is present. Purpura fulminans in the neonate is protein C or protein S deficiency (hereditary or severe acquired) until proven otherwise. Untreated, the lesions result in loss of limb or life.

BIBLIOGRAPHY

Adcock DM et al: Proposed classification and pathologic mechanisms of purpura fulminans and skin necrosis. *Semin Thromb Hemost* 16:333, 1990.

Carpentieri U et al: Clinical experience with an oral anticoagulant in children. *Arch Dis Child* 51:445, 1976.

Corrigan JJ et al: Newborn's fibrinolytic mechanism: Components and plasmin generation. *Am J Hematol* 32:273, 1989.

Doyle JJ et al: Anticoagulation with sodium warfarin in children: Effect of a loading regimen. *J Pediatr* 113:1095, 1988.

Gault DT: Vascular compromise in newborn infants. *Arch Dis Child* 67:463, 1992.

Horgan M et al: Effect of heparin infusates in umbilical arterial catheters on frequency of thrombotic complications. *J Pediatr* 111:774, 1987.

Kennedy LA et al: Successful treatment of neonatal aortic thrombosis with tissue plasminogen activator. *J Pediatr* 116:798, 1990.

Koska J et al: Sucessful use of low-dose tissue plasminogen activator for treatment of thrombosed prosthetic valve in a 22-month-old child. *Am Heart J* 124:783, 1992.

Levy M et al: Tissue plasminogen activator for the treatment of thromboembolism in infants and children. *J Pediatr* 118:467, 1991.

Manco-Johnson MJ et al: Severe protein C deficiency in newborn infants. *J Pediatr* 113:359, 1988.

McDonald MM, Hathaway WE: Anticoagulant therapy by continuous heparinization in newborn and older infants. *J Pediatr* 109:101, 1982.

Payne RM et al: Management and follow-up of arterial thrombosis in the neonatal period. *J Pediatr* 114:853, 1989.

Ryan CA, Andrew M: Failure of thrombolytic therapy in four children with extensive thromboses. *Am J Dis Child* 146:187, 1992.

Schmidt B, Andrew M: Neonatal thrombotic disease: Prevention, diagnosis, and treatment. *J Pediatr* 113:407, 1988.

Schmidt B, Andrew M: Report of scientific and standardization subcommittee on neonatal hemostasis: Diagnosis and treatment of neonatal thrombosis. *Thromb Haemost* 67:381, 1992.

Van Overmeire B et al: Intracardiac thrombus formation with rapidly progressive heart failure in the neonate: Treatment with tissue type plasminogen activator. *Arch Dis Child* 67:443, 1992.

CHAPTER
37

The Adult
with Thrombosis

Twenty years ago, with the possible exception of antithrombin III (AT III) deficiency, little was known about the mechanisms responsible for venous or arterial thromboembolism. Since then, dramatic advances have been made in our understanding of natural anticoagulants, fibrinolytic mechanisms, and platelet reactivity. Many more laboratory tests are now available to help identify hereditary and acquired disorders associated with intravascular thrombosis.

The rationale for pursuing a specific diagnosis in patients with thrombosis is supported by the subsequent modification of treatment programs. For example, patients with recurrent venous thrombosis and deficiency of AT III or other anticoagulant factors are candidates for long-term therapy with oral anticoagulants and will benefit from short-term clotting factor replacement for surgery, childbirth, or trauma. Moreover, intensive antithrombotic prophylaxis should be used for elective surgical procedures. When the defect is hereditary, family studies may identify other individuals at risk for thromboembolism. Lastly, evaluation of patients with acquired thrombotic disorders can lead to the discovery of other diseases such as malignancy or myeloproliferative syndromes that might be amenable to treatment.

The diagnostic evaluation of patients with thromboembolism can be approached in several ways, but one option is to determine whether the underlying disorder is hereditary or acquired and whether the thrombosis involves veins, arteries, or the microvasculature (Tables 37-1, 37-2, and 37-3).

Although there is often some overlap, these distinctions provide direction for further evaluation. For example, an adolescent with recurrent deep venous thrombosis and a strong family history of venous thromboembolism will likely have a deficiency or defect in one of the natural anticoagulants: AT III, protein C, or protein S. Alternatively, an elderly man who has been previously well but who presents to his physician with migratory superficial

TABLE 37-1 Hereditary Hypercoagulable States

Documented Causes	Possible Causes
Antithrombin III deficiency	Heparin cofactor II deficiency
Protein C deficiency	Deficient tissue plasminogen activator
Protein S deficiency	Excess plasminogen activator inhibitor
Dysfibrinogenemia	Elevated lipoprotein (a)
Plasminogen deficiency	Homocystinemia

TABLE 37-2 Acquired Hypercoagulable States

Cancer	Inflammatory states (e.g., systemic lupus erythematosus)
Antiphospholipid antibodies	Nephrotic syndrome
Myeloproliferative disorders/ paroxysmal noctural hemoglobinuria	Heparin-induced thrombocytopenia
Autoimmune hemolytic anemia	Behcet's syndrome

TABLE 37-3 Laboratory Evaluation of Patients with Thrombosis

Venous Thrombosis
CBC, AT III, protein C, free protein S, fibrinogen, thrombin time, reptilase time, lupus anticoagulant, anticardiolipin antibodies (plasminogen, t-PA, PAI—selected patients)

Arterial Thrombosis
CBC, protein S, protein C, AT III, lupus anticoagulant, anticardiolipin antibodies, plasma lipids including lipoprotein (a), (plasma homocysteine—selected patients)

Microvascular Thrombosis
CBC and peripheral blood smear, DIC screen, lupus anticoagulant, anticardiolipin antibodies, (protein C, HAT assay—selected patients)

---

[*]CBC, complete blood count; AT III, antithrombin III; t-PA, tissue plasminogen activator; DIC, disseminated intravascular coagulation; HAT, heparin-associated thrombocytopenia.

thrombophlebitis and an embolic stroke should be carefully evaluated for intra-abdominal or intrathoracic malignancy.

HISTORY

A thorough patient history is needed in all patients who seek medical care for a recent or remote history of thrombosis. Detailed information about the circumstances surrounding prior thromboses must be collected and should include their location, the outcome of diagnostic studies, and the presence of relevant predisposing factors. Inquiries should be made about previous antithrombotic therapy, underlying disease, family history of thrombosis, medications, and habits. A general outline for data collection is included in Table 37-4. Hopefully, sufficient data will be available to determine whether vascular thromboses are hereditary or acquired and whether thrombotic episodes involve veins, arteries, or the microvasculature.

PHYSICAL EXAMINATION

As with the history, a complete general physical examination is warranted in all patients who present with new or remote thromboembolism. Special

TABLE 37-4 Areas of Emphasis in the History of Patients with Thrombosis

Past History of Thromboembolism
Location (e.g., venous, arterial, microvascular)
Diagnostic studies (e.g., venography, scans)
Predisposing factors (e.g., surgery, trauma, pregnancy)
Therapy (e.g., duration, efficacy, complications)

Diseases Associated with Thrombosis

Cancer	Cardiac disease	Hyperlipidemia
Myeloproliferative	Inflammatory	Hemolytic anemia
disorders	disorders	Hereditary thrombotic disorders
Atherosclerosis	Nephrosis	

Family History
Pedigree
Thrombosis (location, diagnosis, therapy)

Medications and Habits
Estrogens, chemotherapy
Tobacco, alcohol, illicit drugs

attention should be directed to certain aspects of the examination, in particular the vascular system, heart, abdominal organs, and skin (e.g., livido reticularis). Occasionally, the physical signs of lower extremity deep venous occlusion are extraordinarily subtle; slight dusky discoloration or increased warmth may be the only findings that suggest diversion of blood flow away from the deep veins toward the skin and superficial veins.

LABORATORY EVALUATION

Extensive batteries of diagnostic laboratory studies are not cost effective for all patients who present with a thromboembolic event. For example, the chance of finding AT III, protein C, or protein S deficiency in an unselected group of patients presenting with venous thrombosis will be < 5 percent (Malm reference). However, if patients with recurrent thrombosis are selected for study, then the rates of positive tests may be as high as 10 to 20 percent. On the arterial side, most instances of myocardial infarction, stroke, or peripheral vascular occlusions occurring in older individuals will be due to atherosclerosis, and additional diagnostic laboratory tests are usually not needed.

One approach to increase the diagnostic yield of these tests is to target the laboratory evaluation of patients with venous thrombosis to those with one or more of the following:

■ Recurrent thrombosis
■ Family history of thrombosis
■ Thrombosis at a young age (e.g., < 45 years)
■ Thrombosis in locations other than the deep veins of the legs

For patients with arterial thromboembolism, the indications for diagnostic studies are even less clear, but laboratory testing could be limited to patients who:

■ Are young (< 45 years)
■ Have multiple thrombotic events
■ Have thrombosis in the absence of obvious atherosclerosis
■ Have both arterial and venous thrombosis

The most useful laboratory assays for hypercoagulable states are not well defined. One approach is to create selected groups of studies for patients with venous, arterial, or microvascular thromboses (see Table 37-3). Obviously, the clinical setting and age of the patient may dictate the addition or subtraction of tests from these general groups.

Venous Thrombosis

A standard battery of tests for patients with venous thromboembolism should include a complete blood count and blood smear (for myeloproliferative disorders), protein C activity, free protein S antigen (or activity measurement if available), AT III activity, and tests for a dysfibrinogenemia (fibrinogen, thrombin time, reptilase time). If the disorder is not clearly hereditary and could be acquired, then tests for antiphospholipid antibodies (APA) should also be included (i.e., lupus anticoagulant and anticardiolipin antibodies). If all tests are normal, then other diagnostic tests could include a functional assay of plasminogen and measurement of plasminogen activator inhibitor (PAI) activity although the yield will be low.

An important consideration in the laboratory evaluation of a patient with thrombosis is the timing of tests relative to thrombotic events and to anti-thrombotic therapy. Ideally, the tests should be obtained at least 2 to 3 weeks after stopping oral anticoagulants to minimize the impact of acute thrombosis or warfarin therapy on test results. Acute thromboembolism produces a rapid fall in AT III (and occasionally protein C and protein S) activity. Therapeutic doses of heparin also decrease AT III activity, but may not affect levels of protein C or protein S. Treatment with warfarin produces a marked drop in protein C and protein S by the inhibition of vitamin K action. Warfarin has also been reported to elevate AT III levels in some patients with AT III deficiency. In general, if levels of AT III, protein C, and protein S are normal immediately following a thrombotic event or during heparin therapy, hereditary deficiencies of these proteins are unlikely. However, low levels may reflect acquired rather than hereditary deficiencies so that tests should be repeated at a later date.

Arterial Thrombosis

Patients who undergo diagnostic evaluation for arterial thromboembolism should also have a complete blood count and scrutiny of the peripheral blood smear for evidence of a myeloproliferative disease or a leukoerythroblastic peripheral blood picture that would suggest marrow infiltration by tumor. Additional laboratory tests to be considered include free protein S, protein C, and AT III, tests for APA, plasma lipids to include lipoprotein(a), and (if available) plasma homocysteine assay by high performance liquid chromatography.

Microvascular Thrombosis

Microvascular thromboses such as ischemia or necrosis of the digits suggest another set of diagnoses. In these patients, a complete blood count and peripheral blood smear to search for evidence of microangiopathic hemolytic anemia (thrombotic thrombocytopenic purpura/hemolytic uremic syndrome) or myeloproliferative disease (erythromelalgia) should be performed. In addition, a disseminated intravascular coagulation (DIC) screen (malignancy, endotoxemia), tests for APA, and when appropriate, assays for protein C (warfarin skin necrosis) and for heparin-associated antiplatelet antibodies should be obtained.

In many instances, the tests described above will not elucidate the mechanisms responsible for the development of thrombosis. Possible explanations for failure include lack of sensitivity of the tests themselves or our lack of knowledge of other plasma defects or deficiencies that predispose to thrombosis. Even more importantly, the currently available plasma-based assays do not identify defects of the vasculature (as opposed to the blood) that could be responsible for thrombosis. For example, an abnormality of thrombomodulin on the vascular surface could lead to inadequate activation of protein C in the vicinity of a vascular injury. Other possibilities include defects or deficiencies in the optimal binding of AT III to the blood vessel or an abnormality of tissue factor pathway inhibitor (TFPI) on the endothelial cell surface. Lastly, many acquired diseases promote the local synthesis of inflammatory cytokines such as interleukin-1, which in turn can stimulate tissue factor synthesis, down-regulate thrombomodulin expression, and enhance PAI release from vascular surfaces.

Currently available tests of fibrinolysis are also inadequate because baseline plasma levels of PAI and tissue plasminogen activator (t-PA) do not reflect the magnitude of the fibrinolytic response in a local area of vascular injury. Measures designed to stimulate the fibrinolytic system such as venous occlusion or infusions of desmopressin (DDAVP) are theoretically attractive but have not yet been shown to be clinically useful. Finally, current laboratory assays are less than optimal for the identification of heightened platelet reactivity, a process likely to play a key role in thrombogenesis. Current tests such as measurement of platelet aggregation, the circulating platelet aggregate ratio, and the plasma levels of platelet-specific proteins lack predictive value for arterial thrombosis.

Research efforts are beginning to focus on new approaches for the identification of patients at risk for thrombosis. Rather than relying only on assessment of deficiencies of antithrombotic factors in the blood, tests are now available for measurement of in vivo activation of coagulation, fibrinolysis, and platelets. Examples of these assays include:

1. *Activation of coagulation*: Activation peptides of prothrombin (F1.2), factor X, factor IX, and protein C are being studied in clinical trials. Other tests include assessments of thrombin production in vivo, including thrombin-antithrombin complexes and fibrinopeptide A.

2. *Activation of fibrinolysis*: In addition to D-dimer, other assays are becoming available to measure the conversion of plasminogen to plasmin. An example is circulating plasmin-antiplasmin complexes. Other fibrin degradation products reflect the action of plasmin on fibrin including the peptide Bβ15–42 (see Chap. 25).

3. *Activation of platelets*: Because plasma levels of β-thromboglobulin (the α-granule-derived platelet specific protein) are often so variable, sensitive flow cytometry assays are now being used to enumerate numbers of platelets that express α-granule-derived activation antigens such as P-selectin on platelet surfaces.

These tests may ultimately prove useful for screening patients at risk of thromboembolism, to identify those who require antithrombotic treatment, and possibly as a guide to the adequacy of antithrombotic therapy. Whether they can be applied in individual patients as well as for the study of larger groups of patients enrolled in clinical trials remains to be seen.

BIBLIOGRAPHY

Abrams C, Shattil SJ: Immunological detection of activated platelets in clinical disorders. *Thromb Haemost* 65:467, 1991.

Bauer KA, Rosenberg RD: The pathophysiology of the prethrombotic state in humans: Insights gained from studies using markers of hemostatic system activation. *Blood* 70:343, 1987.

Comp PC: Hereditary disorders predisposing to thrombosis. *Prog Hemost Thromb* 8:71, 1986.

Gladson CL et al: The frequency of type I heterozygous protein S and protein C deficiency in 141 unrelated young patients with venous thrombosis. *Thromb Haemost* 59:18, 1988.

Haake DA, Berkman SA: Hypercoagulable states and venous thrombosis. *Hosp Pract* December:88c, 1986.

Joist JH: Hypercoagulability: Introduction and perspective. *Semin Thromb Hemost* 16:151, 1990.

Malm J et al: Thromboembolic disease—Critical evaluation of laboratory investigation. *Thromb Haemost* 68:7, 1992.

Mannucci PM, Tripodi A: Laboratory screening of inherited thrombotic syndromes. *Thromb Haemost* 57:247, 1987.

Moake JL: Hypercoagulable states: New knowledge about old problems. *Hosp Pract* March:31, 1991.

Rodgers GM, Shuman MA: Congenital thrombotic disorders. *Am J Hematol* 21:419, 1986.

Samlaska CP, James WD: Superficial thrombophlebitis I. Primary hypercoagulable states. *J Am Acad Dermatol* 22:975, 1990.

Schafer AI: The hypercoagulable state. *Ann Intern Med* 102:814, 1985.

Tabernero MD et al: Incidence and clinical characteristics of hereditary disorders associated with venous thrombosis. *Am J Hematol* 36:249, 1991.

Deep Venous
Thrombosis and
Pulmonary Embolism

Venous thromboembolism is a common clinical problem with a reported incidence of 170,000 to more than 300,000 episodes per year in the United States. Massive pulmonary embolism (PE) accounts for 5 to 10 percent of all hospital deaths. The mortality rate of untreated PE is about 30 percent, but with optimal therapy this figure can be reduced to 8 percent or even less. Effective methods for prevention of venous thrombosis in surgical and medical patients are now available although they are substantially underused.

PATHOGENESIS

Venous thrombi are composed of a fibrin meshwork packed with red blood cells, in contrast to arterial thrombi that usually are white in color and contain large numbers of platelets. As demonstrated many years ago, lower extremity venous thrombi tend to originate in areas of sluggish blood flow behind venous valves and then propagate into the lumen of the vein. Based on data from fibrinogen scans, small clots form frequently following stresses such as surgery and are rapidly destroyed by the fibrinolytic system.

Although venous thrombi often appear to be "spontaneous" in origin, they are associated with one or more predisposing factors in the great majority of instances. Some common situations are venous stasis, endothelial injury, and circulating activated clotting factors. Less often, hereditary or acquired defects of the natural anticoagulants, inadequate fibrinolysis, or circulating activated platelets are involved (Table 38-1).

Fibrin clots, once formed, probably remain highly thrombogenic for up to

TABLE 38-1 Mechanisms of Thrombosis

Mechanism	Examples
Venostasis	Congestive heart failure, obesity
Endothelial injury	Leg or pelvic trauma
Activated clotting factors	Cancer, surgery
Decreased natural anticoagulants	Hereditary protein C deficiency
Inhibition of fibrinolysis	Dysfibrinogenemia
Activated platelets	Myeloproliferative disease

2 weeks. Functional thrombin molecules are present on the surfaces of fresh thrombi where they are protected from inactivation. Consequently, in the absence of effective antithrombotic therapy, newly formed clots are likely to propagate, which increases the risk of embolization. In time (e.g., 3 to 6 months or more), the thrombi gradually diminish in size or become fibrotic and collateral flow develops around regions of venous obstruction.

CLINICAL MANIFESTATIONS

The clinical signs and symptoms of peripheral venous thrombosis reflect obstruction of the deep veins in an extremity and are remarkable because of their variability. On the severe end of the spectrum is massive iliofemoral thrombosis which produces virtually complete obstruction of venous outflow, a condition termed *phlegmasia ceruleum dolens*, a massively swollen blue painful leg. Lesser degrees of venous obstruction in the leg produce pain in the calf or thigh, pitting edema of the ankle or lower leg, and a warm dusky reddish blue discoloration of the skin caused by enhanced superficial venous blood flow. Sometimes these physical signs are subtle, requiring good light and asking the patient to stand for a few minutes to appreciate differences in size, warmth, color, or edema between normal and involved legs. Finally, at least half the time in infants and children as well as adults, deep venous thrombosis (DVT) produces no symptoms whatever, particularly when the clots are small or subocclusive.

Some patients with a past history of severe or recurrent venous thrombosis of the legs develop signs of chronic venostasis. Affected extremities are chronically swollen and painful and show dark discoloration of the skin. Ultimately, cutaneous ulcers develop which are usually located near the malleoli. Recurrent bouts of leg pain and swelling can occur due to hemodynamic obstruction of blood flow but without the formation of new thrombi.

The classic signs and symptoms of PE are well known and include sudden chest pain, dyspnea, anxiety, and cyanosis. Hemoptysis is uncommon. As in DVT, the clinical presentations of PE vary considerably. Over two thirds of patients with PE are completely asymptomatic. Rarely, patients with small but recurrent PE seek medical attention because of chronic pulmonary hypertension, with elevated right heart pressure, dyspnea, and cyanosis.

DIAGNOSTIC STUDIES

Because the diagnosis of DVT or PE by history and physical examination is often misleading (i.e., substantial false positives and false negatives), objective diagnostic methods are required. The venogram remains the gold standard for DVT, but ultrasonography, impedance plethysmography, and Doppler flow studies are now used more commonly. The sensitivity and specificity of these noninvasive procedures are well over 90 percent when compared to venography.

Commonly available tests for the diagnosis of PE include ventilation/perfusion lung scans and pulmonary angiography. Several large clinical trials have critically reviewed the diagnostic usefulness of these studies in groups of patients with and without PE. To summarize these results and current recommendations:

1. A normal lung scan or pulmonary angiogram rules out clinically important PE.
2. A lung scan that is interpreted as "high probability" suggests a probability of PE of 85 percent.
3. The combination of an estimate of the "clinical likelihood" of PE plus the results of the lung scan increases the diagnostic probability of either one alone.
4. The presence of proximal DVT on noninvasive studies of the legs increases the likelihood of PE in patients with nondiagnostic lung scans.

Figure 38-1 depicts a diagnostic strategy for the evaluation of PE.

LABORATORY TESTING

Laboratory tests to identify hereditary or acquired hypercoagulable states in patients with venous thromboembolism are discussed in detail in Chap. 37. In brief, candidates for diagnostic laboratory tests are patients who are young, have recurrent venous thrombosis or a family history of thrombosis, and have

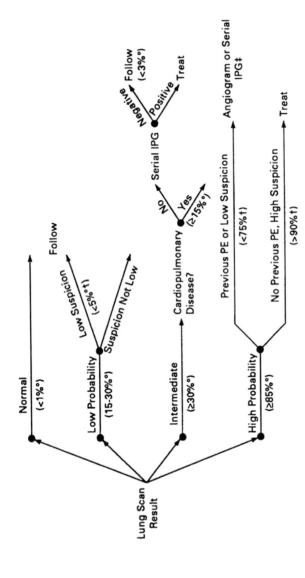

Figure 38-1 A diagnostic strategy for pulmonary embolism (PE). A normal scan result effectively rules out PE. A high probability scan result supports the diagnosis of PE except in the presence of previous PE or low clinical suspicion. Other scan results were less helpful, except for the combination of a low probability scan result and low clinical suspicion. A positive impedance plethysmography (IPG) result supports the diagnosis of thromboembolism. A negative result, when done serially, reliably excludes this disorder only in patients with nondiagnostic scan results and no cardiopulmonary disease. The likelihood of pulmonary embolism is indicated in parentheses. *Strongly supported by clinical studies; †suggested by clinical studies, needs confirmation; ‡a serially negative IPG result may not be sufficient to rule out thromboembolism. (Reproduced with permission from Kelley MA et al: Diagnosing pulmonary embolism: New facts and strategies. Ann Intern Med 114:300, 1991.)

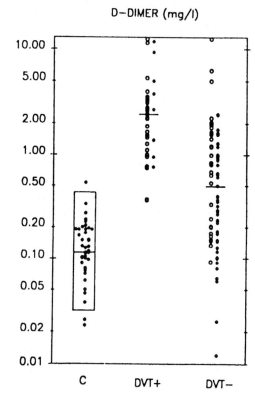

Figure 38-2 Measurement of D-dimer (ELISA) in patients with or without deep venous thrombosis. (Used with permission from Boneau B et al: Thromb Haemost 65:28, 1991.)

thrombi in unusual sites such as the central abdominal veins, the upper extremity, or cerebral sinus veins.

Recently, several cross-sectional clinical studies have been performed to determine whether tests of activation of coagulation or fibrinolysis are diagnostically useful in patients suspected of acute DVT or PE. The most useful of these has proven to be a quantitative ELISA assay for the fibrin degradation product, D-dimer. Its diagnostic value is highest when it is normal (i.e., < 500 ng/mL), with a negative predictive value in both DVT and PE of over 98 percent (Fig. 38-2). Other tests such as the semiquantitative Latex agglutination assay for D-dimer, or tests for thrombin-antithrombin complexes or F1.2 are not useful for diagnosis of thromboembolism.

MANAGEMENT

Thrombolytic Therapy

Thrombolytic therapy with streptokinase, urokinase, or recombinant tissue plasminogen activator (t-PA) is considered the treatment of choice for patients who have massive PE with cardiovascular collapse or for those who have advanced cardiopulmonary disease in which small PE can have major clinical consequences. The use of thrombolytic agents remains controversial in patients with less severe PE. The evidence for short- or long-term benefit in relation to the risks of bleeding is not yet convincing.

Fibrinolytic agents reduce the volume of venous clot as assessed by angiography (e.g., 30 to 40 percent complete clot lysis, 30 percent partial lysis), and several studies have suggested that long-term disability from the postphlebitic syndrome is lessened in treated patients. However, the necessity of 3 or more days of therapy, the risk of bleeding (especially CNS), and the fact that the largest clots are less likely to undergo thrombolysis have tempered enthusiasm for thrombolytic therapy in patients with DVT. Additional clinical trials are needed to determine optimal therapeutic indications, agents and dosing regimens, risks, and long-term benefits in adults, children, and infants.

Anticoagulation

Heparin

Heparin, usually by intravenous infusion, should be started as soon as possible after a diagnosis of DVT or PE is likely (see Chap. 61). Rapid prolongation of the APTT into a therapeutic (e.g., 1.5 to 2 times control) range is essential; suboptimal heparin therapy has been associated with thrombotic recurrence rates of up to 25 percent in the ensuing weeks or months. Heparin administration by subcutaneous injection is also effective provided the APTT is sufficiently prolonged. Several recent prospective randomized clinical trials have shown that low molecular weight heparin administered subcutaneously is as effective and possibly safer than standard heparin for treatment of proximal DVT.

Warfarin

Oral anticoagulation with warfarin should be started shortly after admission in patients with proximal DVT, so that the total duration of heparin therapy will be about 5 days in most patients. A similar strategy is probably appropriate for patients with iliofemoral thrombosis or PE, although clinical trials have not yet been conducted that confirm the efficacy of this regimen in these conditions. Heparin should be continued until oral anticoagulants have become fully effective. Ideally, the PT should be in the therapeutic range for at least 24 h before heparin is stopped.

Warfarin should be given for at least 3 months at low intensity (INR 2 to 3) to patients after a first episode of venous thrombosis, as long as there is no continuing predisposition to thrombosis. Patients who suffer a second thromboembolic event should be treated for at least 12 months, and if more than two thromboses have occurred, lifelong treatment is usually indicated.

Prophylactic Antithrombotic Therapy

Several antithrombotic strategies are now available that can substantially reduce rates of venous thromboembolism following orthopedic, pelvic, or general abdominal surgery. These prophylactic therapies are clearly effective and are substantially underused. Some of these regimens and their success rates in patients having hip surgery are listed in Table 38-2. Low molecular weight heparins or low molecular weight heparinoids are particularly promising and show substantial efficacy with low rates of bleeding.

Special Situations

Calf Vein Thrombosis

Since thromboses limited to the calf veins extend proximally in 20 to 30 percent of patients if left untreated, some form of antithrombotic therapy or ongoing surveillance is indicated. If the facilities are available, repeated leg scanning for up to 5 days to detect proximal extension of the clot has been shown to be a safe and effective strategy. An alternative, and often more practical approach, is to treat patients with calf vein thrombosis for 6 to 12 weeks with anticoagulants (heparin followed by warfarin).

Upper Extremity Thrombosis

Although the risk of PE is low in patients with uncomplicated thrombosis of the axillary or brachial veins, standard anticoagulant therapy is usually indicated to prevent proximal extension of the clot. A recent report suggested that rates of PE are higher in patients who develop upper extremity venous thrombosis as a consequence of central venous catheters.

Pregnancy

Pregnancy confers an elevated risk of venous thromboembolism as a consequence of a hypercoagulable state (see Chap. 3), elevated levels of estrogens, dilatation of the pelvic veins, and obstruction of venous blood flow by the enlarged uterus. The frequency of thrombosis appears to be roughly equal during each of the three trimesters of pregnancy without a marked increase in the third trimester. The thromboembolic risks continue for 4 to 6 weeks postpartum. Intravenous heparin is the mainstay of therapy in pregnant women who develop thromboses and is discussed in Chaps. 31 and 61.

Table 38-2 Venous Thrombosis (VT) Prevention and Elective Hip Replacement: Simple Pooling of Data from Randomized Comparisons Using Routine Venography to Screen for VT

Preventive Method	Trials*	Total No. of Patients	VT (Rate)	95% Confidence Limits	Risk Reduction
Untreated controls	8	394	204 (0.52)	[0.47-0.57]	
Low-dose heparin	6	257	88 (0.34)	[0.28-0.40]	0.34
Adjusted-dose heparin	3	118	13 (0.11)	[0.06-0.18]	0.79
Low-dose heparin/DHE	3	223	83 (0.37)	[0.31-0.44]	0.28
LMW heparins	7	621	100 (0.16)	[0.13-0.19]	0.69
Oral anticoagulants	3	162	30 (0.19)	[0.13-0.26]	0.64
Dextran 70	5	229	68 (0.30)	[0.24-0.36]	0.43
Aspirin	2	141	73 (0.52)	[0.44-0.60]	0.00
Leg compression	2	109	26 (0.24)	[0.16-0.33]	0.54
Elastic stockings	2	137	52 (0.38)	[0.30-0.47]	0.27

SOURCE: Used with permission from Gallus AS: *Baillieres Clin Haematol* 3:651, 1990.

*Number of evaluations for each preventive method.
Risk reduction: Apparent relative risk reduction.
DHE, dihydroergotamine; LMW, low molecular weight.

BIBLIOGRAPHY

Anderson FA et al: Physician practices in the prevention of venous thromboembolism. *Ann Intern Med* 115:591, 1991.

Boneau B et al: D-dimers, thrombin antithrombin III complexes, and prothrombin fragments 1 + 2: Diagnostic value in clinically suspected deep vein thrombosis. *Thromb Haemost* 65:28, 1991.

Bounameaux H et al: Measurement of D-dimer in plasma as diagnostic aid in suspected pulmonary embolism. *Lancet* 337:196, 1991.

Carson JL et al: The clinical course of pulmonary embolism. *N Engl J Med* 326:1240, 1992.

Gallus AS: Anticoagulants in the prevention of venous thromboembolism. *Baillieres Clin Haematol* 3:651, 1990.

Hirsh J: Antithrombotic therapy in deep vein thrombosis and pulmonary embolism. *Am Heart J* 123:1115, 1992.

Hommes DW et al: Subcutaneous heparin compared with continuous intravenous heparin administration in the initial treatment of deep vein thrombosis. *Ann Intern Med* 116:279, 1992.

Hull RD et al: Heparin for 5 days as compared with 10 days in the initial treatment of proximal venous thrombosis. *N Engl J Med* 322:1260, 1990.

Hull RD et al: Subcutaneous low-molecular-weight heparin compared with continuous intravenous heparin in the treatment of proximal-vein thrombosis. *N Engl J Med* 326:975, 1992.

Kelley MA et al: Diagnosing pulmonary embolism: New facts and strategies. *Ann Intern Med* 114:300, 1991.

Lensing AWA et al: Detection of deep-vein thrombosis by real-time B-mode ultrasonography. *N Engl J Med* 320:342, 1989.

Levine MN, Hirsh J: Clinical potential of low molecular weight heparins. *Baillieres Clin Haematol* 3:545, 1990.

Monreal M et al: Upper-extremity deep venous thrombosis and pulmonary embolism. A prospective study. *Chest* 99:280, 1991.

Rich S et al: Pulmonary hypertension from chronic pulmonary thromboembolism. *Ann Intern Med* 108:425, 1988.

Turpie AGG et al: A randomized controlled trial of a low-molecular-weight heparin (enoxaparin) to prevent deep-vein thrombosis in patients undergoing elective hip surgery. *N Engl J Med* 315:925, 1986.

Weitz JI et al: Clot-bound thrombin is protected from inhibition by heparin-antithrombin III but is susceptible to inactivation by antithrombin III-independent inhibitors. *J Clin Invest* 86:384, 1990.

Antithrombin III

Deficiency

Human antithrombin III (AT III) is a 58,000 Mr glycoprotein with a plasma concentration of 150 μg/mL. AT III or heparin cofactor I is a protease inhibitor belonging to the serpin (serine protease inhibitor) superfamily; it functions by forming a 1:1 stoichiometric complex with activated clotting enzymes (thrombin, Xa, IXa, XIa, XIIa) via a reactive site (arginine) on AT III active center (serine) or protease interaction. The relatively slow complex formation is dramatically accelerated in the presence of heparin or when the AT III is activated by cell surface heparan sulfate. The schematic structure of AT III and the residues involved in heparin and thrombin interactions are shown in Fig. 39-1. A deficiency (hereditary or acquired) of the protein is

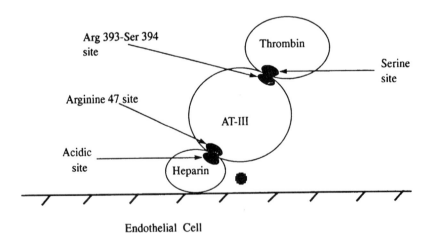

Figure 39-1 The scheme for inhibition of thrombin (or other protease, Xa) by antithrombin (AT III) when bound to heparin (or heparan sulfate) at the endothelial cell surface. The symbol (●) indicates the proposed site for vitronectin, which acts as a noncompetitive inhibitor forming a ternary complex with heparin-AT III and protecting thrombin against rapid inactivation.

associated with a thrombotic tendency as manifested by venous thromboembolism and rarely arterial thrombi.

GENETICS

The 19 kb gene (seven exons, six introns) is located on chromosome 1 (1q23-q25). Mutations resulting in either type 1 (quantitative defects) or type 2 (qualitative defects) are shown in Table 39-1. The common type 1 results in a proportionate decrease in both amount (antigen) and function of AT III and is due to genetic mutations producing silent alleles. The qualitative defects (dysfunctional AT III) are associated with point mutations affecting either the serine protease inhibition site for thrombin, Xa, or the heparin-binding site or both. The heterozygotes for type 1, 2a, 2b display intermediate levels of antithrombin activity associated with a thrombotic tendency; homozygotes are probably not compatible with life. In contrast, the heterozygotes for isolated heparin-binding activity (type 2c) rarely display a thrombotic tendency. How-

TABLE 39-1   Classification of Hereditary Antithrombin III Deficiencies: Molecular Defects

Type I. Low functional and immunoreactive antithrombin III
    1a. Normal molecules synthesized at reduced rate (Frameshift, point mutation)
    1b. Decreased amount of abnormal molecules
        Pro 407–Leu (Utah)
        Arg 406–Met (Kyoto)
        Ala 404–Thr (Oslo)
Type II. Low functional but normal immunoreactive antithrombin III
    2a. Decreased antithrombin activity and heparin-binding activity
        Pro 429–Leu (Budapest)
    2b. Decreased antithrombin activity
        Ser 394–Leu (Denver, Milano 2)
        Ala 384–Pro (Sudbury, Cambridge, Charleville)
        Ala 384–Ser (Cambridge 2)
        Arg 393–Cis (Northwick Park, Milano 1)
        Arg 393–His (Chicago, Glasgow 1, Sheffield)
        Ala 382–Thr (Hamilton, Glasgow 2)
        Gly 392–Asp (Stockholm)
    2c. Isolated low heparin-binding activity
        Arg 47–Cys (Alger, Tours, Toyama, Paris, Amiens, Barcelona 2)
        Pro 41–Leu (Basel, Franconville, Clichy)
        Arg 47–His (Rouen 1)
        Arg 47–Ser (Rouen 2)
        Arg 129–Gln (Geneva)
        Arg 24–Cys (Rouen 4)
        Ile 7–Asn–CHO (Rouen 3)

ever, homozygotes have shown recurrent venous and arterial thrombi, including massive cardiac thromboses and recurrent thrombophlebitis.

The prevalence of hereditary AT III deficiency in the general population has been estimated at 1/2000 to 1/5000. The prevalence of AT III deficiency in consecutive patients being investigated for venous thromboembolism is about 2 to 3 percent. The frequency of AT III deficiency in reported families is as expected for an autosomal dominant heterozygote, about 50 percent; however, the prevalence of thromboses in these heterozygotes is about 25 percent. An age-related incidence of thromboses in affected family members has been noted; the cumulative thrombosis rate ranges from 5 percent at age 0 to 10 years to 95 percent in AT III deficient subjects at 50 to 60 years of age. Although rare before the second decade, thrombotic complications have been reported in infants. The chance that an hereditary deficient individual will have thromboembolic complications depends on other risk factors besides age, including trauma (particularly related to athletic injuries), major surgery, infections, pregnancy, the postpartum period, and the use of oral contraceptive agents (OCA).

CLINICAL MANIFESTATIONS

Measurements of AT III have been by use of two basic types of clinical laboratory assays: immunologic techniques (rocket immunoelectrophoresis) for the AT III antigen and functional assays using chromogenic substrates with and without heparin (AT III activity; progressive antithrombin and heparin cofactor). The most useful assay because it detects abnormalities of both the active serpin center and the heparin-binding center is the AT III heparin cofactor assay using the chromogenic substrate S-2238. A helpful adjunct is the crossed immunoelectrophoretic technique (with heparin in the first dimension) which detects binding to heparin and gross molecular defects. Compared to other coagulation factors, the normal range of AT III in adults is rather narrow (i.e., from 0.8 to 1.2 U/mL). With the exception of the fetus and newborn, physiologic alterations of AT III levels are infrequently seen. Slightly decreased amounts (to approximately 0.9 U/mL) are noted in men over the age of 50 years and in women of childbearing age; pregnancy and exercise have little effect in most studies.

Profound alterations in AT III are seen in the fetus and newborn where levels range from 0.25 U/mL in the 20-week gestation fetus to 0.5 U/mL in the term infant. Adult levels are reached by 6 months of age. Preterm infants with AT III levels < 0.2 U/mL in cord samples have a significantly higher risk for dying of the respiratory distress syndrome or cerebral hemorrhage. In most instances the infant is probably protected against increased thrombotic risk by the physiologically low vitamin K-dependent factors ("warfarin-like effect") and elevated levels of a_2-macroglobulin (inhibits thrombin generation); however, an increased resistance to therapeutic heparin has been observed.

Clinical features of hereditary AT III deficiency include first thrombotic episodes at an early age, family history, recurrent venous thromboembolism, thrombosis during pregnancy, occasional resistance to heparin therapy, and idiopathic venous thrombosis. The clinical manifestations of both hereditary and acquired AT III deficiency are primarily those of thromboses and subsequent embolization-extension of the venous system. The usual vessels involved are deep veins of the lower extremities, iliofemoral, vena caval, renal, axillary and retinal veins. Cerebral venous thrombosis at all ages, mesenteric venous thromboses and Budd-Chiari syndrome are special clinical problems which have been reported. Arterial thromboses may rarely occur.

Acquired deficiencies of AT III may be significant clinical problems and are summarized in Table 39-2. The most common and frequently most severe deficiencies of AT III occur in consumption coagulopathy conditions such as

TABLE 39-2 Acquired Antithrombin III Deficiency

Consumption coagulopathy
    Disseminated intravascular coagulation (shock, sepsis)
    Surgery
    Preeclampsia
Liver dysfunction
    Acute hepatic failure
    Cirrhosis
    Polytransfused thalassemia
    Preterm infants
Renal disease
    Nephrotic syndrome
    Hemolytic uremic syndrome
Malignancies
    Leukemia (acute promyelocytic leukemia)
Malnutrition or gastrointestinal loss
    Vascular reconstruction (diabetes, age)
    Protein-calorie deprivation
    Inflammatory bowel disease
Drugs
    Estrogens-progestins
    Heparin
    L-asparaginase
Other
    Vasculitis
    Infection
    Hemodialysis
    Plasmapheresis
    After prothrombin-complex concentrate infusion

---

disseminated intravascular coagulation (DIC; shock, sepsis), major surgery and its complications, preeclampsia, and malignancies. AT III deficiency associated with failure to synthesize adequate amounts of AT III are seen in cirrhosis, severe thalassemia, malnutrition, and in preterm infants. Both loss and failure to synthesize may be observed in acute hepatic failure and the nephrotic syndrome. The acute use of heparin, L-asparaginase, or after prothrombin-complex concentrate infusions or the chronic use of OCA (related mainly to the estrogen content) are associated with decreases in circulating AT III. The low levels of AT III with OCA, L-asparaginase and after prothrombin-complex concentrate usage have been associated with thrombotic episodes.

MANAGEMENT

In most instances, acute thrombotic episodes in hereditary deficiency of AT III are managed in the usual fashion by heparin therapy followed by chronic warfarin prophylaxis. Older observations suggested that heparin administration may cause adverse clinical effects in patients with AT III deficiency by reducing existing AT III levels and aggravating the hypercoagulable state. Our experience has been that heparin may be used therapeutically for acute thrombotic events without replacement with exogenous AT III (plasma, concentrates) although in clinical situations where bleeding is a risk (parturition or surgery) purified concentrates of AT III have a beneficial role. Intravenous heparin does decrease plasma AT III levels and enhances AT III clearance by increasing uptake in the liver. In patients with acute deep venous thrombosis (DVT), plasma AT III levels fall (by about 20 percent) after therapeutic heparin, but the incidence of DVT recurrence is not related to the lower patient AT III levels. Even so, extensive thrombus formation with heparin resistance may occasionally be seen in familial AT III deficiency.

Warfarin therapy on a chronic basis is usually not associated with an appreciable effect on AT III levels; however, untreated AT III-deficient subjects generate more thrombin than their nondeficient family members and warfarin inhibits this thrombin formation. Hereditary deficient patients who have had a previous thrombotic episode (DVT) are given warfarin prophylaxis indefinitely. Rarely, coumarin-induced skin necrosis may be seen in hereditary AT III deficiency, although most usually it is seen in protein C deficiency. More recently certain androgenic compounds (danazol, stanozolol, oxymetholone) have been shown to increase AT III levels in hereditary deficient patients; however, the benefit in prevention of thrombosis has to be established.

Indications for the use of replacement therapy with AT III concentrates include thrombosis during pregnancy (delivery, postpartum), refractory thrombosis, and major surgery in hereditary deficiency patients. Other potential indications are posttrauma DIC and hemorrhagic shock, acute nephrotic syndrome, fulminant hepatic failure, and persistent DIC in clinical situations where the measured levels are particularly low. AT III concentrate has been used in the sick newborn to prevent thrombotic and hemorrhagic complications although definite clinical benefit has yet to be established. See Chapter 56 for details of concentrate use.

BIBLIOGRAPHY

Blajchman MA et al: Molecular basis of inherited human antithrombin deficiency. *Blood* 80:2159, 1992.

Boyer C et al: Homozygous variant of antithrombin III: AT III Fontainebleau. *Thromb Haemost* 56:18, 1986.

Buller HR, ten Cate JW: Acquired antithrombin III deficiency: Laboratory diagnosis, incidence, clinical implications, and treatment with antithrombin III concentrate. *Am J Med* 87(suppl 3B):44S, 1989.

De Stefano V, Leone G: Antithrombin III congenital defects: Revising classification system. *Thromb Haemost* 62:820, 1989.

Demers C et al: Measurement of markers of activated coagulation in antithrombin III deficient subjects. *Thromb Haemost* 67:542, 1992.

Eyster ME, Parker MD: Treatment of familial antithrombin-III deficiency with danazol. *Haemostasis* 15:119, 1985.

Gallus AS et al: The relative contributions of antithrombin III during heparin treatment, and of clinically recognizable risk factors, to early recurrence of venous thromboembolism. *Thromb Res* 46:539, 1987.

Goodnight SH et al: Measurement of antithrombin III in normal and pathologic states using chromogenic substrate S-2238. *Am J Clin Pathol* 73:639, 1980.

Hathaway WE: Clinical aspects of antithrombin III deficiency. *Semin Hematol* 28:19, 1991.

Pratt CW, Church FC: Antithrombin: Structure and function. *Semin Hematol* 28:3, 1991.

Lane DA et al: Antithrombin III: A database of mutations. *Thromb Haemost* 66:657, 1991.

Manco-Johnson MJ: Neonatal antithrombin III deficiency. *Am J Med* 87(suppl 3B):49S, 1989.

Menache D et al: Evaluation of the safety, recovery, half-life, and clinical efficacy of antithrombin III (human) in patients with hereditary antithrombin III deficiency. Cooperative Study Group. *Blood* 75:33, 1990.

Rosenberg RD: Biochemistry of heparin antithrombin. Interactions and the physiologic role of this natural anticoagulant mechanism. *Am J Med* 87(suppl 3B):2S, 1989.

Thaler E, Lechner K: Antithrombin III deficiency and thromboembolism. *Clin Haematol* 10:369, 1981.

Protein C Deficiency

The description of familial thrombosis in association with protein C (PC) deficiency in 1981 emphasized the clinical importance of PC in controlling the hemostatic system. Since that time, numerous examples of acquired and hereditary PC deficiency have provided convincing evidence of the importance of PC and its cofactor, protein S (PS), in the regulation of thrombin production. PC is a vitamin K-dependent zymogen that on activation by thrombin-thrombomodulin (TM) becomes a serine protease augmented by PS which acts as a potent anticoagulant by destroying activated factors V and VIII and also stimulates the fibrinolytic system (Fig. 40-1).

STRUCTURE AND FUNCTION

Protein C is a vitamin K-dependent glycoprotein with a Mr of 62,000 synthesized in the liver and circulating in a concentration of 5 μg/mL. The molecule

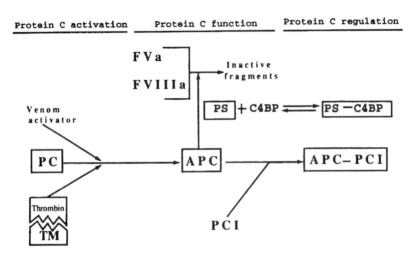

Figure 40-1 Representation of protein C (PC) reactions. APC, activated protein C; PCI, protein C inhibitor; PS, protein S; C4BP, C4b binding protein; TM, thrombomodulin. (Adapted from Preissner reference with permission.)

consists of a heavy chain (serine active site and activation peptide) linked by a disulfide bond to the light chain (γ-carboxylglutamic acid residues and epidermal growth factor region; see Fig. 40-2). PC is activated by thrombin that is bound to endothelial cell-associated TM. TM (Mr 75,000), controlled by an intronless gene on chromosome 20, is found on the endothelial cells (EC) of capillaries, arteries, veins, and lymphatics of various organs. (TM fragments can be found in the circulation in disorders like thrombotic thrombocytopenic purpura and disseminated intravascular coagulation [DIC]). After thrombin binds to TM it fails to act on its usual substrates (VIII, V, fibrinogen XIII), but its capacity to activate PC is enhanced more than 1000-fold.

Activated PC (APC; PC can also be activated in vitro by certain snake venoms) aided by its cofactor PS cleaves factors VIIIa and Va into inactive fragments. These reactions take place on a phospholipid surface in the presence of calcium ions. APC has profibrinolytic activity in vitro by inactivating plasminogen activator inhibitor (PAI); however, no in vivo effect of APC on the fibrinolytic system by infused APC or abnormality in euglobulin lysis in PC-deficient patients has been demonstrated. The natural inhibitors of APC are a Mr 57,000 single chain glycoprotein called PC inhibitor (PCI) and a_1-antitrypsin. PCI (also identical to PAI-3) inhibits thrombin, Xa, XIa, and kallikrein as well as APC; PCI activity is enhanced by heparin (see Fig. 40-1).

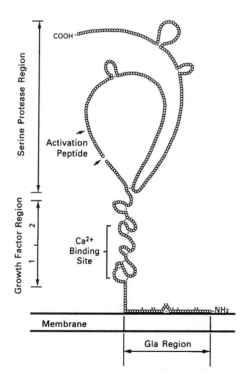

Figure 40-2 Structure-function relationships of the protein C molecule. Activation of protein C by thrombin-thrombomodulin complex depends on the presence of divalent cations; calcium is the most effective. A high affinity binding site for calcium is located in the growth factor region (but probably closer to the heavy chain than depicted in the diagram). The binding of Ca^{++} to the high affinity site (not the Gla domain) induces a confirmational change in the heavy chain allowing activation to a serine protease (see arrows) which subsequently cleaves activated factor V and factor VIII. (Used with permission of the American Society of Biochemistry and Molecular Biology, Inc. From Esmon CT: The roles of protein C and the thrombomodulin in the regulation of blood coagulation. J Biol Chem 264:4743, 1989.)

Protein C is measured in plasma by quantitative or immunologic (rocket, ELISA) assays (PC antigen) or by functional assays which measure the ability of APC to cleave a synthetic substrate (amidolytic assay) or the ability of APC to prolong clotting time assays by destroying VIIIa and Va (APTT or clotting time). Activators of PC in these systems may be thrombin, thrombin-TM, or snake venom (Protac, *Agkristrodon contortrix*). The amidolytic assays evaluate the ability of PC to be activated and the ability to bind and cleave small substrates within the active site pocket, whereas the clotting assays evaluate all anticoagulant functions of the molecule (i.e., activation region, active site pocket, binding domains for clotting factor substrates [Va, VIIa] and cofactor [PS] and phospholipid surface). As noted below the clotting assay is most sensitive to all defects (but is affected by heparin in the sample). The PC antigen assay is least specific for functional activity. For instance, both the antigen assay and the amylolytic assay result in significantly higher values than the clotting assay in patients on warfarin or with type II defects.

GENETICS

The 11.2 kb gene for PC is located on chromosome 2 and is composed of nine exons and eight introns with marked homology with the factor IX gene. Multiple abnormalities such as gross deletions, insertions, nucleotide substitution, promoter gene region substitution, and mRNA splicing defects have been described in hereditary deficiencies. Table 40-1 provides an outline of hereditary PC deficiency based on PC assays and phenotypic expression. Type I deficiencies represent concordant reduction in PC antigen and PC activity levels; type II deficiencies have normal levels of antigen but low activity by functional assays. Type I heterozygotes may be symptomatic with deep venous thrombosis (DVT), pulmonary embolism (PE), arterial strokes and other thrombotic complications (the autosomal dominant type with prevalence of 1/16,000) or "silent" carriers (the autosomal recessive type with a prevalence of 1/300 to 1/1000) who apparently do not have an increased risk for thrombosis. A recent Dutch study (Allaart reference) of PC deficient families identified by molecular studies found that 50 percent of heterozygotes and 10 percent of normal relatives had venous thromboembolism by age 45 years.

The offspring of type I heterozygotic parents may be either severe (PC level < 0.01 U/mL) homozygotes who develop neonatal purpura fulminans, DIC, and other severe thrombotic complications or moderate homozygotes (PC level 0.05 to 0.18 U/mL) with recurrent DVT occurring later in life.

Type II heterozygotes (named after city of origin) represent the dysproteinemic form of PC deficiency and present in an identical clinical manner to

TABLE 40-1 Hereditary Protein C Deficiency. Classification Based on Phenotype and Laboratory Assays*

Type	Phenotype	Protein C Assays (Mean and Lower Limit)		
		Antigen	Amidolytic	Clotting
I (Concordant antigen and activity levels)				
Normal adults		1.0 (0.65)	0.94 (0.61)	0.97 (0.72)
Heterozygote-AD	DVT, PE	0.35–0.63	0.31–0.63	0.34–0.56
Heterozygote-AR	Asymptomatic	0.33–0.65	—	—
Homozygote or compound heterozygote				
Severe	Neonatal purpura fulminans and/or severe thrombosis	<0.01	<0.01	<0.01
Moderate	Recurrent DVT, PE	0.05–0.18	0.05–0.1	—
II (Discordant levels; normal antigen; low activity by amidolytic, clotting assay, or both)				
Heterozygotes				
(Cadiz)	DVT, PE	0.83	0.46	0.36
(Rouen)	DVT, PE	0.98, 1.5	0.98, 0.97	0.36–0.53
(Yonago)	DVT	0.84	0.74	0.43
Homozygotes				
Severe	Neonatal purpura fulminans	0.16–0.23	<0.01	—
Double heterozygotes				
(I and II)	Newborn renal vein thrombosis, DVT, chronic DIC	0.47	0.34	0.14
(I and II Tochigi)	DVT, PE age 14 y	~0.2	<0.01	—

*Examples of values are taken from literature references. DVT, deep venous thrombosis; PE, pulmonary embolism; AD, autosomal dominant; AR, autosomal recessive; DIC, disseminated intravascular coagulation.

the type I heterozygotes; type II homozygotes can present with neonatal purpura fulminans. Double heterozygotes (I and II) are documented with an intermediate phenotypic expression including DVT at an early age and chronic DIC. One of these, PC Tochigi, exhibited an abnormal PC molecule with Arg→Trp substitution at the cleavage site for thrombin-TM. Venous and arterial thromboembolism is rare in the first decade and thereafter increases to approximately 50 percent of PC-deficient individuals by age 45 years.

ACQUIRED DEFECTS

Because PC is consumed in intravascular coagulation states (DIC), is vitamin K dependent, is made in the liver, and has relatively short half-life in the circulation (7 to 9 h), it is not surprising that decreased PC levels are observed in many disease conditions (Table 40-2). In addition, physiologic levels of PC

TABLE 40-2 Acquired Protein C Deficiency

Increased consumption
    Disseminated intravascular coagulation syndromes
    Acquired purpura fulminans (bacterial sepsis, varicella)
    Severe preeclampsia
    Venous thrombosis-induced ulcerations
    Lipodermatosclerosis
    Adult respiratory distress syndrome
    Systemic lupus erythematosus
    Splanchnic venous thrombosis
    Ulcerative colitis
    Colorectal cancer
    IgG paraproteinemia (inhibitor)

Decreased synthesis
    Hepatocellular disease (alcoholic cirrhosis)
    Oral anticoagulant therapy (warfarin)
    Vitamin K deficiency
    Normal newborn infants and children
    L-asparaginase therapy
    Fluorouracil therapy

Both or other
    Renal failure, uremia (inhibitor)
    Homocysteinemia
    Cerebral arterial infarction
    Liver transplantation (postoperative period)
    Hemodialysis
    Plasmapheresis
    Sick newborn infants (idiopathic respiratory distress syndrome, infant of diabetic
        mother)

in the fetus and newborn are low (0.1 to 0.5 U/mL) and may be near zero in the sick preterm infant. Like other coagulation factors, PC level rises rapidly after birth but unlike others does not reach the adult range until age 6 years and does not completely approximate the adult mean until adolescence. Interestingly, the mean PC level increases approximately 4 percent per decade throughout life. Purpura fulminans and skin necrosis, characteristic lesions associated with extremely low levels of PC, have been observed after warfarin administration in PC heterozygotes (both I and II), PC homozygotes, sick preterm infants, severe DIC, and overwhelming bacterial sepsis. Other severe lesions, splanchnic venous thrombosis and cerebral thrombosis, are associated with both hereditary and acquired PC-deficient states. In particular, recurrent coumarin-induced skin necrosis was recently described in three moderate or late onset homozygous PC-deficient adults confirmed by genetic DNA analysis; these patients did not have neonatal purpura fulminans and did have low but detectable PC levels.

An acquired PC inhibitor (IgG paraprotein) was associated with thrombosis and DIC, producing severe and ultimately fatal hemorrhage in a 51-year-old man.

DIAGNOSIS AND MANAGEMENT

The identification of PC heterozygotes is a difficult problem because of the variations of PC levels due to age, concurrent illnesses, and pharmacologic agents. Both heparin and warfarin can interfere with the functional assays; the antigen assay should not be used alone for screening since it will miss all type II heterozygotes. Although variable, mean values for nonhereditary deficient individuals on warfarin are PC antigen, 0.52 U/mL and PC amidolytic activity, 0.36 U/mL.

The low PC level of patients on warfarin, children, and some normal individuals frequently overlap the heterozygote values. A recent multicenter study of known heterozygotes using both antigen and functional assays showed that PC activity assays ranged from 19 to 82 percent and antigen values from 22 to 88.5 percent. Some heterozygote patient values were within the range of the control group (most laboratories use 60 percent as the lower range of normal). Every effort should be made to study a patient before warfarin therapy is instituted or 2 to 3 weeks after the course is completed; repeated samples plus family studies and/or molecular analysis are often necessary in borderline cases and in individuals on warfarin. Comparison of the PC value to factor II and X levels may be helpful as well as use of DNA analysis if available.

Neonatal purpura fulminans, although rare, should be considered due to homozygous PC or homozygous PS deficiency (see Chap. 41) until proven otherwise. The manifestations of the condition are shown in Fig. 40-3. If untreated, the condition will almost surely progress to death. Anticoagulation with heparin has not interrupted the progression in neonatal purpura fulminans, although it has been useful in the acquired form occurring at an older age. The key to successful treatment is the replacement of protein C. Fresh frozen plasma (10 mL/kg) every 12 h is usually required to halt progression of the skin lesions. A PC concentrate (Immuno, Vienna) is available and was used successfully in a term infant where doses of 1 U/kg achieved an increment of 1.2 percent with a biphasic half-life of 6 and 11 h. It appears that a level of 5 to 10 percent will halt the progression of skin lesions but a higher dose is needed to eliminate DIC. The infant should be maintained in a stable state with PC infusion therapy until old enough to begin long-term warfarin therapy (usually about 3 months of age). Warfarin treatment is established with an INR of 3 to 4 and PC infusions are stopped. Recurrences of skin lesions should be treated with further fresh frozen plasma or concentrate. Most patients have been maintained on warfarin alone although the intensity of treatment places them at risk for bleeding. Parents should be studied and counseled accordingly. Most parents have been asymptomatic without history of recurrent thrombosis. Normal levels of PC were maintained in a 20-month-old child with homozygous PC deficiency treated with liver transplantation.

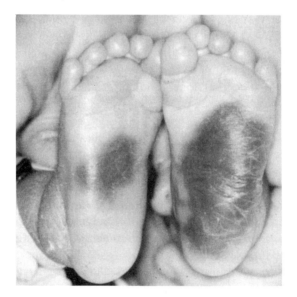

Figure 40-3 Neonatal homozygous protein C deficiency. Infant with purpura fulminans. Manifestations of neonatal homozygous PC deficiency: Purpura fulminans (extremities, buttocks, abdomen, scrotum, scalp); Deep vein thromboses; CNS thromboses (hemorrhage, hydrocephalus); Mental retardation, delayed psychomotor development; Blindness (vitreous or retinal hemorrhage); Disseminated intravascular coagulation; PC levels—extremely low or nondetectable.

About 75 percent of affected PC heterozygotes (from families with thrombosis) have experienced one or more thrombotic events (DVT, mesenteric vein thrombosis, PE); about 63 percent develop recurrent DVT and 40 percent have PE. These individuals and affected family members who are at increased risk for thrombosis should be maintained on prophylactic anticoagulation with warfarin, INR of 2 to 3) indefinitely. Recommendations for children and pregnancy are discussed in Chaps. 36 and 52.

The occurrence of coumarin-induced skin necrosis has been associated with heterozygous (or moderate homozygous) PC deficiency. The syndrome (progressive purpuric, necrotic skin lesions) occurs during the first few days of warfarin therapy usually after large loading doses and is due to rapid depletion of an already low PC (with short half-life) before the other vitamin K-dependent proteins are depressed (except factor VII, also short half-life); thus producing a necrotic and hemorrhagic lesion. The syndrome is best avoided by not using loading doses or by the addition of fresh frozen plasma early in treatment of severely PC-deficient patients. Acute DVT in known PC-deficient heterozygotes is treated by heparinization and gradual institution of warfarin treatment to the desired effect before stopping the heparin (see Chap. 62).

Stanozolol raises the PC level to near normal in heterozygotes (type I) and favors fibrinolysis; however, the long-term effect in preventing thrombosis has not been established.

As noted in Table 40-2 many acquired disorders have been noted to have low PC levels. In those conditions where a low level is associated with DIC or thrombosis, therapeutic intervention is sometimes necessary. Anticoagulation therapy may be adequate for major vessel thrombosis in conditions such as adult respiratory distress syndrome, renal failure, and ulcerative colitis. However, in the acquired purpura fulminans syndrome the sick newborn with thrombosis, in severe hepatocellular disease, and in severe sepsis with skin necrosis, the PC level may be extremely low (< 10 to 20 percent) and the use of heparin anticoagulation alone may be of little help and will increase the risk of bleeding. In such instances, a trial of replacement therapy with PC concentrate or fresh frozen plasma may be warranted.

BIBLIOGRAPHY

Allaart CF et al: Increased risk of venous thrombosis in carriers of hereditary protein C deficiency defect. *Lancet* 341:134, 1993.

Broekmans AW et al: Treatment of hereditary protein C deficiency with stanozolol. *Thromb Haemost* 57:20, 1987.

Casella JF et al: Successful treatment of homozygous protein C deficiency by hepatic transplantation. *Lancet* 1:435, 1988.

Conard J et al: The fibrinolytic system in patients with congenital protein C deficiency. *Thromb Res* 36:363, 1984.

Conard J et al: Homozygous protein C deficiency with late onset and recurrent coumarin-induced skin necrosis. *Lancet* 339:743, 1992.

Dreyfus M et al: Treatment of homozygous protein C deficiency and neonatal purpura fulminans with a purified protein C concentrate. *N Engl J Med* 325:1565, 1991.

Griffin JH et al: Deficiency of protein C in congenital thrombotic disease. *J Clin Invest* 68:1370, 1981.

Marlar RA et al: Diagnosis and treatment of homozygous protein C deficiency. Report of the Working Party on homozygous protein C deficiency of the Subcommittee on protein C and protein S, International Committee on Thrombosis and Haemostasis. *J Pediatr* 114:528, 1989.

Miletich J et al: Absence of thrombosis in subjects with heterozygous protein C deficiency. *N Engl J Med* 317:991, 1987.

Mitchell CA et al: A fatal thrombotic disorder associated with an acquired inhibitor of protein C. *N Engl J Med* 317:1638, 1987.

Pabinger I et al: Hereditary protein C-deficiency: Laboratory values in transmitters and guidelines for the diagnostic procedure. Report on a study of the SSC subcommittee on protein C and protein S. *Thromb Haemost* 68:470, 1992.

Preissner KT: Biological relevance of the protein C system and laboratory diagnosis of protein C and protein S deficiencies. *Clin Sci* 78:351, 1990.

Sugahara Y et al: Protein C deficiency Hong Kong 1 and 2: Hereditary protein C deficiency causd by two mutant alleles, a 5-nucleotide deletion and a missense mutation. *Blood* 80:126, 1992.

Tait RC et al: Age related changes in protein C activity in healthy adult males. *Thromb Haemost* 65:326, 1991.

Tripodi A et al: Asymptomatic homozygous protein C deficiency. *Acta Haematol* 83:152, 1990.

van Teunenbroek A et al: Protein C activity and antigen levels in childhood. *Eur J Pediatr* 149:774, 1990.

Protein S

Deficiency

CHAPTER
41

Protein S (PS) is a vitamin K-dependent plasma glycoprotein that serves as the cofactor for the anticoagulant function of activated protein C (APC) in inactivating factors Va and VIIIa. PS is synthesized in hepatocytes and endothelial cells (EC). An hereditary deficiency of PS is associated with a thrombotic tendency in man.

STRUCTURE-FUNCTION RELATIONSHIP

Protein S (Mr 69,000) is a vitamin K-dependent, nonenzymatic cofactor to APC; PS and APC form a 1:1 stoichiometric complex on the surface of negatively charged phospholipid membranes (platelet, EC). PS, which circulates in plasma in the concentration of 20 to 25 μg/L, is synthesized by vascular EC, hepatocytes, megakaryocytes, and the Leydig cells of human testes. As shown in Fig. 41-1, PS contains multiple domains: from the NH$_2$ terminus, the Gla-containing domain (phospholipid binding), the thrombin-sensitive region, four epidermal growth factor (EGF)-like domains (calcium binding and cofactor function) followed by a region homologous to a sex hormone binding globulin (binding to C4BP).

Protein S exists in two distinct forms in plasma. Approximately 40 percent occurs as free PS, the remainder being bound to a high molecular weight (570 kDa) protein, C4b binding protein (C4BP). Only free PS has cofactor activity for APC; however the binding of PS to C4BP does not directly affect the complement regulatory function of C4BP. C4BP is composed of two types of polypeptide chains, the α chain of Mr 72,000 and the β chain of Mr 45,000. C4BP molecules are heterogeneous; the common oligomer is a spider-like structure with seven α chains and one β chain (only the β chain-containing molecule binds PS). Since C4BP is

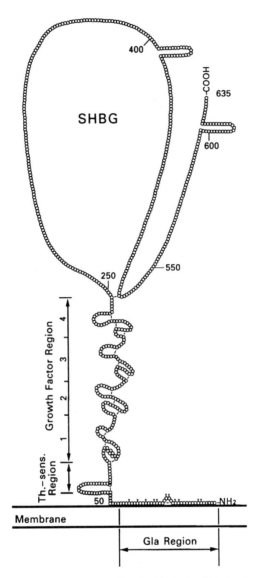

Figure 41-1 Molecular model of protein S. Protein S is depicted binding to phospholipids of the cell membrane by means of the Gla (glutamic acid residues) domain at the NH₂ terminal portion of the molecule.Th–sens, thrombin-sensitive region; the EGF (epidermal growth factor) domains are numbered 1, 2, 3, 4 and represent the calcium binding cofactor function region. The region homologous to a sex hormone binding globulin (SHBG) functions to bind protein S to C4BP. (Used with permission of the American Society of Biochemistry and Molecular Biology, Inc. From Esmon CT: The roles of protein C and the thrombomodulin in the regulation of blood coagulation. J Biol Chem 264:4743, 1989.)

an acute phase reactant, the total amount of PS bound can vary widely according to the total quantity and relative amount of β chain-containing C4BP present in a given condition; the level of free PS may be decreased in inflammatory or related conditions (Table 41-1).

Elevated levels of free PS, which occur in the rare disorder of familial C4BP deficiency, are not associated with increased hemorrhagic tendencies. The existence of PS in the plasma in two forms, free or complexed with C4BP, can complicate laboratory assays. The equilibrium between the two forms depends on the functional integrity of both proteins as well as the concentration of C4BP (especially the β chain molecules). Immunologic assays using treatments to dissociate (dilute plasma; incubation) or remove (polyethylcne glycol adsorption) the complexed form allows quantitative measurements of bound PS, free PS, or both (total PS). Functional assays of PS using PS-depleted plasma and clotting time assays can be used to determine the clotting cofactor function (inactivation of factor Va by APC) of free PS. The clotting time assay usually approximates the free PS. Normal values are given in Table 41-2. Physiologic variations include a lower mean free PS level in normal females than normal males, lower free PS in pregnancy and women on oral contraception, and lower total and free PS in newborn infants.

TABLE 41-1 Conditions Associated with Acquired Protein S Deficiency

Conditions with increased C4BP (acute phase reaction; hormonal)
    Pregnancy
    Oral contraceptive agents
    Diabetes mellitus
    Inflammation (inflammatory bowel disease, stasis ulcers)
    Systemic lupus erythematosus
    Male tobacco smokers
    AIDS
    Renal allograft rejection
    Nephrosis (plus selective urinary loss)
Conditions with decreased synthesis (PS, C4BP, or both)
    Preterm and term infants
    Liver disease
    Vitamin K deficiency
    Coumadin therapy
    Chemotherapy for breast cancer
Conditions with increased cell binding of PS
    Polycythemia vera
    Sickle cell disease
    Essential thrombocythemia

TABLE 41-2 Classification of Hereditary Protein S Deficiency

Type	Phenotype	PS, total (antigen)	PS, free (antigen)	PS, activity (clotting)
Normal	male	82–130%	81–133%	60–150%
Normal	female	50–130%	50–133%	50-125%
I, heterozygote (concordant antigen and free)	DVT, arterial thromboses	low	low	low
I, double heterozygote	DVT, arterial thrombosis	low	very low	very low
I, homozygote	neonatal purpura fulminans	absent	absent	absent
II, heterozygote (discordant antigen and activity)	DVT, arterial thrombosis	normal	normal	low
III, heterozygote (concordant free antigen and activity)	DVT, arterial thrombosis	normal	low	low

GENETICS

The cDNA for human PS has been cloned and fully characterized; there are two copies of the gene, called PSa and PSβ; both are located on chromosome 3. On the basis of multiple base changes in PSβ (termination codons, frameshifts), it is considered a pseudogene.

Protein S deficiency is inherited in an autosomal dominant manner similar to that of protein C (PC) deficiency. The most common heterozygote type I deficiency state is associated with about 50 percent of the normal total PS antigen and decreases of free PS and functional (clotting assay) to about 30 to 40 percent of normal. The usual type II heterozygote (normal level of total PS and free PS but low functional PS) is relatively rare; a more common type has been described with normal total PS, but low free and functional PS and designated as type III. Double heterozygotes with markedly low levels of free and functional PS are known; in addition, data on two infants with homozygous PS deficiency who presented with neonatal purpura fulminans and low or undetectable PS antigen or activity (Fig. 41-2; Table 41-3) have been described. At present the optimal single screening test for hereditary PS deficiency is the functional assay for free PS.

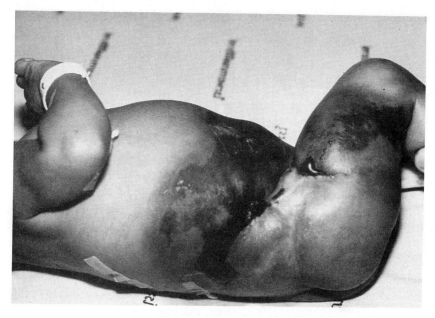

Figure 41-2 Homozygous protein S deficiency. Note purpuric and necrotic skin lesions for Case 1 (see Table 41-3).

TABLE 41-3

	Case 1 (Mahasandana et al)	Case 2 (Pegelow et al)

Clinical Manifestations	Purpura fulminans
	DIC
	Endo-ophthalmitis,
	  blindness
	Cerebral atrophy
		Purpura fulminans
		DIC
		Retinal detachment
		  and hemorrhage
		CNS hemorrhage and
		  infarction

Laboratory		
Total PS	0	0.08 U/mL
Free PS	0	0.012 U/mL
Functional PS	—	0.07 U/mL
Father	Free S = trace	—
Mother	Free S = 10%	Free S = 17%

CLINICAL MANIFESTATIONS OF PROTEIN S DEFICIENCY

A working classification of hereditary PS deficiency (which undoubtedly will be changed when molecular data become available and correlated) is presented in Table 41-2. Events including recurrent deep vein thrombosis (DVT), pulmonary embolism, cerebral and mesenteric thrombosis, superficial thrombophlebitis, and arterial thromboses (cerebral and occlusive disease) are seen most in PS heterozygotes before age 40 but rarely before age 15 years. PS-deficient patients have an increased association with arterial thromboses and may also have cutaneous necrosis even without coumadin therapy. Homozygous PS deficiency is associated with neonatal purpura fulminans (like homozygous PC deficiency; see Fig. 41-2).

As in PC deficiency, the many causes of acquired PS deficiency (see Table 41-1) makes the precise diagnosis and classification of hereditary PS more difficult. The low levels of free PS in inflammatory conditions like systemic lupus erythematosis, nephrotic syndrome, thrombophlebitis, or even diabetes mellitus may be associated with the higher C4BP concentrations (increased bound or complexed PS). Unlike PC, PS is unlikely to be low in disseminated intravascular coagulation (DIC), sepsis, and septic shock.

MANAGEMENT

The heterozygous form of PS deficiency may be discovered at any age; unlike PC deficiency, even newborn infants who have moderately low total PS on a physiologic basis (level about 25 percent) have near normal levels of free or functional PS (level about 75 percent of adult value). This observation is related to near absent levels of C4BP in the fetus and newborn; by 6 months of age adult levels are approximated. Thrombotic events are rare in children and begin to occur at adolescence (like PC deficiency). Our management of heterozygotes who have a thrombotic event is essentially the same for PS as for PC deficiency, i.e., initial heparinization, fibrinolytic therapy if indicated, followed by gradual institution of warfarin therapy which is continued indefinitely. Warfarin-induced skin necrosis has occurred in PS deficiency.

To date, two infants with homozygous PS deficiency have been described (see Table 41-3). Both had purpura fulminans, CNS, and ocular lesions (like homozygous PC deficiency) in association with very low to undetectable PS. The second case could also be a severe double heterozygote (father not available for study). Both infants were successfully managed by administration of fresh frozen plasma and warfarin therapy. Thrombotic episodes and DIC tend to recur without periodic (at least once weekly fresh frozen plasma infusion) administration of PS-containing material. PS has a half-life of 36 to 60 h. PS concentrate is currently under development (Immuno).

BIBLIOGRAPHY

Ceriello A et al: Possible role for increased C4b-binding-protein level in acquired protein S deficiency in type I diabetes. *Diabetes* 39:447, 1990.

Comp PC et al: Familial protein S deficiency is associated with recurrent thrombosis. *J Clin Invest* 74:2082, 1984.

Conlan MG, Haire WD: Low protein S in essential thrombocythemia with thrombosis. *Am J Hematol* 32:88, 1989.

Dahlback B: Protein S and C4b-binding protein: Components involved in the regulation of the protein C anticoagulant system. *Thromb Haemost* 66:49, 1991.

Engesser L et al: Hereditary protein S deficiency: Clinical manifestations. *Ann Inter Med* 106:677, 1987.

Griffin JH et al: Reevaluation of total, free, and bound protein S and C4b-binding protein levels in plasma anticoagulated with citrate or hirudin. *Blood* 79:3203, 1992.

Mahasandana C et al: Homozygous protein S deficiency in an infant with purpura fulminans. *J Pediatr* 117:750, 1990.

Malm J et al: Plasma concentrations of C4b-binding protein and vitamin K-dependent protein S in term and preterm infants: Low levels of protein S-C4b-binding protein complexes. *Br J Haemat* 68:445, 1988.

Mannucci PM et al: Familial dysfunction of protein-S. *Thromb Haemost* 62:763, 1989.

Pegelow CH et al: Severe protein S deficiency in a newborn. *Pediatrics* 89:674, 1992.

Ploos van Amstel HK et al: A mutation in the protein-S pseudogene is linked to protein-S deficiency in a thrombophilic family. *Thromb Haemost* 62:897, 1989.

Preissner KT: Biological relevance of the protein C system and laboratory diagnosis of protein C and protein S deficiencies. *Clin Sci* 78:351, 1990.

Rogers JS et al: Chemotherapy for breast cancer decreases plasma protein C and protein S. *J Clin Oncol* 6:276, 1988.

Wiesel ML et al: Screening of protein S deficiency using a functional assay in patients with venous and arterial thrombosis. *Thromb Res* 58:461, 1990.

Zoppi M et al: Decreased free protein S levels in polycythemia vera. *Thromb Haemost* 64:177, 1990.

Fibrinolytic Defects
and Thrombosis

Defects in the fibrinolytic system have been associated with both venous and arterial thrombosis. Hereditary disorders include deficiencies of plasminogen and tissue plasminogen activator (t-PA), excessive levels of plasminogen activator inhibitor (PAI), and several of the dysfibrinogenemias. Acquired causes of impaired fibrinolysis may be substantially more common, but they have not yet been well characterized. An example is the elevated concentrations of plasma PAI that have been linked to premature myocardial infarction in young men. High levels of the inhibitor also occur following infusions of bacterial endotoxin or the inflammatory cytokine tumor necrosis factor (TNF) into human volunteers.

PATHOGENESIS

Decreased or Dysfunctional Plasminogen

At least 30 families have been reported with hereditary abnormalities of plasminogen synthesis. Half these individuals had decreases in both plasminogen activity and antigen (type I), and the remainder had dysfunctional proteins caused by a variety of defects that usually involved the active center of the protein (type II). All the patients have been heterozygous for the disorder; homozygotes who have very low or absent plasminogen function have not been reported.

Reduced Synthesis of Plasminogen Activators

A few patients have been discovered who have low circulating levels of t-PA or u-PA and a history of thrombosis. Plasma concentrations of plasminogen activator failed to rise following venous occlusion or fibrinolytic stimulation with DDAVP. In one patient, von Willebrand factor increased as expected, which suggested that a general endothelial cell release defect was not responsible for the low post-DDAVP levels of t-PA.

High Resting Levels of Plasma Plasminogen Activator Inhibitor

Because PAI behaves as an acute phase reactant, elevated concentrations of PAI antigen or activity in the blood are rather common. Circulating PAI is bound to vitronectin, which protects the inhibitor from inactivation and perhaps helps to target the fibrinolytic inhibitor to sites of vascular injury. The results of a novel experiment have recently been reported, suggesting that elevated levels of PAI are thrombogenic. Transgenic mice were created that synthesized high levels of plasma PAI-1 shortly after birth. The animals developed venous (but not arterial) thrombi in the tail veins and hind limbs, which later regressed when plasma PAI levels fell back to normal (Fig. 42-1).

The plasma concentration of PAI is directly related to levels of circulating triglyceride. The mechanisms responsible for this association are unknown.

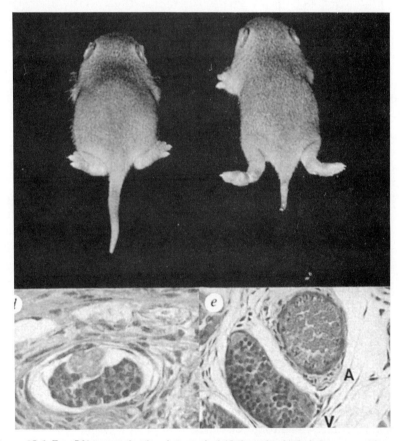

Figure 42-1 Top. PAI transgenic mice photographed 12 days after birth. Left, mouse with normal tail and hind feet; right, transgenic mouse showing necrosis and sloughing of tail and swollen hind feet. Lower left. Histologic cross section through tail vein. Lower right. Section through swollen hind foot. The vein (v) is occluded; the artery (A) appears normal. (Reprinted with permission from Nature 346:74, 1990, copyright 1990 MacMillan Magazines Limited.)

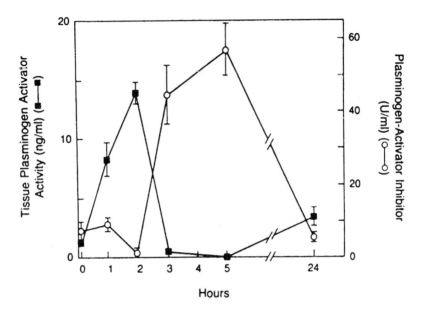

Figure 42-2 Mean levels of t-PA activity and PAI activity in four patients given intravenous endotoxin. (Reprinted with permission of The New England Journal of Medicine, 320:1165, 1989.)

In vitro experiments have suggested that very low density lipoprotein (which is rich in triglyceride) stimulates the release of PAI from cultured human umbilical vein endothelial cells.

Bacterial endotoxin and the cytokine TNF stimulate the release of PAI from vascular endothelial cells in culture. When these agents are infused into human volunteers, PAI levels rise and remain increased for several hours following an early burst of t-PA activity that lasts for < 3 hours (Fig. 42-2). These studies raise the possibility that impaired fibrinolysis might be involved in the thrombotic diathesis that sometimes accompanies sepsis or endotoxin shock.

Dysfibrinogenemias

Hundreds of mutations have been discovered that involve the fibrinogen molecule. Most of the dysfibrinogenemias produce bleeding, but 10 to 15 percent of the defects are associated with thrombosis (see Chap. 19). In a few cases, hemorrhage and thrombosis can both occur if the plasma concentration of the dysfunctional fibrinogen is low.

Some of the dysfibrinogenemias predispose to thrombosis because the abnormal fibrinogen generates fibrin that is resistant to fibrinolysis. One of these abnormal fibrinogens forms plasma clots that fail to lyse when they are placed in a solution that contains plasmin and has been designated fibrinogen Chapel Hill III (Fig. 42-3). Other fibrinogens produce fibrin that is unable to bind t-PA. Yet another fibrinogen (Milano II) cannot bind thrombin, so that higher residual concentrations of thrombin react with normal fibrinogen and accelerate thrombogenesis. Many dysfunctional fibrinogen molecules associated with thrombosis produce fibrin clots that are physically rigid or appear translucent on visual inspection.

Factor XII Deficiency

Fibrinolysis occurs both on the surface of cells (endothelium or platelets) and in the plasma, where it is stimulated by activation of the intrinsic system.

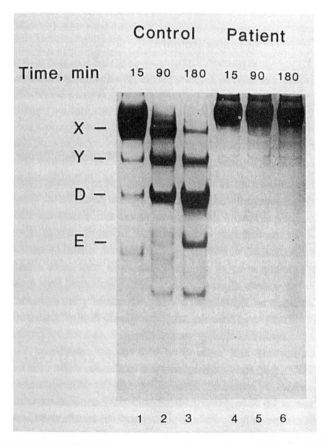

Figure 42-3 Sodium dodecyl sulfate-polyacrylamide electrophoresis of patient and control fibrin samples treated with plasmin. On the left (lanes 1, 2, and 3) multiple fibrin degradation products are formed from normal fibrin. On the right (lanes 4, 5, and 6), fibrinolysis is absent. The patient was a 16-year-old male with recurrent deep and superficial venous thrombosis and a pulmonary embolism. (Used with permission from Carrell N et al: Blood 62:439, 1983.)

Patients with severe (homozygous) deficiencies of factor XII have deficient fluid phase fibrinolysis when measured in vitro and have occasionally been reported to have venous thromboembolism (e.g., Mr. Hageman, the index patient with factor XII deficiency died of a massive pulmonary embolism following a pelvic fracture; see Chap. 17).

LABORATORY STUDIES

Unfortunately, global screening tests are not yet available to detect impairment of the fibrinolytic system. Prolongation of the euglobulin lysis time (ELT) has not proven to be a reliable indicator of defective fibrinolysis. Another approach is to stimulate vascular release of t-PA and measure shortening of the ELT (or accelerated lysis in a fibrin plate) after venous occlusion or DDAVP infusion. Failure to detect enhanced fibrinolysis after the stimulus suggests impaired fibrinolysis.

Enzyme-linked immunosorbent assays (ELISA) are now available for measurement of t-PA activity and antigen, u-PA activity, and PAI activity and antigen. These assays can be performed on plasma from individuals who are in a resting state or following stimulation of fibrinolysis by venous occlusion for 10 to 15 min or an infusion of DDAVP to measure fibrinolytic "capacity." The value of these assays for clinical study of patients with hereditary or acquired thromboembolic disease remains uncertain. Some of the difficulties inherent in these assays include dietary influences, diurnal variations in fibrinolytic activity, and inconsistent results after DDAVP or venous occlusion.

The diagnosis of dysfibrinogenemias that are associated with thrombosis relies on tests that measure the polymerization of fibrinogen. The TCT, Reptilase time, and fibrinogen assays that include both antigen and activity measurements are used to identify defects in fibrinogen function (Table 42-1).

TABLE 42-1 Laboratory Values in a 15-year-old Girl with Cerebral Sinus Vein Thrombosis

Fibrinogen (functional assay) (175–325 mg/dL)	52 mg/dL
Fibrinogen (immunologic assay) (165–350 mg/dL)	317 mg/dL
TCT (20–30 s)	>100 s
Reptilase time (12–21 s)	59.4 s

*Her mother and maternal grandmother had recurrent thrombosis and similar laboratory findings.

CLINICAL MANIFESTATIONS

Hereditary Disorders

Patients with many of the hereditary fibrinolytic defects appear to have lower rates of thromboembolism than individuals who have deficiencies of the natural anticoagulants, antithrombin III, protein C, or protein S. In many instances, a fibrinolytic defect was discovered in the propositus because of one or more episodes of thrombosis, but family members who were later shown to have the same defect have usually been asymptomatic. However, some of the dysfibrinogenemias are more strongly linked with recurrent thromboembolism.

Hereditary abnormalities of plasminogen are very uncommon. In one study from Germany, a plasminogen defect was found in only 1 of 435 patients investigated because of a history of thrombosis. Several patients with reduced generation of t-PA or u-PA after stimulation by venous occlusion or DDAVP have had severe and recurrent venous thromboembolism.

Large numbers of patients have been studied who were found to have elevated resting levels of plasma PAI and a history of thromboembolism. Some of these patients who initially had elevated levels of PAI were normal when retested at a later date. The majority of the subjects with elevated PAI did not have affected family members, and those relatives who did have raised PAI levels did not have thrombosis. In another study of patients with thromboembolism, 9 percent had increased levels of plasma PAI, but so did 9 percent of normal control patients. Lastly, when a cohort of 57 men in the Physicians' Health Study who subsequently developed venous thromboembolism were examined, none of them had elevated resting levels of PAI or decreased t-PA in stored blood samples that had been obtained 4 to 6 years earlier.

Several case reports have suggested a possible relationship between thromboembolism and homozygous factor XII deficiency. In one large study, 8.2 percent of 121 patients with severe factor XII deficiency had thrombosis, but this was similar to rates found in normal subjects. In another report, 15 percent of 103 patients with venous or arterial thrombosis were found to have a deficiency of factor XII (26 to 56 percent of normal). In 67 percent of the affected patients, a positive family history of thrombosis was established.

Acquired Abnormalities

Impaired fibrinolysis, as evidenced by elevated resting levels of plasma PAI, have been noted in several disorders. Clinical studies have shown that patients with impaired fibrinolysis preoperatively subsequently had a higher rate of venous thrombosis after hip surgery. A similar correlation was found when elevated PAI levels were discovered immediately after surgery. Because these findings could be clinically important, additional study is needed to determine if prophylactic antithrombotic therapy would be useful for individual patients with deficient fibrinolysis.

Several provocative reports have suggested that young (< 45 years) male survivors of myocardial infarction have increased PAI levels and a higher rate of subsequent early, but not late, reinfarction. In many of these patients, elevations in PAI were associated with high levels of plasma triglycerides, which raises the question as to whether hypertriglyceridemia might be an important risk factor for atherosclerosis or thrombosis. However, several recent large cross-sectional studies failed to document a relationship between increased resting PAI and the likelihood or extent of coronary heart disease.

MANAGEMENT

Patients with acute thrombosis and evidence of impaired fibrinolysis (e.g., decreased plasminogen, dysfibrinogenemia), should be treated as usual with heparin followed by oral anticoagulants. Sufficient data are not yet available to determine if defects in fibrinolysis pose a long-term risk of thrombosis, and therefore should be considered an indication for indefinite anticoagulant therapy. Until more information is available, it seems prudent to continue anticoagulants in these patients, assuming the risks of therapy are not excessive. If asymptomatic relatives are also found to have laboratory evidence of impaired fibrinolysis, elective anticoagulation is probably not routinely indicated, given the low rates of thrombosis reported in these patients. Prophylactic antithrombotic therapy for surgery is recommended in both patients and their affected relatives.

Little data are available to help decide whether or not to treat patients with acquired defects of fibrinolysis. Aggressive prophylactic therapy (e.g., anticoagulants, leg compression) prior to orthopedic or general surgery in patients with elevated levels of PAI or who have clinical conditions often linked with impaired fibrinolysis seems appropriate (i.e., obesity, smokers, or diabetes). Whether young patients with myocardial infarction and evidence of impaired fibrinolysis might be better treated with long-term anticoagulants than with antiplatelet therapy is unknown.

BIBLIOGRAPHY

Carrell N et al: Hereditary dysfibrinogenemia in a patient with thrombotic disease. *Blood* 62:439, 1983.

Engesser L et al: Elevated plasminogen activator inhibitor (PAI), a cause of thrombophilia? A study in 203 patients with familial or sporadic venous thrombophilia. *Thromb Haemost* 62:673, 1989.

Erickson LA et al: Development of venous occlusions in mice transgenic for the plasminogen activator inhibitor-1 gene. *Nature* 346:74, 1990.

Halbmayer WM et al: The prevalence of factor XII deficiency in 103 orally anti-coagulated outpatients suffering from recurrent venous and/or arterial thromboembolism. *Thromb Haemost* 68:285, 1992.

Lammle B et al: Thromboembolism and bleeding tendency in congenital factor XII deficiency—A study on 74 subjects from 14 Swiss families. *Thromb Haemost* 65:117, 1991.

Levi M et al: Deep vein thrombosis and fibrinolysis. Defective urokinase type plasminogen activator release. *Thromb Haemost* 66:426, 1991.

Levi M et al: Reduction of contact activation related fibrinolytic activity in factor XII deficient patients. *J Clin Invest* 88:1155, 1991.

Nguyen G et al: Residual plasminogen activator inhibitor activity after venous stasis as a criterion for hypofibrinolysis: A study in 83 patients with confirmed deep vein thrombosis. *Blood* 72:601, 1988.

Petaja J et al: Familial hypofibrinolysis and venous thrombosis. *Br J Haematol* 71:393, 1989.

Prins MH, Hirsh J: A critical review of the evidence supporting a relationship between impaired fibrinolytic activity and venous thromboembolism. *Arch Intern Med* 151:1721, 1991.

Prins MH, Hirsh J: A critical review of the relationship between impaired fibrinolysis and myocardial infarction. *Am Heart J* 122:545, 1991.

Ridker PM et al: Baseline fibrinolytic state and the risk of future venous thrombosis. A prospective study of endogenous tissue-type plasminogen activator and plasminogen activator inhibitor. *Circulation* 85:1822, 1992.

Robbins KC: Dysplasminogenemias. *Prog Cardiovas Dis* 34:295, 1992.

Suffredini AF et al: Promotion and subsequent inhibition of plasminogen activation after administration of intravenous endotoxin to normal subjects. *N Engl J Med* 320:1165, 1989.

Winman B, Hamsten A: The fibrinolytic enzyme system and its role in the etiology of thromboembolic disease. *Semin Thromb Hemost* 16:207, 1990.

Antiphospholipid

Antibodies

Antiphospholipid antibodies (APA) are autoantibodies directed against antigens that are composed, at least in part, of negatively charged phospholipids. Clinically important APA include the lupus anticoagulant (LA), anticardiolipin antibodies (ACA), and the antibodies responsible for the false positive VDRL test. The term LA is somewhat misleading because these antibodies occur in many clinical settings other than systemic lupus erythematosus (SLE), and the "anticoagulant" exerts its effect in vitro (e.g., prolongation of the APTT), rather than causing excessive bleeding.

The APA have received considerable attention from the medical community because of their association with a number of serious clinical disorders that include arterial and venous thromboembolism, thrombocytopenia, recurrent pregnancy loss, acute ischemic encephalopathy, and skin lesions such as livido reticularis.

PATHOGENESIS

Although the name APA implies that the antibodies are directed toward phospholipid, the true antigenic determinants are undoubtedly more complex. Laboratory assays for ACA, and possibly the LA as well, require a protein called β_2-glycoprotein I. β_2-glycoprotein I is an apolipoprotein (formerly termed apolipoprotein H) which binds avidly to negatively charged phospholipids and may be involved in a variety of important biochemical pathways in vivo, such as the inhibition of platelet activation and coagulation.

The physical structure of the phospholipids used in the assays is also important. For example, ACA recognize negatively charged phospholipids when they take on a lamellar (platelike) configuration, whereas the LA reacts more strongly with phospholipids when they assume a hexagonal form (Fig. 43-1). ACA and LA are distinct antibodies that can be chromatographically separated. The antigens recognized in vivo by these antibodies (if any) are

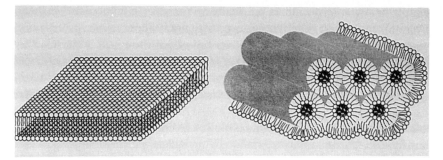

Figure 43-1 Structure of phospholipid antigens for ACA and LA. (Used with permission from Rauch J et al: Thromb Haemost 62:896, 1989.)

unknown. In this regard, it should be recalled that phospholipids with a negative charge are located on the inner surface of intact cell membranes and therefore should not be available to bind to circulating APA in vivo. The origin of APA is also a matter of conjecture; possibilities include: bacterial or viral infections, an abnormal immunoglobulin gene, autoimmune disease, or the exposure of new antigens that arise from cell injury and liberation of acidic phospholipids.

The relationship of APA to vascular thrombosis has been a challenging research problem. Retrospective, cross-sectional, and a few prospective clinical studies have established that the LA and ACA are significantly associated with thromboembolism in patients with SLE. However, the nature of this association is not well understood. For example, APA could *cause* thrombosis (e.g., through interference with a natural anticoagulant or fibrinolytic mechanism), could be a *result* of vascular or other cell injury, or might

TABLE 43-1   Possible Mechanisms of Thrombosis in Patients with Antiphospholipid Antibodies

Defective inhibitors of coagulation
    Decreased conversion of protein C to activated protein C
    Reduced destruction of factors Va and VIIIa by activated protein C
    Low plasma free protein S

Increased platelet reactivity
    Reduced prostacyclin synthesis by endothelial cells (inhibition of phospholipase A$_2$)
    Antibody-induced platelet activation

Impaired fibrinolysis
    Elevated plasma plasminogen activator inhibitor

Activation of coagulation
    Tissue factor synthesis by endothelial cells

simply be a *marker* for an as yet unknown pathologic process that produces both thrombosis and the synthesis of these antibodies.

In an attempt to probe the relationship of APA to thrombosis, investigators have sought evidence that APA blocks normal antithrombotic mechanisms or stimulates thrombogenesis. Proposed mechanisms are listed in Table 43-1. As yet, however, the pathogenesis of thrombosis in patients with APA remains elusive.

LABORATORY TESTING

The ACA are measured by an enzyme-linked immunosorbent assay (ELISA) technique in microtiter plates coated with cardiolipin, a negatively charged phospholipid originally isolated from beef heart. Bovine serum is added to block nonspecific antibody binding and to provide a source of β_2-glycoprotein I. After the addition of diluted patient serum, binding of ACA to the plate is identified by the use of an enzyme linked anti-immunoglobulin antibody. Assay results are usually reported as ACA "units" that are derived from a standard curve. Because of assay variability, test results should be interpreted broadly as either normal or mildly, moderately, or markedly elevated. Antibody isotypes (IgG, IgM, and IgA) are measured and reported individually.

The LA is initially recognized by its ability to inhibit phospholipid-dependent coagulation assays such as the APTT, kaolin clotting time (KCT), or dilute Russell viper venom time (RVVT). The KCT is a sensitive screening test for the LA. It is similar to the APTT but phospholipid is not added to the reaction mixture so that the effect of the LA (an APA) is maximized in the assay. The RVVT uses a snake venom to activate factor X in the presence of bovine brain phospholipid. If the screening tests are abnormal, mixing experiments must then be performed to document the presence of an inhibitor, followed by a test to demonstrate that the inhibitor can be neutralized by excess phospholipid (Table 43-2).

Multiple assays are required (i.e., ACA and three different assays for LA) to identify as many patients as possible with APA. The battery of tests should be performed on at least two occasions 2 to 3 months apart to maximize the predictability of the assays for thrombosis or other pathologic event. Studies have shown that patients with persistently positive tests for APA are significantly more likely to suffer adverse clinical consequences than those with only transiently abnormal tests.

The APA do not cause bleeding, although several hemostatic defects can occur in patients with the LA or ACA. Immune thrombocytopenia, platelet dysfunction (prolonged bleeding time), and isolated prothrombin deficiency (due to antiprothrombin antibodies with rapid clearance of the prothrombin-antiprothrombin complexes) have all been reported in patients with APA.

TABLE 43-2 Laboratory Identification and Characterization of the Lupus Anticoagulant

The following three steps should be satisfied for a definitive diagnosis:

Step 1: Phospholipid-dependent screening tests are used to detect the presence of the LA. Examples include the APTT, KCT, and RVVT.

Step 2: A mixing study (using normal plasma) must be performed to show that the abnormal screening test is due to an inhibitor rather than a clotting factor deficiency (see Chap. 4).

Step 3: The inhibitor must be neutralized by an excess of phospholipid. Disrupted platelets (the platelet neutralization test) or hexagonal phospholipids may be used.

Prothrombin deficiency should be suspected when the PT is > 1.4 times control.

A special problem in laboratory management arises in patients with the LA who are being treated with heparin for acute thrombosis, since the APTT does not reflect the intensity of anticoagulation. In this circumstance, a heparin assay (Xa inhibition) can be used to monitor heparin therapy (target range of 0.35 to 0.7 U/mL).

CLINICAL MANIFESTATIONS

The APA are found in two broad categories of patients. Thrombosis, thrombocytopenia, and pregnancy loss are common in one group of patients (sometimes called the APA syndrome), whereas APA are usually of little clinical consequence in other individuals (e.g., normal blood donors, children with histories of infections, AIDS patients, and as a reaction to drugs, particularly phenothiazines). Nonpathologic APA are frequently low in titer, transient, and are more often IgM. In contrast, antibodies found in patients with thromboembolic disease tend to be high titer, persistent, and consist of IgG or IgA isotypes.

The medical literature is replete with case reports and small series of patients that associate APA with thrombosis. These reports can be grouped into several more or less distinct clinical scenarios.

Primary Antiphospholipid Antibody Syndrome

These patients do not have evidence of SLE or other well-defined autoimmune disorder. The syndrome often occurs in young males with high titers of APA, thrombocytopenia, and recurrent arterial and venous thromboses. Livido reticularis of the skin is common, and many patients have CNS infarction.

Recurrent Venous Thromboembolism

Deep venous thrombosis (DVT) is often associated with APA. Retrospective studies in large numbers of patients with SLE found thrombosis to be associated with APA in 42 percent of patients compared to only 13 percent of lupus patients without the antibody. A more recent cross-sectional study used multiple sensitive assays for APA and objective evidence for the presence of venous thrombosis. SLE patients with APA had a high rate of DVT (72 percent), which was significantly higher than in patients without APA (47 percent). Venous thrombosis is also common in patients with APA who do not meet criteria for a diagnosis of SLE.

Arterial Thromboembolism

The APA are frequently discovered in young patients who are evaluated for stroke or transient ischemic attacks (TIA) (Fig. 43-2). In one study, 47 percent of patients < 45 years of age who were treated for acute stroke or TIA had either LA or ACA, compared to only 8 percent of patients who were seen for other neurologic disease. CNS infarcts are frequently small (Fig. 43-3) and show no evidence of vasculitis on biopsy. The cardiac valves may be a source of cerebral emboli (see below). In some patients, recurrent CNS thrombosis leads to multi-infarct dementia (see Chap. 51).

Cardiac Valvular Disease

Vegetations composed of fibrin and platelets occur frequently on the mitral and aortic cardiac valves in patients with APA. For example, studies using transthoracic echocardiography have documented vegetations in approximately 25 percent of patients with SLE who had APA on laboratory testing. Similar findings have been reported in non-SLE patients with high titers of antibody. Transesophageal echocardiography may identify even larger numbers of patients with valvular lesions.

Recurrent Pregnancy Loss

First trimester spontaneous abortion and second trimester fetal loss have been associated with increased levels of APA in large clinical studies. The mechanisms that promote pregnancy loss are not entirely clear, but fetal wastage is most likely due to placental insufficiency as a result of thrombosis or other vascular dysfunction. Pregnancy loss is more common when APA are persistent (over 3 to 4 months) and high in titer.

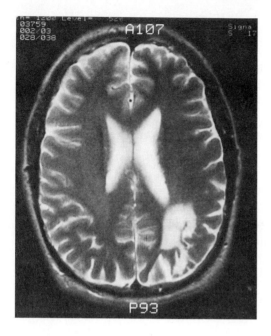

Figure 43-2 MRI scan showing a large infarct in a young man with APA.

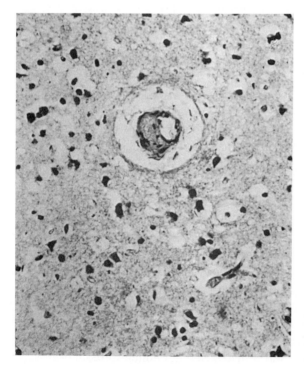

Figure 43-3 Section of brain frontal cortex obtained at autopsy that shows a platelet-fibrin thrombus within a small cerebral artery. There is no evidence of vasculitis. (H & E; $\times$ 40 before 2 percent enlargement.) (Used with permission from Briley DP et al: Ann Neurol 25:221, 1989.)

Other Associations

The APA have been associated with a wide variety of other clinical disorders caused by vascular disease including Addison's disease (adrenal cortical infarction), central abdominal vein thrombosis, primary pulmonary hypertension, livido reticularis of the skin, retinal artery occlusion, migraine headache, acute ischemic encephalopathy, and myocardial infarction in young men.

MANAGEMENT

Optimal management of patients with APA-associated thrombosis or pregnancy loss is controversial because of the lack of prospective trials of antithrombotic or other therapies. However, until more data are available, recommendations for treatment include:

1. Patients with APA who do not have a history of thrombosis should not be treated.
2. No data suggest that immunosuppressive therapy (e.g., prednisone, cyclophosphamide) protects against thrombosis.
3. Prolonged antithrombotic therapy should be strongly considered for patients who have a history of thrombosis (arterial or venous) and who have persistently elevated levels of APA.
4. The best antithrombotic agents for long-term therapy remain to be defined. One nonrandomized cohort study of 70 patients suggested that low doses of aspirin or very low intensity warfarin (INR < 2.6) did not prevent recurrent thromboembolic events in patients with APA (see Rosove reference). In contrast, higher intensity warfarin to prolong the INR to > 2.6 protected against both venous and arterial thromboembolism.
5. The optimal therapy for the prevention of recurrent pregnancy loss is also a subject of ongoing clinical trials. At present, low-dose aspirin and prednisone appear ineffective, whereas the use of heparin throughout pregnancy may be of value. However, the possibility of osteopenia or heparin-associated thrombocytopenia must be considered. Heparin therapy should not be recommended to asymptomatic patients who have APA without a history of fetal loss.
6. Immune thrombocytopenia is relatively common in patients with APA and thrombosis and usually responds to standard approaches such as corticosteroids, intravenous gamma globulin, or splenectomy. In some cases, severe thrombocytopenia must be treated before antithrombotic therapy with heparin or warfarin can be safely administered.

7. Patients with APA and a history of thrombosis who require surgery should receive prophylactic anticoagulants (see Chap. 61).

BIBLIOGRAPHY

Asherson RA et al: The "primary" antiphospholipid syndrome: Major clinical and serological features. *Medicine* 68:366, 1989.

Bajaj SP et al: A mechanism for the hypoprothrombinemia of the acquired hypoprothrombinemia-lupus anticoagulant syndrome. *Blood* 61:684, 1983.

Brey RL et al: Antiphospholipid antibodies and cerebral ischemia in young people. *Neurology* 40:1190, 1990.

Briley DP et al: Neurological disease associated with antiphospholipid antibodies. *Ann Neurol* 25:221, 1989.

Feinstein DI: Lupus anticoagulant, anticardiolipin antibodies, fetal loss, and systemic lupus erythematosus. *Blood* 80:859, 1992.

Galli M et al: Anticardiolipin antibodies (ACA) directed not to cardiolipin but to a plasma protein cofactor. *Lancet* 335:1544, 1990.

Ginsberg JS et al: Relationship of antiphospholipid antibodies to pregnancy loss in patients with systemic lupus erythematosus: A cross-sectional study. *Blood* 80:975, 1992.

Ingram SB et al: An unusual syndrome of a devastating noninflammatory vasculopathy associated with anticardiolipin antibodies: Report of two cases. *Arthritis Rheum* 30:1167, 1987.

Long AA et al: The relationship of antiphospholipid antibodies to thromboembolic disease in systemic lupus erythematosus: A cross-sectional study. *Thromb Haemost* 66:520, 1991.

Love PE, Santoro SA: Antiphospholipid antibodies: Anticardiolipin and the lupus anticoagulant in systemic lupus erythematosus (SLE) and in non-SLE disorders. *Ann Intern Med* 112:682, 1990.

McNeil HP et al: Immunology and clinical importance of antiphospholipid antibodies. *Adv Immunol* 49:193, 1991.

McNeil HP et al: Antiphospholipid antibodies are directed against a complex antigen that includes a lipid-binding inhibitor of coagulation: β_2-Glycoprotein I (apolipoprotein H). *Proc Natl Acad Sci USA* 87:4120, 1990.

Rosove B: Antiphospholipid thrombosis: Clinical course after the first thrombotic event in 70 patients. *Ann Intern Med* 117:303, 1992.

Shi W et al: Prevalence of lupus anticoagulant and anticardiolipin antibodies in a healthy population. *Aust NZ J Med* 20:231, 1990.

Triplett DA, Brandt J: Annotation. Laboratory identification of the lupus anticoagulant. *Br J Haematol* 72:139, 1989.

Myeloproliferative

Disorders and

Paroxysmal Nocturnal

Hemoglobinuria

The clinical course of patients with myeloproliferative disease (MPD) is often complicated by thrombosis or excessive bleeding. The thrombotic complications of the myeloproliferative disorders are discussed in this chapter; hemorrhagic events are covered in Chap. 34. Thrombosis is more common than bleeding in these patients. For example, in a large group of subjects with essential thrombocythemia (ET), thromboembolism occurred at a rate of 6.6 events/patient-year (compared to 1.2 in normal individuals), whereas 0.33 episodes of serious bleeding were observed per patient-year. The MPD commonly associated with thromboembolism include ET, polycythemia rubra vera (PRV), and myelofibrosis with myeloid metaplasia (MM). In contrast, chronic granulocytic leukemia (chronic phase) is not usually accompanied by thrombosis or bleeding. Peripheral and central abdominal vein thrombosis is a prominent cause of death in patients with paroxysmal nocturnal hemoglobinuria (PNH), a myeloid stem cell disorder.

PATHOGENESIS

Myeloproliferative Disorders

For the most part, thrombotic events in patients with MPD are platelet mediated, rather than a result of pathologic activation of coagulation or insufficient fibrinolysis. Although all of the MPD are commonly accompanied by thrombocytosis, abnormal function (rather than increased numbers) of platelets is more likely to be the cause of vascular occlusion. Patients with reactive thrombocytosis and normally functioning platelets (e.g., as a result of splenectomy) rarely develop thromboembolism. A wide spectrum of platelet function defects, some seemingly predictive of bleeding and others of thrombosis, have been described in patients with MPD; several of these are depicted in Fig. 44-1. Which, if any, of these disorders are responsible for arterial or venous thrombosis is not clear. The elevated concentration of red blood cells and increased blood viscosity in patients with PRV magnifies the risk of thrombosis. Erythrocytes may also enhance platelet reactivity and platelet vascular interactions.

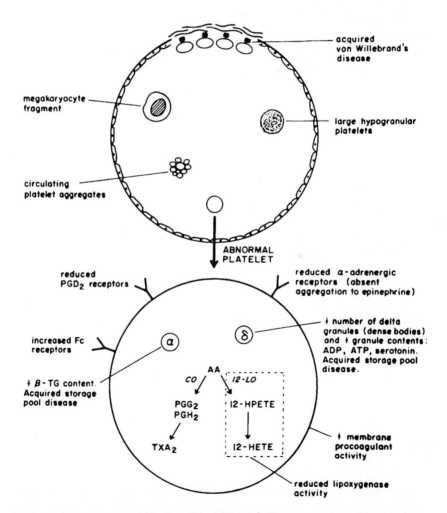

Figure 44-1 Structural, biochemical, and metabolic abnormalities in essential thrombocythemia. (Used with permission from Mitus AJ, Schafer AI: Thrombocytosis and thrombocythemia. Hematol Oncol Clin North Am 4:157, 1990.)

Notably, excessive amounts of platelet-derived growth factor (PDGF) in both plasma and urine have been found in patients with MPD, although it is uncertain whether the growth factor is released from platelets or megakaryocytes. PDGF could be involved in the genesis of marrow fibrosis seen so commonly in MPD, and may also be responsible for the vascular proliferation that occurs in the digits of patients with severe erythromelalgia (see below).

Paroxysmal Nocturnal Hemoglobinuria

The thrombotic complications of PNH are likely to be mediated by increased platelet reactivity. PNH platelets are extremely sensitive to certain aggregating agents; for example, only 1/1000 as much thrombin is required for maximal platelet aggregation in PNH as compared to normal controls. Recently, a membrane defect (related to the glycolipid anchor) has been described in peripheral blood leukocytes. PNH patients have a deficient receptor for urokinase-type plasminogen activator on monocytes and granulocytes, which could be responsible for impaired fibrinolysis and thrombosis.

CLINICAL MANIFESTATIONS

Myeloproliferative Disorders

Thromboses complicating ET, PRV, or MM involve almost all levels of the vascular tree including peripheral or abdominal veins, large arteries, and distal arterioles. Vascular occlusion occurs at some point during the course of the illness in 20 to 40 percent of patients. Although the disease is most common in older subjects, MPD occurs in younger patients as well. In one series of young adults (age < 40 years) followed for 4.5 years, half had a thrombotic episode during the course of their illness, but the event was life-threatening in < 5 percent. Certain thromboses merit special mention.

 1. *Central abdominal vein thrombosis:* Some of the vasculature in the abdomen represents a special target for thrombosis and includes the hepatic veins (Budd-Chiari syndrome) and the portal, mesenteric, and splenic veins. On occasion, thromboses of these vessels predate the diagnosis of MPD by several years. In one study of patients who presented with portal vein thrombosis, MPD was identified in 50 percent of them using erythroid colony assays as a marker (see below).
 2. *Arterial occlusion:* Patients with MPD have suffered thrombotic occlusions of almost every major artery, including myocardial infarction, peripheral artery thrombosis, and stroke. Other CNS symptoms of a vascular origin include transient ischemic attacks, amaurosis fugax, central retinal artery

thrombosis, and headache (which has been ascribed to platelet thrombi within the cerebral microcirculation).

3. Erythromelalgia: This syndrome often occurs in a subgroup of patients with MPD and consists of recurrent episodes of painful red feet (75 percent), hands (9 percent), or both (16 percent). Erythromelalgia has been associated with all forms of MPD, particularly when the platelet count is elevated. Vascular occlusion is almost certainly due to platelet clumping within the arterioles of the distal extremities. When the disorder is prolonged or severe, arteriolar inflammation, fibromuscular hyperplasia, and irreversible thrombosis can occur, culminating in necrosis of the digits (Fig. 44-2). As will be discussed later, low doses of aspirin or indomethacin often dramatically relieve symptoms of pain and erythema.

Paroxysmal Nocturnal Hemoglobinuria

The thromboses of PNH often involve peripheral veins, but frequently affect the veins of the portal and hepatic circulation as well. In one series, about 30 percent of young patients with PNH developed venous thrombosis, which included occlusion of the inferior vena cava, renal, and pelvic veins and the cerebral venous sinuses. In another report, 12 percent of 40 patients with PNH had Budd-Chiari syndrome. Thrombosis, along with infection, is a major clinical problem in patients with PNH and accounts for up to half the deaths in this disorder.

LABORATORY TESTING

The diagnosis of MPD is usually not difficult when a patient has elevation of peripheral blood counts, splenomegaly, and hypercellularity of the myeloid elements of the bone marrow. However, in some instances, thrombosis is the presenting symptom and a diagnosis of MPD is much more difficult. An examination of the peripheral blood may be normal or show only a mild elevation in platelet count, slightly abnormal platelet morphology, or a minimal left shift in the granulocyte series. In difficult cases, a peripheral blood or bone marrow erythroid colony assay can be used to establish the correct diagnosis. Erythropoietin-independent erythroid colony formation is a sensitive and specific marker for ET and PRV and is often present before changes in peripheral blood counts or enlargement of the spleen.

Other laboratory procedures such as the platelet count, platelet aggregation tests, bleeding time, spontaneous platelet aggregation, circulating platelet aggregates, or plasma levels of platelet-specific proteins (β-thromboglobulin) are rarely predictive of thrombosis. In several large series of

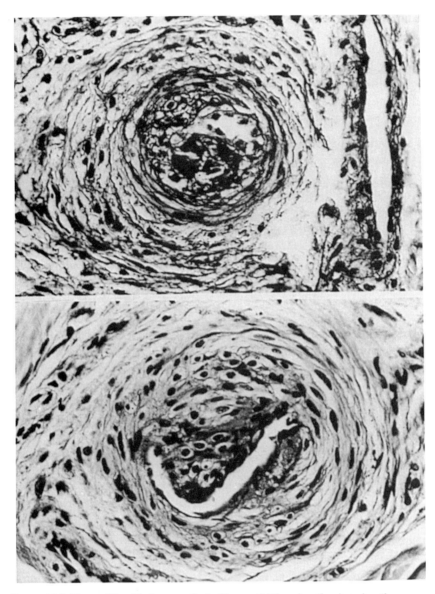

Figure 44-2 Biopsy of the skin from a patient with essential thrombocythemia and erythromelalgia. Top. Arteriole with pronounced cell proliferation of the inner layer of the media and degenerative cytoplasmatic swelling. Bottom. Thrombotic occlusions of an arteriole with proliferative vessel wall changes. (Hematoxylin and azophyloxine; original magnification × 380.) (Reproduced with permission from Michiels JJ et al: Erythromelalgia caused by platelet-mediated arteriolar inflammation and thrombosis in thrombocythemia. Ann Intern Med 102:466, 1985.)

patients, a prior history of thromboembolism was the single best indicator of future vascular occlusion.

MANAGEMENT

Myeloproliferative Disorders

Two therapeutic strategies have been used for the treatment or prevention of thromboembolism in patients with MPD: antithrombotic agents and measures to reduce the platelet count and hematocrit.

Antithrombotic Therapy

Acute thrombosis in patients with MPD is treated as usual with intravenous heparin followed by oral anticoagulants for long-term management. Early thrombolytic therapy has been successful in selected patients for lysis of thrombi that involve the hepatic or portal veins. Platelet inhibition with aspirin is often useful for treatment of microvascular thrombotic events, particularly in patients with erythromelalgia. Low doses of aspirin (e.g., 325 mg daily) can provide dramatic relief of symptoms. Aspirin is also used for treatment of transient ischemic attacks, amaurosis fugax, or sometimes headache, all of which may be due to intermittent clumping of platelets within the CNS.

Aspirin has been used for antithrombotic prophylaxis in PRV, although some patients developed upper gastrointestinal bleeding. The bleeding time has been used as a screening test to identify patients who are at increased risk of bleeding with aspirin therapy. A subgroup of patients with mild MPD have normal bleeding times before aspirin therapy, but develop prolonged bleeding times after aspirin treatment (Fig. 44-3). If aspirin is used in patients with MPD, pharmacologic measures to prevent gastric injury should be considered along with careful monitoring to detect early gastrointestinal bleeding.

Cytoreductive Therapy

A second therapeutic strategy for the prevention of vaso-occlusive events in patients with MPD is to lower elevated platelet counts. Unfortunately, the benefits (and risks) of this approach are uncertain because of the lack of controlled therapeutic trials. However, some general guidelines for management of patients with MPD are listed below.

1. Patients who are admitted to the hospital with acute vascular thrombosis and marked thrombocytosis (e.g., a platelet count > 1,000,000/μL) should receive urgent platelet apheresis to reduce platelet counts to < 500,000/μL,

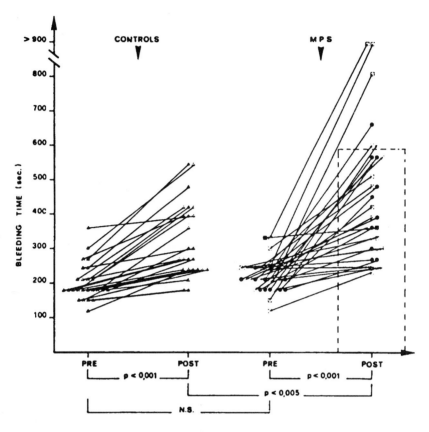

Figure 44-3 Bleeding times in 25 control subjects and 32 patients with chronic myeloproliferative syndromes (MPS) measured before (pre) and 2 h after (post) 500 mg aspirin administered intravenously. ●, polycythemia vera; ○, chronic myelogenous leukemia; □, essential thrombocythemia; ■, idiopathic myelofibrosis. Dashed line represents the normal range (mean ± 3 SD).
(Reprinted with permission from Barbui T et al: Am J Med 83:265, 1987.)

followed by hydroxyurea or other suppressive therapy to prevent rebound
thrombocytosis.

2. Patients with thrombocytosis who have a past history of thrombosis
associated with MPD should probably be treated to maintain platelet counts
at < 600,000/μL. However, it must be emphasized that there is no firm
evidence as yet that a long-term reduction in platelet count prevents future
thromboembolism.

3. Patients with known atherosclerosis or those who are at high risk for
coronary, cerebral, or peripheral vascular disease should probably be treated
to reduce platelet counts to 600,000/μL or less.

4. Young patients with MPD (i.e., < 45 years) pose an even greater
therapeutic dilemma. Thromboembolic events are known to occur in un-

treated young patients with marked thrombocytosis, but it is not known whether cytoreductive therapy prevents future thrombosis. Since cytoreductive therapy must be given for many years, side effects or complications of the medications are of major concern. Children are not usually treated because of the long-term risks of therapy and because spontaneous remissions have been reported.

Therapeutic Agents

In the past, alkylating agents such as busulfan or radionuclides such as radioactive phosphorus (^{32}P) were used to lower platelet counts in patients with MPD. These modalities are rarely used because of their leukemogenic potential. Oral hydroxyurea is now commonly recommended in doses of 500 to 1500 mg daily. Rates of malignancy (particularly acute leukemia) are not known to be increased in patients treated with hydroxyurea as compared to control populations with similar MPD. However, longer follow-up in treated and control populations is needed. Some patients become refractory to hydroxyurea and others develop painful skin lesions as a complication of therapy.

Two new drugs are currently under study for treatment of patients with thrombocytosis due to MPD. Anagrelide impairs megakaryocyte maturation and platelet production, and in clinical trials, reduced the platelet count in 93 percent of patients. Anagrelide does not decrease white blood cells, but lowers the hematocrit by about 10 percent in one third of patients. Other side effects include cardiac palpitations (36 percent), fluid retention (24 percent), and gastrointestinal symptoms (35 percent). In one large series, 16 percent of patients discontinued the medication because of side effects. Anagrelide may be useful for patients who fail treatment or who develop unacceptable side effects with hydroxyurea.

Interferon-a (IFN-a) lowers the platelet count in up to 85 percent of patients with MPD, but in contrast to anagrelide, regularly reduces leukocyte counts and hematocrit. IFN-a impairs platelet production and also shortens platelet survival. Side effects include flulike symptoms which limit treatment in about 25 percent of patients.

Paroxysmal Nocturnal Hemoglobinuria

Anticoagulants are the mainstay of therapy for venous thrombosis in patients with PNH. Early thrombolytic treatment has been successful in some patients who present with acute hepatic vein thrombosis. In others, portal-systemic shunting will be required to lower portal vein pressures and reduce bleeding from esophageal varices. Peritoneal-venous shunts for treatment of ascites often fail in PNH because of repeated thrombotic occlusion of the catheter.

BIBLIOGRAPHY

Anagrelide Study Group: Anagrelide, a therapy for thrombocythemic states: Experience in 577 patients. *Am J Med* 92:69, 1992.

Barbui T et al: Aspirin and risk of bleeding in patients with thrombocythemia. *Am J Med* 83:265, 1987.

Gersuk GM et al: Platelet-derived growth factor concentrations in platelet-poor plasma and urine from patients with myeloproliferative disorders. *Blood* 74:2330, 1989.

Kurzrock R, Cohen PR: Erythromelalgia: Review of clinical characteristics and pathophysiology. *Am J Med* 91:416, 1991.

Mazur EM et al: Analysis of the mechanism of anagrelide-induced thrombocytopenia in humans. *Blood* 79:1931, 1992.

McIntyre KJ et al: Essential thrombocythemia in young adults. *Mayo Clin Proc* 66:149, 1991.

Michiels JJ et al: Erythromelalgia caused by platelet-mediated arteriolar inflammation and thrombosis in thrombocythemia. *Ann Intern Med* 102:466, 1985.

Mitus AJ et al: Hemostatic complications in young patients with essential thrombocythemia. *Am J Med* 88:371, 1990.

Ploug M et al: The receptor for urokinase-type plasminogen activator is deficient on peripheral blood leukocytes in patients with paroxysmal nocturnal hemoglobinuria. *Blood* 79:1447, 1992.

Schafer AI: Essential thrombocythemia. *Prog Hemost Thromb* 10:69, 1991.

Silver RT: Interferon in the treatment of myeloproliferative diseases. *Semin Hematol* 27:6, 1990.

Silverstein MN et al: Anagrelide: A new drug for treating thrombocytosis. *N Engl J Med* 318:1292, 1988.

Valla D et al: Primary myeloproliferative disorder and hepatic vein thrombosis. *Ann Intern Med* 103:329, 1985.

Valla D et al: Hepatic vein thrombosis in paroxysmal nocturnal hemoglobinuria. A spectrum from asymptomatic occlusion of hepatic venules to fatal Budd-Chiari syndrome. *Gastroenterology* 93:569, 1987.

Wadenvik H et al: The effect of a-interferon on bone marrow megakaryocytes and platelet production rate in essential thrombocythemia. *Blood* 77:2103, 1991.

Other Potential Causes
of Thrombosis

HEREDITARY DISORDERS

Heparin Cofactor II Deficiency

Heparin Cofactor II (HCII) is a glycoprotein of the serpin (serine protease inhibitor) family that inhibits thrombin, but in contrast to antithrombin III (AT III), has little activity against factor X_a or other activated clotting factors. Both dermatan sulfate and the high molecular weight fractions of heparin are capable of dramatically increasing the antithrombin activity of HCII (i.e., more than 1000-fold). Plasma levels of HCII are low at birth (approximately 50 percent) but reach adult levels of 100 percent by 6 months of age. Reduced concentrations are found in patients with liver disease and disseminated intravascular coagulation, whereas elevated levels are observed in renal disease with proteinuria, pregnancy, and women using oral contraceptive agents. Plasma HCII is not altered by heparin or warfarin therapy.

Data have been reported on several patients who had reduced (e.g., 50 percent) levels of HCII activity in their plasma in association with venous thromboembolism. In some cases, close family members also had low levels of the anticoagulant along with a history of thrombosis. Large screening studies of patients with recurrent thromboembolism have yielded an incidence of HCII deficiency of 1 to 2 percent, but a similar rate (1 percent) was found in normal blood donors. Therefore, it is not clear that HCII deficiency poses a major risk for thrombosis. Based on this data, routine screening of thrombosis patients for HCII deficiency is probably not warranted.

Histidine-rich Glycoprotein

Histidine-rich glycoprotein (HRG) is a single chain plasma protein with a molecular weight of 75 kd that is enriched in the amino acids histidine and proline (12 percent by weight). It is synthesized in the liver and behaves as a "negative" acute phase reactant; plasma concentrations fall during stress or inflammation. The glycoprotein binds to highly charged molecules such as heparin, thrombospondin, and perhaps most importantly, to lysine binding sites of plasminogen. Plasma levels (normal, 10 mg/dL) are reduced in patients with sepsis, systemic lupus erythematosus, pregnancy, oral contraceptive agents, acute myocardial infarction, and severe liver disease. Newborns have low plasma concentrations of HRG which can be 20 to 30 percent of normal in preterm infants, with an increase to adult levels by 6 months of age.

Because it binds to plasminogen, elevated levels of HRG could inhibit fibrinolysis by preventing the interaction of plasminogen with fibrin. HRG also binds heparin so that less of the anticoagulant might be available to activate AT III. One patient has been reported with abnormally high levels of HRG who suffered recurrent venous thromboembolism and a myocardial infarction. Elevated levels were found in family members, some of whom also had thrombosis. Stressed newborns have increased concentrations of HRG in their plasma although this finding has not been directly related to thrombosis.

Tissue Factor Pathway Inhibitor

Tissue factor pathway inhibitor (TFPI; previously termed extrinsic pathway inhibitor [EPI] and lipoprotein-associated coagulation inhibitor [LACI]) is a lipoprotein (most likely synthesized by endothelial cells) that inhibits factor VIIa in the presence of factor Xa (which acts as a cofactor; Fig. 45-1). TFPI is found in plasma (54 to 142 ng/mL), in platelets (8 ng/mL), and on the surfaces of vascular endothelium in much larger amounts. Following an injection of heparin, plasma levels of TFPI rapidly increase to 220 to 800 ng/mL (Fig. 45-2). Heparin-released TFPI is structurally different from the protein usually found in plasma and normally exists bound to glycosaminoglycans on endothelial cell surfaces.

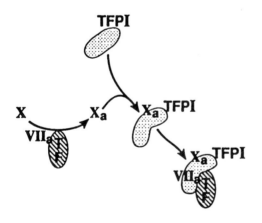

Figure 45-1 A schematic representation of how the beginning catalytic activity of factor VIIa/tissue factor complexes may initiate a two-step reaction that inhibits further factor VIIa/tissue factor catalytic activity. (Used with permission from Rapaport SI: Thromb Haemost 66:6, 1991.)

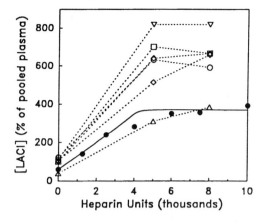

Figure 45-2 Dose-response curves for lipoprotein-associated coagulation inhibitor (tissue factor pathway inhibitor) for seven healthy adult males injected with varying doses of intravenous heparin on different days. Plasma samples were drawn before injection and 6 min after heparin injection. (Used with permission from Novotny WF et al: Blood 78:387, 1991.)

Plasma concentrations of TFPI are normal in patients with end-stage liver disease, acute thrombosis, the lupus anticoagulant, primary pulmonary hypertension, and during warfarin therapy. Some, but not all patients with gram-negative sepsis and disseminated intravascular coagulation have reduced plasma levels. Since TFPI is a lipoprotein, patients with homozygous abetalipoproteinemia have very low plasma levels of the inhibitor, and yet do not have thrombosis, suggesting that plasma TFPI is not an important circulating anticoagulant. Elevated levels of TFPI have been found in women during the early stages of labor, in patients during intravenous infusion of tissue plasminogen activator (t-PA), and as mentioned, following intravenous heparin.

Screening of large series of patients with thromboembolism for low levels of TFPI has been unrewarding. However, since most TFPI is located on the vascular endothelium, it may be more appropriate to study this pool of the lipoprotein, perhaps by stimulation of its release with heparin and measurement of its appearance in the plasma.

Homocysteinemia

Homocysteine (HC) is a thiol-containing amino acid that is produced by demethylation of methionine. Its concentration in body fluids is regulated by an enzyme, cystathionine β-synthase, which converts HC to its breakdown products, mixed disulfides. An autosomal recessive condition, homocysteinuria, is most often due to a severe deficiency of this enzyme, and results in premature atherosclerosis and arterial or venous thromboembolism as well as mental retardation, ectopic lens, and skeletal abnormalities.

The mechanisms underlying the predisposition for vascular disease in homocysteinuria are not entirely clear, but research studies have suggested that HC can damage vascular endothelium, accelerate platelet consumption, and stimulate vascular smooth muscle cell proliferation. In vitro, HC has been shown to activate clotting factors on the surface of endothelial cells, inhibit both the cell surface expression of thrombomodulin and the activation of protein C, and to oxidize low-density lipoproteins (LDL). The homozygous disorder, homocysteinuria, is rare, but laboratory tests are now sufficiently sensitive (high performance liquid chromatography) to accurately measure HC in plasma samples and to identify patients who are heterozygous for deficiency of cystathionine β-synthase.

Recently, a series of cross-sectional studies in patients with atherosclerotic vascular disease have found that substantial proportions of these individuals have elevated plasma levels of HC (Fig. 45-3). Representative frequencies of elevated HC concentrations in these disorders are 42.5 percent of patients with cerebrovascular disease, 28 percent of patients with peripheral vascular disease, and 30 percent of patients with cardiovascular disease. These figures should be compared to uniformly normal HC levels in large groups of control subjects. Measurement of cystathionine β-synthase activity and family studies have documented the enzymatic defect and hereditary nature of this disorder in subsets of these (heterozygous) subjects. The finding of elevated plasma levels of HC in patients with atherosclerosis is intriguing. Additional research must determine whether affected patients have more rapid progression of vascular occlusive disease, whether rates of thrombosis relative to atherosclerosis are increased, and whether therapeutic agents such as folic acid or pyridoxine, known to lower plasma levels of HC, will be of benefit.

Not all increases in plasma HC are due to hereditary defects of cystathionine β-synthase. High levels can also occur as a result of abnormalities in other enzyme systems responsible for HC metabolism: less than optimal intakes of folate, vitamin B_{12}, or vitamin B_6; abnormal renal function; and following therapy with bile acid sequestrants plus niacin.

At present, it has not been established whether the screening of patients for elevated levels of HC is useful. However, since simple, safe, and low-cost therapy (folic acid, pyridoxine) is available to lower plasma levels of HC, testing might be considered in individual patients with premature arterial occlusive disease.

Lipoprotein(a)

Lipoprotein(a) [LP(a)] is a macromolecular complex composed of an LDL-like particle that contains a high molecular weight protein, apo(a), bound to apolipoprotein B. Apo(a) has a remarkable molecular similarity to plasminogen, since it contains numerous copies (e.g., 37) of the characteristic kringle 4 domains of plasminogen (Fig. 45-4). Elevated levels of LP(a) are under genetic control and have been strongly associated with accelerated athero-

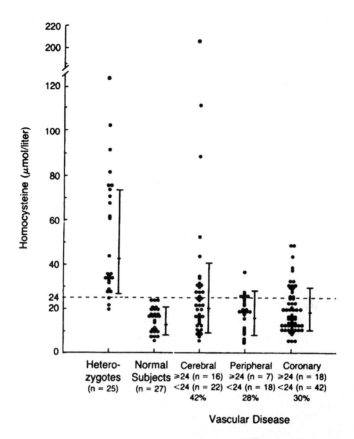

Figure 45-3 Serum homocysteine concentrations following methionine loading in obligate hetero-zygotes for cystathionine β-synthase deficiency, normal subjects, and patients with atherosclerosis. (Reprinted by permission of the New England Journal of Medicine 324:1149, 1991.)

genesis, particularly when associated with high concentrations of LDL or decreased high density lipoprotein (HDL) cholesterol. LP(a) is not present in the normal arterial wall but is abundant in atherosclerotic lesions.

Laboratory studies have shown that LP(a) inhibits fibrinolysis. Because of its similarity to plasminogen, it effectively competes with plasminogen for binding to fibrin or endothelial cells. LP(a) also binds to t-PA and, in one study, was shown to stimulate the expression and release of plasminogen activator inhibitor 1 (PAI-1) from vascular endothelial cells. Inhibition of fibrinolysis could promote fibrin deposition within or on the surface of atherosclerotic lesions, with acceleration of the atherogenic process and promotion of thrombosis on the surface of atherosclerotic plaques. However, the links between impaired fibrinolysis and atherosclerosis or thrombosis remain to be proved in man.

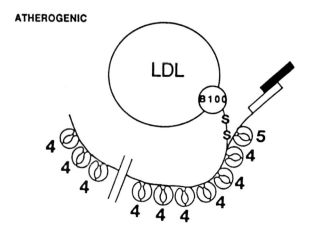

ATHEROGENIC

THROMBOGENIC

Figure 45-4 Schematic of lipoprotein(a) structure. Low-density lipoprotein (LDL) sites postulated to be atherogenic and the apolipoprotein(a) [apo(a)] sites postulated to be thrombogenic are shown. Apolipoprotein(a) is bound to apolipoprotein B-100 (B100) by disulfide (S-S) linkage. Numbers 4 and 5 refer to the types of kringles. (Reproduced with permission from Scanu AM et al: Lipoprotein(a) and atherosclerosis. Ann Intern Med 115:209, 1991.)

Few therapies are available for reduction of elevated levels of LP(a) in the plasma, since hydroxymethylglutaryl coenzyme A reductase inhibitors (e.g., lovastatin) and fibric acid derivatives are ineffective. High doses of nicotinic acid and extracorporeal apheresis may be of some benefit in selected subjects. Before routine screening for elevated LP(a) in patients with atherosclerotic or thrombotic disease can be recommended, assays need to be standardized, treatment programs devised, and evidence obtained that therapy modifies the course of the disease. In patients found to have elevated levels, therapy for other atherosclerotic risk factors is warranted and should include aggressive lowering of elevated levels of LDL cholesterol; increasing HDL cholesterol; and treating hypertension, diabetes, tobacco abuse, or obesity.

ACQUIRED DISORDERS

Behçet's Syndrome

Behçet's syndrome is an unusual disorder of unknown etiology that produces recurrent oral and genital ulceration and relapsing iridocyclitis. Small vessel vasculitis is frequent and 25 to 35 percent of patients develop large vessel vasculopathies. Some of the vascular complications include arterial aneurysms, particularly of the aorta, but also pulmonary, femoral, popliteal and carotid arteries. Aneurysmal rupture is the leading cause of death in these patients. Venous thromboembolism is common and develops in 30 to 40 percent of patients. In addition to classic deep venous thrombosis of the extremities, unusual venous thromboses such as cerebral sinus vein thrombosis (in up to 10 percent of patients), superficial thrombophlebitis, and occlusion of the inferior vena also occur. On occasion, clots extend from the inferior vena cava into the hepatic vein producing an acute Budd-Chiari syndrome. Thrombosis is caused in part by inflammation of the blood vessels.

Additional mechanisms have been invoked to help explain the predisposition to thrombosis in these patients. Some investigators have found impaired fibrinolysis, elevated levels of plasma clotting factors (e.g., fibrinogen, von Willebrand factor), abnormal platelet function including increased platelet aggregation to adenosine diphosphate, decreased vascular production of prostacyclin on venous biopsy, and decreased platelet sensitivity to prostacyclin. Although chronic anticoagulant therapy is of help in some patients, others fail to respond, perhaps as a result of severe vascular inflammation.

Inflammatory Bowel Disease

Patients with inflammatory bowel disease such as ulcerative colitis or Crohn's disease have been reported to have increased rates of venous and arterial thrombosis which are more common when the disease is active or in the presence of other precipitating events (e.g., surgery). A variety of hematologic abnormalities reflecting acute inflammation such as thrombocytosis and elevated levels of fibrinogen and von Willebrand factor have been noted in these patients. A few patients have AT III deficiency, which appears to correlate with disease activity.

Recent studies have found evidence of impaired fibrinolysis, such as elevated circulating plasma levels of PAI. Another report described a patient with an acquired deficiency of free protein S. However, these findings could simply reflect chronic inflammation because PAI is an acute phase reactant and inflammation elevates C4b-binding protein with a shift of free protein S to the bound form.

Management of these patients involves standard anticoagulation therapy with aggressive antithrombotic prophylaxis with anticoagulants and leg compression during surgical procedures such as bowel resection. Since thrombotic events are often associated with disease activity, consideration should be given to stopping antithrombotic therapy if the disease enters remission.

Nephrotic Syndrome

Thrombosis is a common complication of the nephrotic syndrome. In one reported series, renal vein thrombosis occurred in 35 percent and venous thromboembolism in 20 percent of patients with membranous nephropathy (Llach reference). Arterial occlusions have also been reported. The causes of the hypercoagulable state associated with nephrosis are not known with certainty. However, two likely mechanisms are AT III deficiency (due to loss in the urine) and lowered levels of free protein S (due to loss of functional protein in the urine and elevated C4b-binding protein in the plasma). Other possibilities include high plasma concentrations of fibrinogen and factor VIII, increased platelet reactivity, and hyperlipidemia. Hemoconcentration, lower extremity edema, and physical inactivity may also predispose to thrombosis. Management involves treatment of the renal disease and standard anticoagulation therapy.

BIBLIOGRAPHY

Bertina RM et al: Hereditary heparin cofactor II deficiency and the risk of development of thrombosis. *Thromb Haemost* 57:196, 1987.

Broze GJ et al: The lipoprotein-associated coagulation inhibitor. *Prog Hemost Thromb* 10:243, 1991.

Clarke R et al: Hyperhomocysteinemia: An independent risk factor for vascular disease. *N Engl J Med* 324:1149, 1991.

Conlan MG et al: Prothrombotic abnormalities in inflammatory bowel disease. *Digest Dis Sci* 34:1089, 1989.

Corrigan JJ Jr, Jeter MA: Tissue-type plasminogen activator, plasminogen activator inhibitor, and histidine-rich glycoproteins in stressed human newborns. *Pediatrics* 89:43, 1992.

Engesser L et al: Familial elevation of plasma histidine-rich glycoprotein in a family with thrombophilia. *Br J Haematol* 67:355, 1987.

Hayashi T et al: An atherogenic stimulus homocysteine inhibits cofactor activity of thrombomodulin and enhances thrombomodulin expression in human umbilical vein endothelial cells. *Blood* 79:2930, 1992.

Koc Y et al: Vascular involvement in Behçet's disease. *J Rheumatol* 19:402, 1992.

Lentz SR, Sadler JE: Inhibition of thrombomodulin surface expression and protein C activation by the thrombogenic agent homocysteine. *J Clin Invest* 88:1906, 1991.

Llach F: Hypercoagulability, renal vein thrombosis, and other thrombotic complications of nephrotic syndrome. *Kidney Int* 28:429, 1985.

Nachman RL: Thrombosis and atherogenesis: Molecular connections. *Blood* 79:1897, 1992.

Peterson CB et al: Histidine-rich glycoprotein modulation of the anticoagulant activity of heparin. Evidence for a mechanism involving competition with both antithrombin and thrombin for heparin binding. *J Biol Chem* 262:7567, 1987.

Rapaport SI: The extrinsic pathway inhibitor: A regulator of tissue factor-dependent blood coagulation. *Thromb Haemost* 66:6, 1991.

Scanu AM et al: Lipoprotein(a) and atherosclerosis. *Ann Intern Med* 115:209, 1991.

Wechsler B et al: Cerebral venous thrombosis in Behçet's disease: Clinical study and long-term follow-up of 25 cases. *Neurology* 42:614, 1992.

Heparin Associated

Thrombocytopenia

Heparin-associated thrombocytopenia (HAT) is an uncommon but some-times devastating clinical syndrome that consists of an immune-mediated fall in the platelet count in patients treated with heparin. The incidence of HAT is unknown, but it probably occurs in 1 to 3 percent of adult patients receiving heparin for a week or more. Approximately 10 to 15 percent of patients with the disorder develop arterial or venous thromboses, and of these, at least 30 percent will die or require amputation as a result of vascular occlusion. Whether HAT is increasing in frequency or whether it is simply being recognized more readily is a matter of debate. Early recognition is important because appropriate treatment may reduce both morbidity and mortality.

PATHOGENESIS

Slight drops in the platelet count occur frequently in patients given heparin; this is a benign process that is probably due to a direct interaction of some component of the heparin with platelets. However, in other patients, heparin administration incites the formation of IgG antibodies that react with heparin to form immune complexes that bind to platelet Fc receptors triggering platelet aggregation, the release reaction, and a subsequent fall in the circu-lating platelet count (Fig. 46-1). The etiology of the vascular thromboses that occur in a subgroup of patients with HAT is less well understood. Occlusion of the microvasculature by platelet aggregates is one likely cause but other mechanisms may also be involved. For example, one laboratory study sug-gested that the HAT antibody binds to heparan on the endothelial surface and stimulates the synthesis and expression of tissue factor by the endothelial cells. Why some patients only become thrombocytopenic, whereas others develop life-threatening thromboses, is not clear.

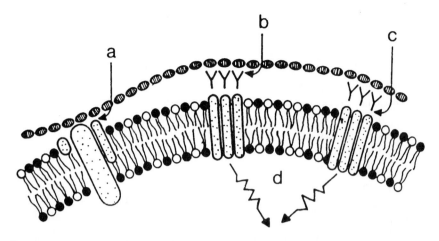

Figure 46-1 A model of heparin-platelet antibody interaction in heparin-induced thrombocyto-penia: (a) heparin becomes localized to the platelet surface by binding to platelet proteins; (b) anti-heparin IgG then binds to the repeating antigenic determinants on the heparin molecule; (c) the IgG in turn binds to platelets via the 40 kd Fc receptors, which (d) initiates platelet activation. (Used with permission from Warkentin TE, Kelton JG: Heparin and platelets. Hematol Oncol Clin North Am 4:243, 1990.)

CLINICAL MANIFESTATIONS

The fall in the platelet count associated with HAT usually develops after about 8 days (4 to 14 days) when a patient is given heparin for the first time. However, the syndrome can occur in only 1 to 3 days in patients who have had prior exposure to heparin. Reductions in platelets are variable; counts sometimes drop to rather low levels (e.g., 10,000 to 20,000/μL); but in other instances more moderate thrombocytopenia is seen especially when the platelet count was previously elevated. Although somewhat arbitrary, an abrupt decrease in the platelet count to < 100,000/μL or the sudden fall in a high platelet count by half should raise the possibility of HAT. Once heparin is stopped, the platelet count usually recovers in 2 to 5 days.

The HAT syndrome occurs not only after full therapeutic doses of heparin, but also after minidose heparin prophylaxis (e.g., 5000 U bid), or even as a consequence of the very small amounts of heparin used for flushing intravenous lines. Whether the frequency of HAT is less in patients who receive lower doses of heparin is unclear, but even small quantities may sensitize patients to the early onset of HAT after subsequent heparin exposure.

The most dramatic clinical manifestations of HAT are bleeding and thrombosis. In fact, bleeding is rather unusual, probably because the thrombocytopenia is seldom profound. Activation of platelets by the immune complexes might also transiently augment their hemostatic capacity. In contrast, the effects of thrombosis are usually sudden and devastating. Arterial, venous, and microvascular thrombosis have all been described. Arterial occlusion is the most frequent (i.e., two thirds of patients). A particularly common clinical scenario is one of microvascular occlusion of the extremities with gradually progressive gangrene that begins in the digits, progresses proximally, and ultimately leads to amputation. Peripheral arterial pulses can be intact despite the extensive tissue injury. Other thrombotic events include stroke, myocardial infarction, and mesenteric artery occlusion.

Heparin-associated thrombocytopenia has rarely (see Potter reference) been documented in infants and children even though the use of heparin, especially in sick infants and after cardiopulmonary bypass, has been substantial. Reasons for this clinical observation include (1) infrequent use of heparin for more than a few days; (2) failure to monitor the platelet count; (3) underdeveloped immune system in infants; and (4) lack of other risk factors for complicating thrombosis in children.

LABORATORY TESTING

A recent unexpected fall in the platelet count in patients treated with heparin is usually the first indication of the HAT syndrome. Clinical criteria for a diagnosis of HAT based on the magnitude, incremental fall, or timing of thrombocytopenia are not well established. Because thrombocytopenia is so common in acutely ill hospitalized patients who are receiving heparin, guidelines are needed for diagnosis. One approach is to consider the possibility of HAT in patients receiving heparin who either have a fall in platelet count to < 100,000/μL or who have decreased their platelet counts by half in a period of 24 to 48 h.

Several laboratory tests have been devised to confirm the diagnosis of HAT. Most are based on the initiation of platelet aggregation or the platelet release reaction after the addition of patient plasma (as a source of HAT antibody) plus heparin to freshly isolated normal platelets. The end point of the assay is platelet aggregation in the platelet aggregometer or the release of ^{14}C-serotonin from platelet dense granules. Whatever the assay, appropriate controls must be included to avoid both false-positive and false-negative results. If available, these assays should be used to confirm the diagnosis, but additional information on test sensitivity and specificity is needed. Alternatively, clinical criteria for diagnosis can be used, although overdiagnosis is likely, given the frequency of thrombocytopenia in hospitalized patients.

Finally, another clue to the presence of HAT is an unexpected shortening of the APTT in patients receiving therapeutic concentrations of heparin for treatment of thrombosis. An explanation for this finding is the release of the a-granule protein, platelet factor 4 (PF4), into the plasma as a consequence of platelet aggregation in vivo. PF4 avidly binds heparin and neutralizes its anticoagulant activity.

MANAGEMENT

Prevention

Prevention of HAT will probably not be possible as long as heparin remains the standard parenteral anticoagulant. However, several measures can be taken to reduce the frequency of the syndrome or limit its morbidity. The use of heparin in the treatment of deep venous thrombosis should be restricted to approximately 5 days by beginning oral anticoagulants on the first day of treatment if at all possible. Secondly, many studies have shown that normal saline is equally effective as dilute heparin to maintain patency of peripheral intravenous lines, except in infants and small children where the addition of heparin to the infusate does increase the duration of patency of the indwelling catheters. The use of saline as a flush solution instead of heparin (in adults) should substantially reduce the primary exposure of patients to heparin. Finally, daily platelet counts are now being recommended for hospitalized patients who are treated with full therapeutic doses of heparin. Early identification of HAT should allow the heparin to be stopped promptly and alternative therapies instituted.

Therapy

Once a diagnosis of HAT is suspected, all sources of heparin (including flush solutions) should be immediately stopped. If the only manifestation of the disorder is mild to moderate thrombocytopenia, with no evidence of thrombosis, then simply stopping the heparin will allow the platelet count to return to normal over the next several days. If bleeding should occur (e.g., in a postoperative patient), platelet transfusions might be necessary, but they should be given only after all heparin has cleared (e.g., normal TCT) from the circulation to prevent further platelet aggregation.

If the indication for anticoagulants is strong, either as a consequence of a prior thromboembolism or because of new arterial, venous, or microvascular thrombosis accompanying HAT, then several therapeutic options should be considered. Patients with lower extremity venous thrombosis may benefit from the insertion of an inferior vena caval filter to prevent pulmonary emboli. Additional antithrombotic measures (described below) include the use of intravenous dextran, and, if available, low molecular weight heparinoid, or the snake venom, ancrod. Warfarin should be started (or continued) to provide long-term anticoagulation.

Dextran may be of some help, although no prospective clinical trials have been performed with this drug. Two new agents are currently being studied to determine their safety and efficacy for treatment of thrombosis due to HAT. A low molecular weight heparinoid (ORG 10172) has a different chemical composition than standard heparin and cross-reacts with heparin antibodies only 20 percent of the time when tested in vitro (Fig. 46-2). Alternatively, ancrod, a snake venom that exerts its antithrombotic effect by reducing plasma fibrinogen, is effective in some patients with HAT-related thrombosis. Other measures tried in a few patients include plasmapheresis to remove circulating antiheparin antibodies or immune complexes and high-dose intravenous gamma globulin. Documentation of efficacy in the form of controlled clinical trials is not yet available for these modalities.

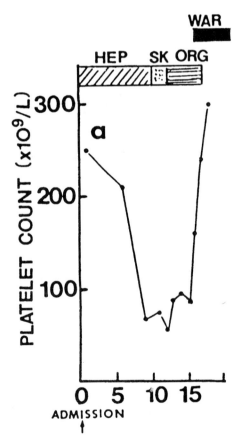

Figure 46-2 Serial platelet counts in a patient with HAT and thrombosis treated with Org 10172 (ORG). The heparinoid was given in a dose of 2400 anti-Xa U as a bolus followed by 200 U hourly for 5 days. HEP, heparin; SK, streptokinase; WAR, warfarin. (Used with permission from Chong BH et al: Blood 73:1592, 1989.)

BIBLIOGRAPHY

Anderson GP: Insights into heparin-induced thrombocytopenia. *Br J Haematol* 80:504, 1992.

Brady J et al: Plasmapheresis. A therapeutic option in the management of heparin-associated thrombocytopenia with thrombosis. *Am J Clin Pathol* 96:394, 1991.

Chong BH et al: Heparin-induced thrombocytopenia: Mechanism of interaction of the heparin-dependent antibody with platelets. *Br J Haematol* 73:235, 1989.

Chong BH et al: Heparin-induced thrombocytopenia: Studies with a new low molecular weight heparinoid, Org 10172. *Blood* 73:1592, 1989.

Cola C, Ansell J: Heparin-induced thrombocytopenia and arterial thrombosis: Alternative therapies. *Am Heart J* 119:368, 1990.

Demers C et al: Rapid anticoagulation using ancrod for heparin-induced thrombocytopenia. *Blood* 78:2194, 1991.

Kelton JG et al: Heparin-induced thrombocytopenia: Laboratory studies. *Blood* 72:925, 1988.

Ortel TL et al: Parenteral anticoagulation with the heparinoid lomoparan (Org 10172) in patients with heparin induced thrombocytopenia and thrombosis. *Thromb Haemost* 67:292, 1992.

Potter C et al: Heparin-induced thrombocytopenia in a child. *J Pediatr* 121:135, 1992.

Walls JT et al: Heparin-induced thrombocytopenia in open heart surgical patients: Sequelae of late recognition. *Ann Thorac Surg* 53:787, 1992.

Warkentin TE, Kelton JG: Heparin-induced thrombocytopenia. *Prog Hemost Thromb* 10:1, 1991.

Thrombosis and Cancer

In a widely cited paper published in 1865, Trousseau highlighted the association of malignancy and vascular thrombosis. Since then, cancer has been recognized as one of the most common acquired causes of venous and arterial thrombosis. Although thromboembolism most often accompanies advanced malignancy, superficial or deep venous thrombosis (DVT) can be an early sign of the disease.

PATHOGENESIS

The cause of the thrombosis in cancer patients is most likely related to the procoagulant activity of the malignant cells. For example, neoplastic cells can activate factor VII by a mechanism involving tissue factor, and tumor-associated mucin or cysteine proteases can directly activate factor X. Tumor cells have also been reported to shed plasma membrane vesicles that promote clot formation. Lastly, malignant cells may secrete cytokines or other products capable of activating macrophages or endothelial cells. Chemotherapeutic regimens (e.g., cyclophosphamide, methotrexate, fluorouracil) or hormonal manipulations (tamoxifen) used in the treatment of breast cancer have also been associated with increased rates of thromboembolism during early cycles of drug administration. Plasma levels of protein C and protein S are reduced in some of these patients.

Hypercoagulability in cancer patients varies widely. The majority of patients have minimal activation of hemostasis which is usually asymptomatic and is discovered only by laboratory tests such as fibrinopeptide A, a marker of thrombin generation. Moderate activation of hemostasis may present clinically as episodic venous or arterial thromboembolism, and marked stimulation could produce overt disseminated intravascular coagulation.

CLINICAL MANIFESTATIONS

Several thrombotic syndromes occur in patients with malignancy.
Migratory superficial phlebitis: The onset of thrombosis that involves the

superficial veins of the extremities, chest, or abdomen was prominent in Trousseau's patients, and is strongly suggestive of malignancy.

Classic DVT: Venous thrombosis or pulmonary embolism can occur at any time during the course of patients with cancer. One large study of patients with DVT found that 8 percent developed a malignancy at some time in the next 2 years (Fig. 47-1). Venous thrombosis is often recurrent and refractory to anticoagulation therapy.

Arterial thromboembolism: Arterial thrombosis often presents as stroke or acute peripheral artery occlusion. Vascular obstruction results either from in situ thrombosis at sites of preexisting atherosclerotic plaques or from emboli originating in the heart (see below).

Microvascular thrombosis: Small vessel occlusion of the distal extremities can result in peripheral gangrene of the fingers and toes. Although digital ischemia can be due to large vessel occlusion by thrombosis or embolism, disseminated intravascular coagulation (DIC) can also produce in situ microvascular thrombosis. Microangiopathic hemolytic anemia is common.

Nonbacterial thrombotic endocarditis: Vegetations composed of platelets and fibrin can form on mitral and aortic cardiac valves and embolize to the

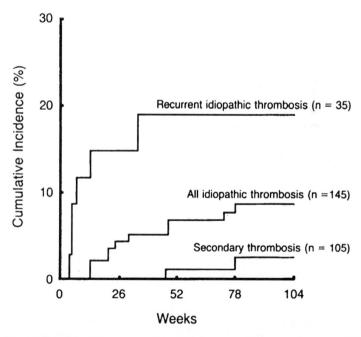

Figure 47-1 Cumulative incidence of cancer in patients with secondary thrombosis (predisposing factor), idiopathic thrombosis (no predisposing factor), and recurrent idiopathic thrombosis. (Reprinted by permission of The New England Journal of Medicine 327:1131, 1992.)

brain or other organs ("marantic endocarditis"). The kidney, spleen, liver, or extremities are other targets of the emboli.

Some cancers are more thrombogenic than others. In general, lymphoproliferative disease (e.g., lymphomas, Hodgkin's disease) rarely provoke thrombosis. Acute myeloid disorders (e.g., acute promyelocytic leukemia) are often associated with DIC, brisk fibrinolysis, and bleeding, but clinically evident venous or arterial thromboembolism is unusual. In contrast, the chronic myeloproliferative disorders are more frequently associated with thrombosis than bleeding. Most dramatic, however, are adenocarcinomas of abdominal organs such as the pancreas, stomach, or biliary tract. Small cell carcinoma of the lung is also frequently complicated by thrombosis. Advanced prostate cancer has commonly been linked to hemostatic abnormalities such as chronic DIC or systemic fibrinolysis, but arterial or venous thrombosis is rare in the early stages of the disease.

Malignancy is often advanced with metastases to the liver or other organs when it is associated with thrombosis. Less commonly, superficial venous thrombosis or DVT can be an early sign of cancer, particularly in malignancies that involve the tail of the pancreas or the biliary tract. In children, unexplained (acquired rather than hereditary) large vessel thrombosis suggests malignancies such as neuroblastoma, histocytosis, or Hodgkin's disease.

Opinions vary as to whether previously healthy patients who present to their physicians with an acute thrombosis should be examined for malignancy. Some generally accepted guidelines are as follows:

1. If a thrombosis is associated with systemic symptoms such as weight loss or new complaints that involve the chest or abdomen, additional diagnostic tests are indicated.

2. Patients with new-onset migratory superficial venous thrombosis or recurrent DVT deserve further investigation.

3. An extensive evaluation for malignancy is not warranted in other subjects who simply have an uncomplicated first episode of DVT. However, in children secondary causes should always be considered.

If investigation for malignancy is warranted, a chest radiograph, a computed tomography scan of the abdomen (and perhaps the chest in a smoker), stool for occult blood, and laboratory tests to include a carcinoembryonic antigen and α-fetoprotein should be considered. In addition, a complete blood count should be obtained and the peripheral blood smear scrutinized for signs of marrow invasion by malignant cells (e.g., circulating nucleated red blood cells or immature leukocytes). Unfortunately, little data exist to show that evaluation for malignancy in thrombosis patients will be cost effective or prolong survival.

LABORATORY TESTING

Screening tests of hemostasis in cancer patients often show elevated fibrinogen concentrations (Fig. 47-2), thrombocytosis, and a short APTT which
occurs as a result of circulating activating clotting factors or elevated levels
of factor VIII. These abnormalities often become more pronounced as the
tumor progresses. More sensitive tests that reflect activation of coagulation
and fibrinolysis are frequently abnormal. Mild to moderate elevations of
fibrinopeptide A and D-dimer are common, although markedly high levels

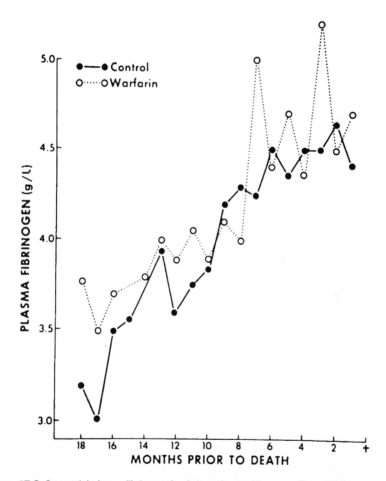

Figure 47-2 Sequential plasma fibrinogen levels in patients with cancer. The solid line represents
the mean fibrinogen level for all patients in the control group who had fibrinogen determinations
at the indicated time before death. The dashed line represents the mean fibrinogen level for anticoagulated patients (PT > 18 s) at the same time points. Plasma fibrinogen levels increased in
both groups of patients as disease progressed. (Used with permission from Edwards RL et al: Am J
Clin Pathol 88:596, 1987.)

are usually found only in patients with overt DIC. In general, tests of thrombin activation such as fibrinopeptide A and thrombin-antithrombin complexes tend to be relatively higher than those that reflect secondary fibrinolysis such as the D-dimer assay. This imbalance between thrombin and plasmin activity might help explain the predisposition to thrombosis in patients with cancer. Sophisticated tests of coagulation such as those discussed above are not useful in the diagnosis or treatment of malignancy and are usually reserved for clinical research purposes.

A leukoerythroblastic picture with circulating nucleated red blood cells or immature white cells on the peripheral blood smear often reflects marrow invasion by tumor. Fragmented red blood cells are commonly seen in patients with DIC or disseminated tumor cell emboli in the microvasculature. Echocardiography, either transthoracic or transesophageal, can be used to identify vegetations on the mitral or aortic valves.

MANAGEMENT

The initial treatment for thrombosis in patients with cancer is intravenous heparin in full therapeutic doses. Most patients with venous thrombosis will respond promptly although a few may be refractory. A substantial proportion of patients develop recurrent thromboemboli when they are subsequently treated with oral anticoagulants. In fact, some patients may have had an intensification of their hypercoagulable state shortly after warfarin was administered as evidenced by an acute rise in fibrin degradation products; the mechanism is unknown (Fig. 47-3). Patients with cancer who are refractory to oral anticoagulants usually require long-term outpatient antithrombotic therapy with subcutaneous heparin. Doses are given subcutaneously every 12 h to increase the APTT to 1.5 to 2 times control when measured 4 to 6 h after an injection.

Superficial venous thromboses are often resistant to anticoagulants, antiplatelet agents, or anti-inflammatory drugs and must be treated symptomatically. Optimal therapy for nonbacterial thrombotic endocarditis is not established. Intravenous heparin is probably a preferable choice despite the possibility of hemorrhagic transformation of a cerebral infarction. Intensive chemotherapy provokes recurrent thromboembolic events in some patients, possibly as a result of tumor cell stimulation or lysis and the release of procoagulant substances into the circulation. Prophylactic heparin started before each cycle of treatment may be useful in this situation.

Because the hemostatic system is commonly activated in malignancy and since fibrin formation has been shown to support the implantation of metastases, several clinical trials have been conducted in humans to determine if anticoagulant therapy can slow tumor progression. Some benefit has been

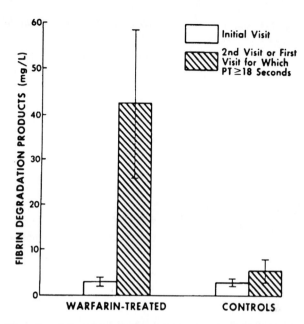

Figure 47-3 Effect of warfarin anticoagulation on the level of plasma fibrinogen degradation products (FDP). The height of the bars represents the mean (±1 SEM) FDP level in the indicated patient group. The panel at the left represents results in the warfarin-treated group before (clear bar) and after (cross-hatched bar) initiation of anticoagulation. The panel at the right represents FDP levels obtained at the same time points in the control group. FDP levels were significantly elevated after anticoagulation with sodium warfarin. (Used with permission from Edwards RL et al: Am J Clin Pathol 88:596, 1987.)

observed following warfarin treatment in patients with small cell carcinoma of the lung. Recently, a review of clinical trials in which low molecular weight heparin was used for treatment of thrombosis suggested that the number of cancer deaths was lower among patients treated with low molecular weight heparin compared to those who received standard (unfractionated) heparin.

BIBLIOGRAPHY

Drewinko B et al: Untreated prostatic carcinoma is not associated with frequent thrombohemorrhagic disorders. *Urology* 30:11, 1987.

Edwards RL et al: Abnormalities of blood coagulation tests in patients with cancer. *Am J Clin Pathol* 88:596, 1987.

Goldberg RJ et al: Occult malignant neoplasm in patients with deep venous thrombosis. *Arch Intern Med* 147:251, 1987.

Goodnight SH: Bleeding and thrombosis in hematologic neoplasia. In: Wiernik PH,

Canellos GP, Kyle RA, Schiffer CA (eds): *Neoplastic Diseases of the Blood*, 2d ed., New York, Churchill Livingstone, 1991, pp 967–982.

Gordon B et al: High frequency of antithrombin III and protein C deficiency following autologous bone marrow transplantation for lymphoma. *Bone Marrow Transplant* 8:497, 1991.

Green D et al: Lower mortality in cancer patients treated with low-molecular-weight versus standard heparin. *Lancet* 339:1476, 1992.

Griffin MR et al: Deep venous thrombosis and pulmonary embolism. Risk of subsequent malignant neoplasms. *Arch Intern Med* 147:1907, 1987.

Gugliotta L et al: Hypercoagulability during *l*-asparaginase treatment: The effect of antithrombin III supplementation in vivo. *Br J Haemat* 74:465, 1990.

Levine MN et al: The thrombogenic effect of anticancer drug therapy in women with stage II breast cancer. *N Engl J Med* 318:404, 1988.

Monreal M et al: Occult cancer in patients with deep venous thrombosis. A systematic approach. *Cancer* 67:541, 1991.

Nand S et al: Hemostatic abnormalities in untreated cancer: Incidence and correlation with thrombotic and hemorrhagic complications. *J Clin Oncol* 5:1998, 1987.

Patterson WP et al: Coagulation and cancer. *Semin Oncol* 17:137, 1990.

Prandoni P et al: Deep-vein thrombosis and the incidence of subsequent symptomatic cancer. *N Engl J Med* 327:1128, 1992.

Ratnoff OD: Hemostatic emergencies in malignancy. *Semin Oncol* 16:561, 1989.

Rogers JS et al: Chemotherapy for breast cancer decreases plasma protein C and protein S. *J Clin Oncol* 6:276, 1988.

Rogers LR: Cerebrovascular complications in cancer patients. *Neuro Clin* 9:889, 1991.

Sack GH et al: Trousseau's syndrome and other manifestations of chronic disseminated coagulopathy in patients with neoplasms: Clinical, pathophysiologic, and therapeutic features. *Medicine* 56:1, 1977.

Zurborn KH et al: Investigations of coagulation system and fibrinolysis in patients with disseminated adenocarcinomas and non-Hodgkin's lymphomas. *Oncology* 47:376, 1990.

Atherosclerosis
and Thrombosis

Myocardial infarction and stroke due to atherosclerosis are major causes of disability and death in Western societies. Acute arterial occlusion is rarely due to progressive luminal narrowing but is usually caused by the formation of a fresh thrombus overlying a ruptured atherosclerotic plaque. Evidence for coronary artery thrombosis is based on pathologic examination at autopsy, the results of thrombolytic therapy, and direct visualization of thrombi by angioscopy. A major research effort is underway to learn more about the pathogenesis of atherosclerosis and thrombosis along with large controlled clinical trials to determine the most effective methods for prevention and treatment of the disorder.

PATHOGENESIS

Atherosclerosis is the culmination of a complex process involving vascular injury, lipid deposition, and the activation or proliferation of macrophages, smooth muscle cells, and platelets. As the plaque enlarges, fissures can develop that expose intensely thrombogenic substances that attract platelets and generate thrombin, which culminates in a localized platelet/fibrin thrombus. If the thrombus is sufficiently large, acute vascular occlusion and tissue infarction ensue. However, if the clot is smaller and subocclusive, fibrinolytic resolution occurs followed by incorporation of any remaining thrombus into the atherosclerotic lesion, which may then culminate in further luminal narrowing (Fig. 48-1).

The atherosclerotic vessel is not only morphologically abnormal but also has functional defects that predispose to thrombosis or excessive vasoconstriction. The endothelium overlying an atherosclerotic lesion synthesizes reduced amounts of prostacyclin (which inhibits platelet function and produces vasodilatation), tissue plasminogen activator (t-PA), and endothelium-derived relaxing factor (EDRF). Moreover, blood flowing over vascular stenoses causes increased shear forces which promote platelet activation. In addition to vascular dysfunction, abnormalities of the blood have been

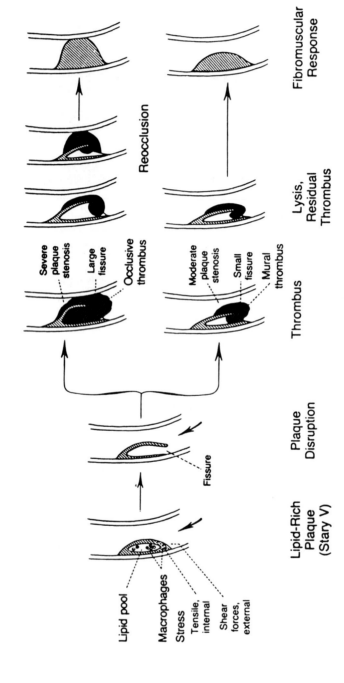

Figure 48-1 Typical dynamic evolution of the complicated disrupted plaque. (Reprinted by permission of the New England Journal of Medicine 326:242, 1992.)

Lipid pool

Macrophages

Stress

Tensile, internal

Shear forces, external

Fissure

Lipid-Rich Plaque (Stary V)

Plaque Disruption

Severe plaque stenosis

Large fissure

Occlusive thrombus

Reocclusion

Moderate plaque stenosis

Small fissure

Mural thrombus

Thrombus

Lysis, Residual Thrombus

Fibromuscular Response

reported to predispose patients to arterial thrombosis; they are discussed below.

Coagulation Factors

Elevated levels of plasma fibrinogen have been repeatedly and strongly linked to an increased risk of myocardial infarction; the predictive value of fibrinogen for vascular disease approaches or exceeds that of low-density lipoprotein (LDL) cholesterol. Whether high fibrinogen concentrations are pathogenetically related to atherogenesis or thrombosis or whether the protein is a marker for an underlying pathologic (e.g., inflammatory) process is unknown. Variations in fibrinogen genotype have recently been described that are associated with an increased risk of peripheral atherosclerosis.

Epidemiologic studies have also suggested that elevated plasma levels of activated factor VII (VII_a) are associated with increased morbidity and mortality rates when patients are followed for the ensuing 5 years. Again, factor VIIa was more strongly associated with future coronary heart disease than total cholesterol. More work is needed to learn if elevated concentrations of activation peptides of prothrombin such as F1.2 (suggesting thrombin formation) also predict future vascular ischemic events.

Fibrinolytic Factors

Some clinical studies have described a link between elevated levels of plasminogen activator inhibitor (PAI) and myocardial infarction, although other reports have been less definitive. The interpretation of these data is made difficult because of the direct association of PAI levels with plasma triglyceride, and the possibility that PAI may be released from vascular endothelium as a result of a thromboembolic event or low-grade chronic inflammation. Evidence that elevated plasma PAI levels reflect significantly decreased fibrinolytic activity in vivo is not yet available.

Elevated levels of lipoprotein(a) [LP(a)] have been associated with accelerated atherosclerosis especially when linked with high concentrations of LDL cholesterol. LP(a) has structural homology to plasminogen and acts as a competitive inhibitor of fibrinolysis in vitro. These data suggest that patients with high levels of LP(a) could be predisposed to thrombosis as well as premature atherosclerosis.

Platelets

High platelet counts and increased mean platelet volume (MPV) have recently been directly related to increased rates of coronary heart disease in clinical studies, although the nature of this relationship is unknown. Various aspects of platelet reactivity have been examined to seek links to atherosclerosis or platelet-mediated thrombus formation. For example, a diurnal variation in platelet reactivity has been described, with peak reactivity that occurs in the early morning hours, a time period when there is an increased frequency of acute myocardial infarction. Smoking has been implicated in accelerated platelet accumulation at sites of coronary artery constriction in experimental animals, which may be mediated by smoking-induced release of catecholamines. Finally, fatty acid composition and content of the diet affect platelet function. Saturated fatty acids have been reported to increase platelet reactivity, whereas monounsaturated fatty acids and n-3 fatty acids from marine sources suppress platelet function.

Other Plasma Factors

The homozygous inborn error of metabolism, homocystinuria, has long been associated with premature atherosclerosis and recurrent venous thrombosis. However, in recent years, assays have improved to the point that heterozygotes with homocysteinemia can be identified using sensitive measurements for homocysteine and related substances in the plasma. Strong relationships between increased levels of plasma homocysteine and coronary artery, cerebral vascular, and peripheral vascular disease have now been reported in a series of cross-sectional studies. Homocysteine could promote atherogenesis or thrombosis via chronic perturbation or injury of vascular endothelial cells, or possibly by augmenting the antifibrinolytic effects of LP(a).

CLINICAL MANIFESTATIONS

The clinical expressions of atherothrombotic disease are diverse but fall into four general categories of vascular events.

1. The most dramatic and serious complication of atherosclerosis is *plaque rupture* with acute thrombotic vascular occlusion and organ infarction. The best clinical example of this sequence of events is a coronary artery thrombosis producing a massive (Q wave) myocardial infarction. A large hemispheric stroke due to carotid artery occlusion is an example that involves the CNS.

2. If plaque injury is less severe, *subocclusive platelet-mediated thrombosis* may be of sufficient size to temporarily slow blood flow and produce reversible ischemia, but then regress, only to recur at a later time. Intermittent vasoconstriction could augment the ischemic symptoms. A classic clinical

example of this lesion is unstable angina or perhaps stroke-in-evolution when it involves the cerebral vasculature.

3. Even smaller degrees of vascular injury permit *accumulation of small platelet thrombi* at sites of plaque irregularities which do not disrupt blood flow but may embolize to the distal circulation with intermittent occlusion of the microvasculature. A clinical example of this phenomenon is a transient ischemic attack or amaurosis fugax in patients with carotid artery atherosclerosis. In addition to platelet emboli, atheromatous cholesterol crystals can embolize and produce similar signs and symptoms. Common origins of cholesterol emboli include the carotid artery and ascending aorta for cerebrovascular events, and the descending or distal aorta as origins for emboli to the toes (e.g., "the purple toe syndrome" in some patients given warfarin).

4. Lastly, *progressive narrowing of an atherosclerotic artery* without major surface disruption can reduce blood flow to a point where intermittent oxygen deficits produce reversible organ ischemia. Examples include angina on exertion and exercise-induced ischemia in the legs of patients with extensive iliofemoral atherosclerosis.

LABORATORY TESTING

Unfortunately, blood tests are not available to detect or localize atherosclerosis, measure its extent, or identify plaques that are likely to rupture. However, as previously discussed, some laboratory tests involving coagulation, fibrinolysis, or platelet function might ultimately prove helpful as predictors of future atherosclerotic complications. Whether these tests can be applied to individual patients as well as groups of patients enrolled in large epidemiologic studies remains to be seen. Assays that could be of value are fibrinogen, factor VII_a, plasminogen activator inhibitor, platelet count and MPV, measures of platelet reactivity, plasma homocysteine, and LP(a).

Several sophisticated tests have been used to detect increased platelet-vascular interactions that result from atherosclerosis, including radioisotopic measurements of platelet survival, the excretion of metabolites of thromboxane A_2 (platelets) and prostacyclin (vessels) in the urine, and the content of platelet specific proteins (β-thromboglobulin) in the plasma. To date, these tests are not sufficiently sensitive or specific to be of value in individual patients.

Clinical investigators are now beginning to examine the possibility that measurement of activation peptides of various clotting factors might be useful in the diagnosis or therapy of patients with arterial disease. Tests under study include the prothrombin activation peptide, F1.2, but also activation peptides of factor X, factor IX, and protein C. In one study, levels of F1.2 progressively rose after age 40. Whether this increase reflects more extensive atherosclerosis in an older population or whether coagulation is activated via factor VIIa or another mechanism is not yet clear.

MANAGEMENT

Therapy of Atherosclerosis

Regression of established atherosclerosis has recently been documented by quantitative coronary angiography in groups of patients extensively treated for 2 years or more with pharmaceutical agents (e.g., lovastatin) to lower blood cholesterol. Nonpharmacologic approaches have also been successful in a small cohort of patients who were treated with a very low-fat diet, a moderate exercise regimen, and relaxation therapy. Further studies will be required to show that lifestyle modification can also reduce rates of myocardial infarction or prolong life.

Fibrinolytic Therapy for Acute Thrombosis

The rationale behind thrombolytic therapy for acute arterial occlusion is that prompt resumption of blood flow allows salvage of the tissue served by the vessel and ultimately improves survival. This approach has been successful in patients with acute coronary artery occlusion treated within 6 h of onset of the chest pain. Vascular surgeons and interventional radiologists have also had some success in the reestablishment of blood flow in peripheral arteries using low-dose, catheter-directed thrombolytic therapy for lesions that are not amenable to surgery or for thrombosis that occurs in patients who are not operative candidates. Finally, multicenter clinical trials are now underway to evaluate the safety and efficacy of intravenous fibrinolytic agents in patients with the recent onset of thrombotic stroke.

Anticoagulation Therapy

Anticoagulants for prevention of thrombosis in arterial disease are once again gaining acceptance. Therapeutic doses of heparin are commonly used in the initial treatment of unstable angina with or without the addition of low-dose aspirin. However, a recent report suggested that reactivation of angina can occur following cessation of therapy when heparin is used without the antiplatelet agent. Two studies have suggested that oral anticoagulants given at high intensity (INR 3 to 4.5) following myocardial infarction significantly reduces rates (by 30 to 50 percent) of death, recurrent myocardial infarction, and stroke. Additional trials are needed to compare anticoagulants to aspirin alone, to learn whether lower intensities of anticoagulation

TABLE 48-1 Clinical Conditions in Which Antiplatelet Therapy Has Been Shown to be of Benefit for Treatment of Atherosclerosis

Coronary Heart Disease
- Primary prevention of myocardial infarction
- Secondary prevention of myocardial infarction
- Unstable angina
- Chronic stable angina
- Following coronary thrombolysis
- Coronary artery bypass grafts
- Percutaneous transluminal coronary angioplasty (early occlusion)

Cerebrovascular Disease
- Primary prevention of stroke in patients with coronary artery disease
- Secondary prevention of stroke following transient ischemic attack

Chronic Lower Extremity Ischemia
- Infrainguinal arterial bypass grafts

will be equally effective, and whether low intensity warfarin combined with low doses of aspirin is safe and effective.

Antiplatelet Therapy

Aspirin is the most commonly used antiplatelet agent for treatment of patients with atherosclerotic vascular disease. Clinical trials have been conducted in patients with various atherosclerotic lesions, and have shown substantial efficacy in some conditions, but little or no effect in others. Indications for aspirin use are listed in Table 48-1. A slight increase in the risk of central nervous hemorrhage with chronic low-dose aspirin therapy must be balanced with the benefits of therapy. Patients who are unable to take aspirin may benefit from a new antiplatelet agent with a different mechanism of action, ticlopidine. However, high cost and several side effects including neutropenia, diarrhea, and cutaneous sensitivity limit its use to patients who are intolerant of aspirin.

BIBLIOGRAPHY

Brown G et al: Regression of coronary artery disease as a result of intensive lipid-lowering therapy in men with high levels of apolipoprotein B. *N Engl J Med* 323:1289, 1990.

Fowkes FGR et al: Fibrinogen genotype and risk of peripheral atherosclerosis. *Lancet* 339:693, 1992.

Fuster V et al: The pathogenesis of coronary artery disease and the acute coronary syndromes. Parts 1 and 2. *N Engl J Med* 326:242, 310, 1992.

Goodnight SH: Fish oil and vascular disease. *Trends Cardiovasc Med* 1:112, 1991.

Goodnight SH et al: Recommendations for the use of aspirin in cardiac, cerebral and peripheral vascular disease. Parts 1 and 2. *West J Med* 1993.

Manson JE et al: The primary prevention of myocardial infarction. *N Engl J Med* 326:1406, 1992.

Meade TW et al: Haemostatic function and ischaemic heart disease: Principal results of the Northwick Park Heart Study. *Lancet* 2:533, 1986.

Mizuno K et al: Angioscopic evaluation of coronary-artery thrombi in acute coronary syndromes. *N Engl J Med* 326:287, 1992.

Ornish D et al: Can lifestyle changes reverse coronary heart disease? *Lancet* 336:129, 1990.

Scheffer MG et al: Thrombocythemia and coronary artery disease. *Am Heart J* 122:573, 1991.

Theroux P et al: Reactivation of unstable angina after the discontinuation of heparin. *N Engl J Med* 327:141, 1992.

Tofler GH et al: Concurrent morning increase in platelet aggregability and the risk of myocardial infarction and sudden cardiac death. *N Engl J Med* 316:1514, 1987.

Trip MD et al: Platelet hyperreactivity and prognosis in survivors of myocardial infarction. *N Engl J Med* 322:1549, 1990.

Waters D, Lesperance J: Regression of coronary atherosclerosis: An achievable goal? Review of results from recent clinical trials. *Am J Med* 91:1S-10S, 1991.

Willard JE et al: The use of aspirin in ischemic heart disease. *N Engl J Med* 327:175, 1992.

Vascular Disorders
Associated
with Thrombosis

Vasculitis (angiitis) can be produced by inflammation, infection, metabolic disease, immunologic disorders, and degenerative processes in the vascular wall which often result in vascular insufficiency and thrombosis. This chapter discusses vascular disorders which may be associated with changes in hemostasis or which should be considered in the differential diagnosis of arterial (and sometimes venous) thrombosis.

Most of the disorders affect large and medium-sized vessels, whereas, the small vessel or cutaneous vasculitis syndromes more commonly produce palpable purpura or petechiae and are considered in Chap. 22. In general, most of the vasculitic syndromes are either directly caused by or closely associated with an immunopathogenetic mechanism. Circulating immune complexes (CIC) can be deposited in the vascular wall, producing an increased permeability (via platelet-derived vasoactive amines) with trapping of CIC along basement membranes of the vessel wall and activation of the complement system. The complement-derived chemotactic factors can cause release of lysosomal enzymes (collagenases, elastase) from polymorphonuclear cells which in turn produce necrosis, thrombotic occlusion, and hemorrhage in the vessel wall. Table 49-1 lists the vasculitic syndromes associated with thrombotic disease; each is discussed below. The thrombotic complications noted include thrombosis in arterial aneurysm, coronary arterial disease, cerebral vascular lesions (ischemic and hemorrhagic strokes), and peripheral gangrene.

TAKAYASU'S DISEASE

Aortoarteritis (Takayasu's disease) is a rare chronic inflammatory disorder of unknown etiology affecting all races and involving the aorta, arteries

TABLE 49-1 Vasculitides Associated with Thrombotic Disease

Disorder	Major Thrombotic Manifestations
Takayasu's arteritis	Stroke, pulmonary hypertension, peripheral arterial insufficiency: coronary artery disease
Giant cell arteritis	Ocular involvement
Polyarteritis nodosa	Necrotizing glomerulonephritis, necrotic skin lesions, spontaneous visceral hemorrhage, myocardial infarction
Kawasaki syndrome	Coronary artery thrombosis, peripheral gangrene
Moyamoya disease	Cerebral vascular accident
Behcet's syndrome	Venous and arterial thromboses
Connective tissue disorders (RA, SLE, scleroderma)	Venous and arterial thromboses
Buerger's disease	Superficial thrombophlebitis; claudication, ulceration, gangrene

arising from the aorta, and pulmonary and coronary arteries. The inflammation leads to stenosis or aneurysm formation or both. Four major complications are hypertension, retinopathy, aortic regurgitation, and arterial aneurysm. Upper extremity claudication and gradual obliteration of peripheral pulses are seen in most cases ("pulseless disease"). Histopathology includes both granulomatous arteritis and sclerosing arteritis. Other complicating events during progression of the disease include dissecting aneurysm, cerebral thrombosis-embolism, subarachnoid hemorrhage, massive hemoptysis (pulmonary hypertension); blindness, and coronary artery disease. Treatment has included corticosteroids and anticoagulation therapy. In one series of 88 patients, the overall survival and event-free survival rates at 20 years after onset were 80 percent and 60 percent, respectively.

GIANT CELL ARTERITIS (TEMPORAL ARTERITIS)

Although temporal arteritis characteristically involves one or more branches of the carotid artery, particularly the temporal artery, the disease may be widespread and any medium-sized or large artery may be involved. The syndrome of temporal arteritis is common and easily recognized by the classic picture of fever, anemia, elevated sedimentation rate, and polymyalgia rheumatica syndrome (stiffness; aching; pain in muscles of neck, shoulders, back, hips, and thighs), headache, and jaw claudication. A serious complication is ocular involvement (central retinal artery occlusion) leading to sudden blindness in some patients. The disease must be differentiated from Takayasu's disease, another giant cell arteritis. Diagnosis is confirmed by temporal artery biopsy. Corticosteroids are highly effective and treatment should be started early to preserve vision.

POLYARTERITIS NODOSA

The pathologic lesion characteristic of polyarteritis nodosa (PAN) is a focal segmental vasculitis and fibrinoid necrosis of medium and small arteries associated with microaneurysm. Sometimes arterioles and even venules are involved. Large vessel (aorta involvement) is virtually unknown. The key clinical features suggestive of PAN include skin lesions (palpable purpura, livedo reticularis, necrotic lesions, infarcts of tips of digits), peripheral neuropathy, and renal involvement (proteinuria, sediment abnormalities). These features and evidence of other organ involvement in a patient with vague constitutional symptoms of fever, fatigue, anorexia, weight loss, joint and muscle pain, and laboratory evidence of anemia of chronic disease with acute phase reaction (high fibrinogen, thrombocytosis) are suggestive of PAN. Diagnosis is confirmed by biopsy of involved tissue (usually skin, sural nerve, skeletal muscle).

KAWASAKI SYNDROME

Kawasaki syndrome or mucocutaneous lymph node syndrome is a distinctive multisystem vasculitis which occurs in children (80 percent < 4 years of age). Epidemic and endemic groups of cases have been reported in Japan, Korea, Europe, and the United States, although a racial predisposition is striking (Oriental), suggesting a genetic predisposition. The etiology is unknown, but the epidemiology, age susceptibility, evidence for immune complex formation, and elevated DNA polymerase activity in patients strongly suggest an infectious agent. About 30 percent of patients develop evidence for cardiac disease (frequently coronary artery aneurysm), and death from myocardial infarction has occurred in about 2 percent of cases.

The principal diagnostic criteria include: (1) fever for 5 or more days; (2) rash (scarlatiniform, morbilliform, or erythema multiforme); (3) conjunctival injection; (4) changes in mouth (erythema, fissures of lips, strawberry tongue, diffuse oropharyngeal redness); (5) acute cervical lymphadenopathy; and (6) changes in peripheral extremities (erythema of palms and soles, induration of hands and feet, desquamation of fingertips and toe tips 2 weeks after onset). At least five of the six should be present for the diagnosis of Kawasaki syndrome; however, infants have developed complicating coronary aneurysms with only 4 of the signs present. The acute phase of the illness lasts about 11 days (untreated). Complications include urethritis, abdominal pain and diarrhea, myocarditis, myocardial infarction, obstructive jaundice, hydrops of the gallbladder, and formation of aneurysms in medium-sized arteries (usually in coronary arteries).

Laboratory abnormalities include leukocytosis and a striking thrombocytosis (may last for 3 to 4 weeks); a rare patient may have thrombocytopenia. In addition, acute phase reactants (factor VIII, fibrinogen, von Willebrand factor) are elevated acutely; low antithrombin III (AT III) levels and decreased fibrinolytic activity are seen in about half the patients initially. Plasma β-thromboglobulin may be elevated. Thus, a hypercoagulable state is present in many patients during the acute phase of the disease and can be correlated with the formation of coronary aneurysm and thrombosis in a few patients.

Current recommendations for treatment include intravenous gamma globulin as soon as the disease is recognized. The dose is 2 g/kg given in a 10- to 12-h infusion or 400 mg/kg per day for 5 consecutive days. Aspirin, in an anti-inflammatory dose of 100 mg/kg per day is given until fever has abated (or to day 14) followed by ASA 5 to 10 mg/kg daily for about 2 months until all laboratory signs are normal. Patients with transient or small aneurysms are treated with low doses of ASA until resolution of lesions or indefinitely; patients with large aneurysms, myocardial infarction, or coronary artery thromboses may be anticoagulated with heparin followed by warfarin therapy until stabilization of lesions. Maintenance therapy (after heparin-warfarin) is individualized but has frequently been ASA and dipyridamole. Prognosis and follow-up are discussed in the article by Melish and Hicks.

Another complication which may require anticoagulation is severe peripheral ischemia with resultant gangrene which has occurred in infants < 7 months of age.

MOYAMOYA DISEASE

Moyamoya disease is a chronic cerebral arterial occlusive disorder involving bilateral stenosis or occlusion of the terminal portion of internal carotid arteries. This occlusion is associated with the formation of an abnormal collateral vascular network resulting in an angiographic appearance to which the Japanese expression for "something hazy such as a puff of cigarette smoke drifting in the air" or "moyamoya" has been applied. The disorder is most often seen in children. Childhood moyamoya presents with ischemic cerebrovascular episodes, whereas in adults, subarachnoid and intracranial hemorrhage from the small arteries is the prevailing presentation. The possibility of moyamoya disease should be considered in any young child with transient ischemic attacks or stroke and in the older child with cerebral hemorrhage.

The etiology of moyamoya disease is unknown although the characteristic angiographic signs (but unilateral) may appear in other conditions such as neurofibromatosis, tuberous sclerosis, PAN, congenital heart disease, and after radiation therapy.

Treatment has been mostly surgical to improve perfusion. Anticoagulation has not been consistently applied except as an adjunct to surgery or in the acute management of acute hemiplegia or childhood stroke.

BEHCET'S SYNDROME

Behcet's syndrome is discussed in Chapter 45.

CONNECTIVE TISSUE DISORDERS

Connective tissue or collagen-vascular disorders such as systemic lupus erythematosus (SLE), rheumatoid arthritis (RA), and scleroderma have long been associated in the literature with thrombotic complication. In addition, a large but often anecdotal literature indicates that antiphospholipid antibodies (APA) are found in many of these patients with thrombosis. Certainly, other mechanisms for triggering a thrombosis are operative in these patients, including vasculitis and endothelial cell damage, platelet activation by immune complexes and acquired deficiencies of coagulation regulatory proteins (AT III, protein C, protein S). In a recent series of SLE in children with no other risk factors for thrombosis, 73 percent of patients with SLE and thrombotic (arterial or venous) episodes had APA, as compared to 14 percent of SLE patients without thrombotic events in the same age group; that is, a few patients had thrombosis without APA. Activation of coagulation (mild to severe disseminated intravascular coagulation) has been demonstrated in systemic-onset juvenile RA.

BUERGER'S DISEASE

Thromboangiitis obliterans is a vasculitic process of medium- and small-sized arteries leading to gangrene which involves mainly the legs and arms (rarely cerebral and visceral vessels). It usually affects men under 50 years of age and is considered an autoimmune reaction triggered and made worse by tobacco use. The disorder was previously thought to be more common because of the young individuals with premature atherosclerosis in this diagnostic category. Patients with hematologic disorders, connective tissue disease, ergot overuse, thoracic outlet syndromes, embolic disease, and cold injury may have vascular disease features resembling Buerger's disease. The disease is discussed in more detail in the reference by Joyce.

BIBLIOGRAPHY

Burns JC et al: Coagulopathy and platelet activation in Kawasaki syndrome: Identification of patients at high risk for development of coronary artery aneurysms. *J Pediatr* 105:206, 1984.

Chafa O et al: Behcet syndrome associated with protein S deficiency. *Thromb Haemost* 67:1, 1992.

Fauci AS et al: The spectrum of vasculitis. *Ann Intern Med* 89:660, 1978.

Gordon N, Isler W: Childhood moyamoya disease. *Dev Med Child Neurol* 31:103, 1989.

Hall S, Buchbinder R: Takayasu's arteritis. *Rheum Dis Clin North Am* 16:411, 1990.

Joyce JW: Buerger's disease (thromboangiitis obliterans). *Rheum Dis Clin North Am* 16:463, 1990.

Krowchuk DP: Kawasaki disease presenting with thrombocytopenia. *Am J Dis Child* 144:19, 1990.

Melish ME, Hicks RV: Kawasaki syndrome: Clinical features, pathophysiology, etiology and therapy. *J Rheumatol* 17(suppl 24):2, 1990.

Montes de Oca MA et al: Thrombosis in systemic lupus erythematosus: A French collaborative study. *Arch Dis Child* 66:713, 1991.

Scott JP et al: Evidence for intravascular coagulation in systemic onset, but not polyarticular, juvenile rheumatoid arthritis. *Arthritis Rheum* 28:256, 1985.

Subramanyan R et al: Natural history of aortoarteritis (Takayasu's disease). *Circulation* 80:429, 1989.

Cardiac Disease
and Thrombosis

The most frequent cause of thrombosis that involves the heart in adults is coronary artery disease, whereas congenital heart defects and Kawasaki syndrome are more common in infants and children (see Chaps. 48 and 49). Advanced cardiac disease also predisposes to other forms of thrombosis (Fig. 50-1). Left ventricular thrombi occur in patients with cardiomyopathy, ventricular aneurysm, and transmural myocardial infarction. Thrombosis can complicate mechanical or tissue cardiac valves, and systemic emboli are common in patients with chronic atrial fibrillation. Thromboembolism related to cardiac disease is an important clinical problem and can be treated successfully with oral anticoagulants or other antithrombotic agents.

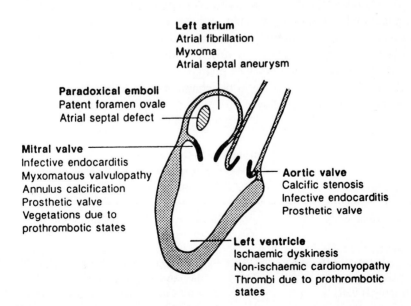

Figure 50-1 Sources of cardiogenic emboli. (Used with permission from Hart RG: Cardiogenic embolism to the brain. Lancet 339:589, 1992.)

PATHOGENESIS

The pathogenesis of cardiac thromboembolism is complex but is likely to involve one or more of the following: endocardial injury, stasis of blood, the generation of activated clotting factors, or defects in fibrinolysis (Table 50-1).

Damage to the endothelium that covers the interior surface of the left ventricle is important in the pathogenesis of mural thromboses following a full-thickness myocardial infarction. Endothelial cell injury creates a thrombogenic surface due to the synthesis and expression of tissue factor and the loss of protective mechanisms from the cardiac surface such as the platelet inhibitor prostacyclin, the effects of anticoagulants such as protein C and antithrombin III, and the fibrinolytic enzyme, tissue plasminogen activator. In children, damage to the heart can also occur as a consequence of endocardial tissue injury from long-term indwelling parenteral nutrition catheters.

Stasis of blood due to cardiac chamber enlargement or abnormal cardiac rhythms allows the accumulation of circulating prothrombotic substances, which overwhelms local concentrations of antithrombotic proteins and leads to thrombosis. In many instances, recently formed thrombi are not firmly attached to cardiac surfaces, thus facilitating systemic embolization to the brain or other organs. Prime examples of disturbed cardiac blood flow include chronic rheumatic or nonrheumatic atrial fibrillation, advanced cardiomyopathy with stasis of blood in the dilated ventricles, and congenital heart disease in infants and children.

Activated coagulation factors (e.g., thrombin, factor Xa) or platelets can be generated in the heart, particularly at sites of tissue damage (e.g., following myocardial infarction or on the surface of a damaged heart valve in subacute bacterial endocarditis). Alternatively, activated clotting factors may be activated at sites of inflammatory or malignant disease elsewhere in the body and subsequently accumulate in the chambers of a failing heart because of stasis or disturbed blood flow.

TABLE 50-1 Mechanisms of Thrombosis in Cardiac Disease

Mechanism	Example
Endocardial injury	Transmural myocardial infarction with mural thrombus
Sluggish or disturbed blood flow	Atrial fibrillation with embolic stroke
Activated clotting factors or platelets	Pancreatic cancer with nonbacterial thrombotic endocarditis
Fibrinolytic defects	Coronary artery disease and myocardial infarction

Preliminary evidence suggests that some patients with premature coronary artery disease have impaired fibrinolysis due to elevated circulating levels of plasminogen activator inhibitor which in some cases is associated with increased concentrations of plasma triglyceride. Local fibrinolysis may be impaired in individuals with coronary artery disease who have high levels of lipoprotein(a) (see Chap. 45).

CLINICAL MANIFESTATIONS

Cardiomyopathy.   Advanced cardiac muscle dysfunction of any cause is frequently associated with intracardiac thrombi. In one series, 75 percent of patients had thrombi discovered in the heart at autopsy. Systemic emboli occur at a rate of approximately 4 to 5 percent per year in cardiomyopathy patients. After a recent systemic embolus, rates of subsequent emboli may be as high as 10 to 20 percent per year. Deep venous thrombosis and pulmonary emboli are common in both children and adults with advanced cardiac failure (e.g., awaiting cardiac transplantation).

Transmural Myocardial Infarction.   As many as 50 percent of patients suffering a large anterior transmural myocardial infarction develop left ventricular thrombi. The clinical course in about 10 percent will be complicated by cerebral embolization. Half of these take place during the first week following infarction, and the remainder occur in the next 2 to 12 weeks.

Atrial Enlargement and Atrial Fibrillation.   Patients with dilated left atria (e.g., > 5 cm in diameter) or chronic atrial fibrillation due to rheumatic heart disease, coronary artery disease, or other cardiac disorder have a high incidence of systemic embolization. For example, untreated patients with chronic nonrheumatic atrial fibrillation have been found to have embolic complication (usually associated with stroke) at a rate of 6 to 8 percent per year.

Valve Replacement.   Patients who require artificial (mechanical) heart valves are almost always treated with anticoagulants to prevent valvular thrombosis and subsequent systemic embolization. Despite these precautions, mechanical valves in the mitral position continue to generate emboli at a rate of approximately 2 to 3 percent per year, whereas aortic valves have a lower risk (e.g., approximately 1 percent per year). Heterotopic tissue valves (e.g., of porcine origin) have lower rates of embolic complications, particularly when implanted in the aortic position.

Chronic Congestive Heart Failure.   Patients with severely impaired cardiac function and left ventricular ejection fractions of < 35 percent also are at high risk of systemic emboli, although few clinical trials or epidemiologic surveys are available. Deep venous thrombosis and pulmonary emboli are likely as a result of physical inactivity and chronic lower extremity edema from congestive heart failure.

LABORATORY TESTING

As of yet, laboratory tests are not available that will predict thrombosis in patients with advanced cardiac disease. Studies are needed to determine if tests reflecting activation of coagulation such as F1.2, thrombin-antithrombin complexes, fibrinopeptide A, or plasmin-antiplasmin complexes will prove to be of clinical value. Careful monitoring of oral anticoagulant therapy using the INR as a guide is essential to avoid recurrent thrombosis or excessive bleeding.

MANAGEMENT

Cardiomyopathy. Patients with severe dilated cardiomyopathy are usually treated with low-intensity warfarin (INR 2 to 3). The management of antico-agulant therapy is often a challenge in patients with chronic congestive heart failure because of poor diet, congestive hepatomegaly with liver dysfunction, and interactions of warfarin with the multitude of other drugs that are required for the treatment of advanced heart disease.

Transmural Myocardial Infarction. Patients with large anterior myocardial infarctions should be promptly treated with heparin, either in doses of 1250 U/h intravenously or 17,500 U every 12 h by subcutaneous injection to maintain the APTT in a therapeutic range (e.g., 1.5 to 2 times control). Oral anticoagulants should be started early with a target INR of 2–3 and continued for a period of 3 months. If myocardial function is adequate, whether or not a left ventricular aneurysm is present, anticoagulants can then be stopped. However, if ejection fractions are low (e.g., < 35 percent), long-term low-in-tensity therapy is probably required.

Rheumatic Heart Disease. Patients with rheumatic heart disease compli-cated by a large left atrium, chronic atrial fibrillation, a history of emboliza-tion, or advanced congestive heart failure should be treated with warfarin at low intensity (INR 2 to 3). If a recent embolus has occurred, then the INR should probably be higher (i.e., 2.5–3.5) for the next year, with subsequent reduction to a ratio of 2 to 3. Alternatively, asprin (160 mg daily) could be added to low-intensity warfarin.

Non-Rheumatic Atrial Fibrillation.   Several recent large prospective clinical trials have now unequivocally demonstrated the benefits of anti-thrombotic therapy in patients with chronic (and perhaps intermittent) non-rheumatic atrial fibrillation (Fig. 50-2). Controversy exists as to the best form of treatment. Until additional data are available, patients with advanced cardiac disease, a history of embolization, or who are elderly (e.g., over 74 years of age), should receive warfarin at a low-intensity range (INR 2 to 3). Other patients can either be treated with warfarin or low doses of aspirin until clinical trials directly comparing the two therapies are completed. Young patients with atrial fibrillation who have no known heart disease ("lone" atrial fibrillation) do not require antithrombotic agents.

Mechanical or Tissue Valves.   Adults and children with artificial (mechanical) cardiac valves should be treated indefinitely with oral anticoagulants. The optimal INR range for the lowest risks of embolization and bleeding is currently being reevaluated. In the past, all patients were given high intensity warfarin (INR 3 to 4.5), but now some authorities have recommended lower

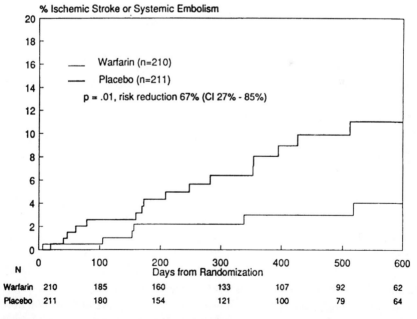

Figure 50-2 Cumulative rate of primary events (stroke or systemic embolization) for warfarin versus placebo in patients with nonrheumatic atrial fibrillation. (Used with permission from Stroke Prevention in Atrial Fibrillation Investigators, Circulation 84:527, 1991.)

levels (e.g., an INR of 2.5–3.5) for adults with mechanical valves and no history of emboli. Alternatively, low doses of aspirin (160 mg daily) or dipyridamole (400 mg daily) may be added to low-intensity warfin. Similar ranges are probably appropriate for children although applicable clinical trials are not available. When tissue valves are inserted in the mitral position, low-intensity warfin is usually given for a period of 3 months and then stopped. Anticoagulation is optional for aortic bioprostheses. Some patients with valve prostheses require long-term warfin therapy, especially if the left atrium is dilated or if atrial fibrillation is present.

BIBLIOGRAPHY

Chesebro JH et al: Trial of combined warfarin plus dipyridamole or aspirin therapy in prosthetic heart valve replacement: Danger of aspirin compared with dipyridamole. *Am J Cardiol* 51:1537, 1983.

Dalen JE, Hirsh J: Third ACCP Consensus Conference on Antithrombotic Therapy. *Chest* 102:303S, 1992.

Fuster V et al: Prevention of thromboembolism induced by prosthetic heart valves. *Semin Thromb Hemost* 14:50, 1988.

Fuster V, Halperin JL: Left ventricular thrombi and cerebral embolism. *N Engl J Med* 320:392, 1989.

Goodnight SH: Pathogenesis and therapy of thrombosis in patients with congestive heart failure. In: Hosenpud JD, Greenberg BH (eds): *Congestive Heart Failure: Pathophysiology, Differential Diagnosis and Comprehensive Approach to Therapy,* New York, Springer Verlag (in press).

Hamsten A et al: Increased plasma levels of a rapid inhibitor of tissue plasminogen activator in young survivors of myocardial infarction. *N Engl J Med* 313:1557, 1985.

Hsu DT et al: Acute pulmonary embolism in pediatric patients awaiting heart transplantation. *J Am Coll Cardiol* 17:1621, 1991.

Meltzer RS et al: Intracardiac thrombi and systemic embolization. *Ann Intern Med* 104:689, 1986.

Roberts WC et al: Idiopathic dilated cardiomyopathy: Analysis of 152 necropsy patients. *Am J Cardiol* 60:1340, 1987.

Saour JN et al: Trial of different intensities of anticoagulation in patients with prosthetic heart valves. *N Engl J Med* 322:428, 1990.

Stein B et al: Antithrombotic therapy in cardiac disease. An emerging approach based on pathogenesis and risk. *Circulation* 80:1501, 1989.

Stratton JR et al: Fate of left ventricular thrombi in patients with remote myocardial infarction or idiopathic cardiomyopathy. *Circulation* 78:1388, 1988.

Stroke Prevention Atrial Fibrillation Investigators: Stroke prevention in atrial fibrillation study: Final results. *Circulation* 84:527, 1991.

Tsevat J et al: Warfarin for dilated cardiomyopathy: A bloody tough pill to swallow? *Med Decis Making* 9:162, 1991.

Turpie A et al: Randomised comparison of two intensities of oral anticoagulant therapy after tissue heart valve replacement. *Lancet* 1:1242, 1988.

Turpie AGG et al: Comparison of high-dose with low-dose subcutaneous heparin to prevent left ventricular mural thrombosis in patients with acute transmural anterior myocardial infarction. *N Engl J Med* 320:352, 1989.

Cerebrovascular
Disease and Thrombosis

Causes of stroke include cerebral thrombosis due to atherosclerosis, cardiac emboli, thrombosis of the cerebral veins, and intracranial hemorrhage. This chapter emphasizes abnormalities of the blood that are associated with thrombotic stroke (Table 51-1). Cardiac emboli are covered elsewhere (see Chap. 50), and thrombosis due to atherosclerosis is discussed in Chap. 48.

TABLE 51-1 Hematologic Disorders Associated with Ischemic Stroke

Deficiencies of coagulation inhibitors
   Antithrombin III
   Protein C
   Protein S

Impaired fibrinolysis
   Dysfibrinogenemia
   Plasminogen deficiency

Antiphospholipid antibodies

Myeloproliferative disease
   Essential thrombocytosis
   Polycythemia rubra vera

Hyperlipidemia
   Elevated lipoprotein(a)

Homocystinemia

Hemoglobinopathies
   Sickle cell disease
   S-C disease

Heparin-associated thrombocytopenia

Hemolytic uremic syndrome–thrombotic thrombocytopenic purpura

PATHOGENESIS AND CLINICAL MANIFESTATIONS

Most thrombotic strokes in older individuals are a consequence of athero-sclerosis of the carotid or cerebral arteries. However, in young adults and children a larger proportion of CNS vascular occlusive events are associated with abnormalities of the blood rather than blood vessels. The hematologic disorders that predispose to stroke can be hereditary or acquired.

Hereditary Disorders

Deficiencies of Protein S, Protein C, Antithrombin III, and Plasminogen

Most reports of stroke associated with deficiencies of the anticoagulant or fibrinolytic proteins are individual case reports or small clinical series, so that the prevalence of these disorders is unknown. Transient ischemic attacks (TIA), amaurosis fugax, and cerebral vein thrombosis have also been asso-ciated with hematologic disorders. Although case reports can be misleading, protein S deficiency appears to be associated with stroke more frequently than deficiencies of other natural anticoagulants in adults. In contrast, pro-tein C deficiency is more common in children with CNS thrombosis.

Elevated Lipoprotein(a) and Homocystinemia

Patients with persistently elevated plasma concentrations of lipoprotein(a) (Lp(a)) or homocysteine have increased rates of stroke and myocardial infarction as well as other manifestations of atherosclerotic vascular disease. Whether the vascular occlusion in these patients is the result of atheroscle-rosis, or whether inhibition of fibrinolysis (due to LP(a)) or vascular injury (due to homocystinemia) could also promote thrombosis is not yet certain. In one series of patients with stroke, 42 percent had elevated plasma levels of homocysteine.

Sickle Cell Disease

Stroke is a relatively common and often devastating sequela of homozygous sickle cell disease that occurs in 8 to 17 percent of patients at some time during their lives. The rate of cerebrovascular thrombosis is even higher if a sensitive test such as magnetic resonance imaging (MRI) is used for screening pur-poses. Stroke has also been reported to occur in 2 to 5 percent of patients with hemoglobin S-C disease. The vascular pathology involves the major cerebral vessels with segmented narrowing of the distal internal carotid artery, the vessels of the circle of Willis, and the proximal branches of other major vessels of the brain. Pathologic studies describe a large vessel arterio-pathy with intimal proliferation that includes large numbers of smooth muscle cells and fibroblasts. In addition, microvascular obstruction by sickled cells occurs. Stroke is very rare in hemoglobin S heterozygotes (sickle cell trait) and has only been reported in extreme circumstances of hypoxia, infection, or acidosis. MRI is useful for the diagnosis of cerebral infarction, and transcranial Doppler studies are helpful for evaluation of distal cerebral arteriopathy.

Acquired Disorders

Antiphospholipid Antibodies

Antiphospholipid antibodies (APA) for example, anticardiolipin antibodies (ACA) or the lupus anticoagulant (LA), are frequently discovered in patients with thrombotic or embolic stroke. In one series, 8.2 percent of a group of stroke patients of all ages were found to have APA, as compared to only 1.6 percent of an age-matched population of blood donors. Rates of APA are even higher (10 to 45 percent) if young patients with stroke are selected for study. Cerebral vascular events either reflect in situ cerebral vascular thrombosis or are the result of emboli that originate from vegetations on the mitral or aortic cardiac valves. In a few cases, pathologic studies have shown bland thrombi in the small vessels of the brain without evidence of vasculitis (see Chap. 43).

A wide spectrum of vessels have been involved, ranging from large and medium-sized arteries to very small vessels with multiple tiny punctate white matter lesions visualized on MRI scan (Fig. 51-1). Cerebral sinus vein throm-

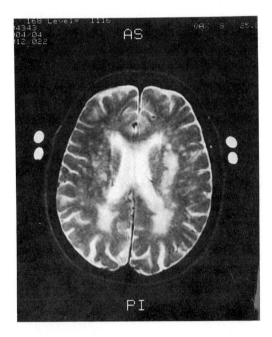

Figure 51-1 MRI scan showing punctate lesions in a patient with high titer APA.

bosis and retinal occlusion have also been reported. Two clinical constellations deserve mention:

1. Sneddon's syndrome is the association of stroke, livido reticularis of the skin, and (often) Raynaud's symptoms. A large percentage of these patients have high titer APA.
2. Multi-infarct dementia is a common sequelae in patients with APA and stroke. Higher cortical function often progressively declines in the absence of overt neurologic signs or symptoms; multiple infarcts are found on neuroradiologic studies.

Myeloproliferative Disease and Cancer

Stroke is one of the spectrum of thrombotic events that complicates the clinical course of patients with myeloproliferative disease or malignancy. Cerebral vein thrombosis has also been reported. Thrombosis in patients with myeloproliferative disease is most likely due to increased numbers or reactivity of platelets or both, whereas activation of coagulation is more prominent in the coagulopathies of malignancy.

Heparin-Associated Thrombocytopenia

When patients with heparin-associated thrombocytopenia develop thrombosis, acute thrombotic stroke as well as myocardial infarction or peripheral artery occlusion can occur. The CNS pathology is due to either microvascular occlusion or thrombosis of the major cerebral arteries.

Other

Several other diseases associated with CNS thrombosis are discussed elsewhere: hemolytic uremic syndrome–thrombotic thrombocytopenic purpura (see Chap. 29); vascular disorders (see Chap. 49); oral contraceptives (see Chap. 52); and the nephrotic syndrome (see Chap. 28).

LABORATORY TESTING

Routine laboratory tests to detect hereditary or acquired thrombotic disorders are not warranted in older patients with stroke due to atherosclerosis of the carotid or cerebral arteries. In younger adults (e.g., < 45 to 50 years of age and in children) in whom there is no obvious reason for stroke, a search for an underlying predisposition to thrombosis can be fruitful and could alter therapy. In addition to general laboratory screening tests (e.g., complete blood count and review of the peripheral blood smear), the evaluation should include some or all of the assays listed in Table 51-2.

In general, the focus in children will be on hereditary causes of thrombosis such as protein C, protein S, antithrombin III, and perhaps plasminogen

TABLE 51-2 Laboratory Assays in Children and Young Adults with Thrombotic Stroke

Antithrombin III
Protein C (especially in children)
Protein S (especially in young women)
Plasminogen
Fibrinogen (also TCT, Reptilase time)
Antiphospholipid antibodies
Lipoprotein(a) (when associated with premature atherosclerosis)
Plasma homocysteine

deficiencies. In young adults, antiphospholipid antibodies and a free protein S assay are most likely to be abnormal. In patients who are older and who have evidence of accelerated atherosclerosis, Lp(a) and plasma homocysteine levels may be useful.

Diagnostic yields from these studies vary and in some instances will be quite low (e.g., hereditary abnormality of plasminogen). Positive findings may be substantially higher in other situations, such as a teenager with a spontaneous cerebral vein thrombosis or a child with acute thrombotic stroke. However, most of these diagnoses carry major implications for therapy, so that the laboratory tests are justified.

ANTITHROMBOTIC MANAGEMENT OF STROKE

Acute Embolic Stroke

When an acute stroke is caused by a cardiac embolus, anticoagulants are usually administered to prevent a recurrence. The risk of a second embolic event has been estimated to be approximately 1 percent per day for the next 2 weeks. Since most hemorrhagic transformations of an embolic infarct occur in the first 48 h, a delay of anticoagulation therapy for 1 to 2 days followed by a CT scan is usually warranted to reduce the risks of CNS bleeding. If hemorrhagic transformation of the infarction has not occurred and its size is < 4 to 5 cm in diameter, heparin can then be started without a loading dose. Oral anticoagulation therapy is usually needed for long-term prophylaxis.

Acute Thrombotic Stroke

Thrombotic vascular occlusions with brain infarction (completed stroke) are not treated with anticoagulants. However, almost all of these patients are candidates for long-term antiplatelet therapy with aspirin for secondary prevention of stroke and prevention of myocardial infarction (see Chap. 64). Clinical trials are underway to assess the safety and efficacy of prompt (< 4 to 6 h) thrombolytic therapy to preserve neurologic function in patients with thrombotic stroke. The preliminary results appear encouraging, but much more information is needed before fibrinolytic therapy can be recommended for general use.

Stroke-in-Evolution

Patients with repeated and progressive neurologic deficits that are most likely due to intermittent thrombotic cerebral vascular occlusion are candidates for heparin anticoagulation, provided neuroradiologic scans do not show evidence of CNS bleeding.

Transient Ischemic Attacks

Defined as reversible CNS thrombotic events lasting < 24 h, TIAs are treated with antiplatelet therapy, usually with low or moderate doses of aspirin, based on the encouraging results from recent clinical trials (see Chap. 64). Ticlopidine is also effective if aspirin cannot be used.

Acute Cerebral Vein Thrombosis

A recently reported clinical trial has strongly supported the use of intravenous heparin in patients with spontaneous cerebral vein thrombosis (Einhaupl reference). In many instances, the sinus vein thrombi cleared over the ensuing several weeks. The risk of CNS bleeding was low. A retrospective analysis of cerebral venous thrombosis in children that were due to hypercoagulable states and were not associated with major cerebral infarction suggested that outcomes were good without acute anticoagulation therapy. An alternative and more aggressive treatment involves catheter-directed thrombolysis to lyse cerebral vein thrombi, but additional data are needed to confirm the efficacy and safety of this approach as compared to anticoagulation therapy.

Central Retinal Artery Thrombosis

Antithrombotic therapy is usually of no avail in patients with acute central retinal artery obstruction. However, some patients have recently been treated with catheter-guided thrombolytic therapy of the affected retinal artery shortly after the onset of acute monocular blindness. Some of these patients were reported to regain partial or complete vision in the affected eye.

Treatment of Hypercoagulable States Associated with Stroke

Stroke patients with hereditary deficiencies of protein C, protein S, anti-thrombin III, and plasminogen are usually treated with long-term oral anticoagulants rather than antiplatelet therapy. Patients with thrombotic or embolic stroke associated with APA also may benefit from anticoagulants, although definitive controlled clinical trials are not available. One recent retrospective study suggested that warfarin given at moderate intensity (INR ~3) was useful (see Rosove reference). Effective treatment to lower elevated levels of Lp(a) is not available, but aggressive management of other atherosclerotic risk factors may be helpful. Folic acid or pyridoxine can be tried in patients with elevated levels of plasma homocysteine (see Chap. 45).

BIBLIOGRAPHY

Amarenco P et al: The prevalence of ulcerated plaques in the aortic arch in patients with stroke. *N Engl J Med* 326:221, 1992.

Barron TF et al: Cerebral venous thrombosis in neonates and children. *Pediatr Neurol* 8:112, 1992.

Brattstrom L et al: Hyperhomocysteinaemia in stroke: Prevalence, cause, and relationships to type of stroke and stroke risk factors. *Eur J Clin Invest* 22:214, 1992.

Briley DP et al: Neurological disease associated with anticardiolipin antibodies. *Ann Neurol* 25:221, 1989.

Brott T: Thrombolytic therapy. *Neurol Clin* 10:219, 1992.

Coull BM, Goodnight SH: Hematological abnormalities in stroke. In: Barnett H (ed): *Stroke*, vol 2, New York, Churchill Livingstone, 1993 (in press).

del Zoppo GJ et al: Recombinant tissue plasminogen activator in acute thrombotic and embolic stroke. *Ann Neurol* 32:78, 1992.

Einhaupl KM et al: Heparin treatment in sinus venous thrombosis. *Lancet* 338:597, 1991.

Furlan AJ et al: Stroke in a young adult with familial plasminogen disorder. *Stroke* 22:1598, 1991.

Green D et al: Protein S deficiency in middle-aged women with stroke. *Neurology* 42:1029, 1992.

Hart RG, Kanter MC: Hematologic disorders and ischemic stroke. A selective review. *Stroke* 21:1111, 1990.

Kohler J et al: Ischemic stroke due to protein C deficiency. *Stroke* 21:1077, 1990.

Rosove MH et al: Antiphospholipid thrombosis: Clinical course after the first thrombotic event in 70 patients. *Ann Intern Med* 117:303, 1992.

Sacco RL et al: Free protein S efficiency: A possible association with cerebrovascular occlusion. *Stroke* 20:1657, 1989.

Sandercock P, Willems H: Medical treatment of acute ischaemic stroke. *Lancet* 339:537, 1992.

Thrombosis

---

in Pregnancy

Venous thromboembolism is the most serious vascular complication that can arise during pregnancy and parturition. Pulmonary embolism (PE) is the leading cause of death in many obstetric services. The incidence of thromboembolic complications varies between 2 and 5/1000 deliveries, and in women who have had a previous thrombotic episode (excluding superficial thrombophlebitis), the mean chance for recurrence is 15 percent. Predisposing factors for thrombosis in obstetric patients besides the "hypercoagulable" state of pregnancy (see below) include method of delivery (more deep vein thrombosis-PE [DVT-PE] after cesarean-section), excessive weight gain, associated illnesses (diabetes, hypertension, heart disease, multiple pregnancy, placenta previa) requiring restricted activity, hormone suppression of lactation, and postpartum use of oral contraceptives (use should be delayed for at least 5 weeks after delivery), presence of lupus anticoagulant, and presence of hereditary thrombotic disorder (most frequently antithrombin III [AT III], protein C, and protein S deficiencies). The increased risk for thrombotic disease is present throughout pregnancy and the puerperium (up to 6 weeks postpartum). This chapter also considers the increased risk for thrombotic disease associated with the use of oral contraceptive agents (OCA).

PATHOPHYSIOLOGY OF PREGNANCY-RELATED THROMBOSIS

Major changes in the hemostatic system occur during pregnancy, presumably in preparation for the hemostatic challenge of delivery. The platelet count remains steady with mildly increased reactivity and enhanced platelet destruction near term. Major increases of several clotting factors are seen: von Willebrand factor; factors VII, VIII, and X; the contact factors, factor XIII and fibrinogen. The marked increase of factor VII is associated with parallel increases in both antigen and activity. Other factors remain normal

430

(factor IX, II, V, AT III, protein C) or fall (factor XI and total protein S). Overall fibrinolytic activity decreases with striking changes in the fibrinolytic system—threefold increase of plasminogen activator inhibitor (PAI-1) and urokinase, 30-fold increase of PAI-2, 1.5-fold increase of tissue plasminogen activator (t-PA), and normal or slightly decreased levels of plasminogen and histidine-rich glycoprotein. The balance of these changes favors hypercoagulability and decreased fibrinolysis. Along with these physiologic alterations, one would expect a higher incidence of thrombosis based on the altered venous hemodynamics and vascular flow produced by the gravid uterus.

At least two mechanisms are probably protective in the pregnant woman as she nears term: placental-derived anticoagulants, such as dermatan sulfate proteoglycan, circulate in the pregnant woman and the lowered viscosity of maternal blood due to hemodilutional anemia. In fact, a fivefold increase in thrombotic complication is seen in the immediate postpartum period when these factors are abruptly restored to the normal state.

DIAGNOSIS OF VENOUS THROMBOEMBOLIC DISEASE

The clinical manifestations of DVT occur as a consequence of deep venous outflow obstruction and inflammation of the venous walls and surrounding tissues and result in pain, swelling, warmth, redness, and cyanosis of the extremities. The most severe form, phlegmasia caeruleae dolens (massive swelling of leg; distended, bursting appearance with cyanotic, tight, shiny skin), occurs in 1 percent of cases. The clinical diagnosis of DVT is unreliable and can be confused with arthritis, cellulitis, lymphoedema, tendinitis, superficial thrombophlebitis, primary varicose veins, leg trauma, muscle hemorrhage, and pregnancy-associated swelling or stasis. Patients with pain and swelling in the right leg rarely have venous thrombosis. The diagnosis must be confirmed by Doppler ultrasound or impedance plethysmography (IPG); venography or isotopic methods are seldom used in pregnancy because of radiation exposure risks.

The clinical diagnosis of PE is also unreliable mainly because of the varied manifestations and severity and the wide differential diagnosis including heart disease (pericarditis, mitral stenosis), pleuritis, pneumonia, pneumothorax, sepsis, and physiologic dyspnea of pregnancy. An approach to clinically suspected PE during pregnancy is shown in Figure 52-1.

Cerebral venous and arterial thrombosis can occur during pregnancy and is usually diagnosed by CT. Other rare thrombotic complications include septic pelvic vein thrombophlebitis and ovarian vein thrombosis. These lesions are usually treated with systemic anticoagulation with heparin

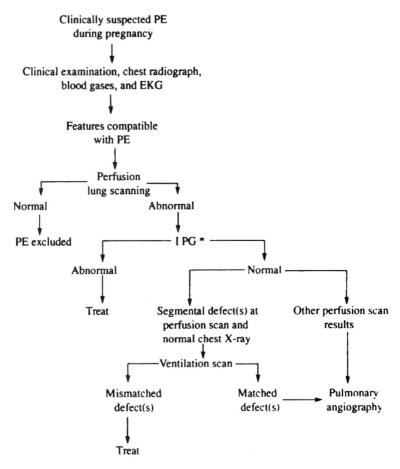

Figure 52-1 Approach for diagnosis of pulmonary embolism during pregnancy. IPG, impedance plethysmography or Doppler ultrasound. (Adapted from Le Clerc and Roy reference.)

(if CNS CT shows an ischemic pattern without hemorrhage in cerebral lesions).

Coagulation Laboratory Testing

Hereditary and acquired coagulopathies are particularly apt to be found in women with pregnancy-associated DVT. One recent study which investigated DVT diagnosed by IPG in 32 consecutive obstetric patients noted that 20 percent were subsequently found to have a coagulation or fibrinolytic abnormality (de Boer reference). In another study of known hereditary deficient families, 44 percent of AT III-, 25 percent of protein C-, and 17 percent of protein S-deficient women had thromboses during pregnancy or the postpartum period (Conard reference). Women with AT III deficiency are particularly at risk for thrombotic complications after abortion, during pregnancy, and especially in the postpartum period. These considerations and the known association of antiphospholipid lupus anticoagulant (see Chap. 43) with recurrent abortion and thromboses during pregnancy suggests that all women with newly diagnosed pregnancy-associated thrombotic complication (DVT-PE) should have coagulation testing to include the basic screen (platelets, fibrinogen, APTT, PT, TCT) plus assays for AT III, protein C, and protein S. In women with a positive family history, additional evaluation for fibrinolytic system defects may be considered if the above tests are non-revealing (see Chap. 42).

MANAGEMENT

Pregnant women with venous thrombosis should be heparinized by continuous intravenous administration acutely, followed by intermittent subcutaneous heparin for the remainder of pregnancy. (Heparin does not cross the placenta and is not associated with harm to the fetus.) Because of the teratogenic potential of warfarin in the first trimester and the risk of fetal bleeding in the third trimester, we do not recommend using coumarin compounds during pregnancy. Prophylactic subcutaneous heparin should be used in patients with hereditary thrombotic disorders and in women with previous major thromboembolic disease. Warfarin can be used after delivery in the standard manner. Table 52-1 presents details of heparin use during pregnancy. Specific problems with management are discussed below.

Hereditary Thrombotic Defects

Women with known hereditary thrombotic defects (see above) should be maintained on prophylactic anticoagulation throughout pregnancy. If the patient is on warfarin at time of conception, the drug is stopped and subcutaneous heparin is started (see Table 52-1); ideally the switch to heparin prophylaxis could be accomplished before conception in a successfully planned pregnancy. Within 24 h of delivery, the heparin is stopped and an appropriate replacement concentrate is begun (both AT III concentrate and protein C concentrates have been used; see Chap. 56). After delivery, the replacement infusion is continued for 3 days and the woman's standard anticoagulation prophylaxis is restarted (usually warfarin). If clotting factor concentrate is not available, the heparin dose should be reduced and maintained by continuous intravenous infusion so that heparin levels are not > 0.3 U/mL; fresh frozen plasma may be used for partial replacement during major surgery (cesarean-section) as indicated.

TABLE 52-1 Heparinization During Pregnancy

A. Acute heparinization (acute DVT)
Sodium heparin 50–75 U/kg IV bolus injection followed by 15–25 U/kg per h by continuous infusion to prolong APTT to 1.5–2 times normal; continue therapy for 5–7 days.

B. Chronic heparinization for remainder of pregnancy
Sodium heparin 12,500 U SC every 12 h to keep APTT at 4 h 1.5–2 times normal or heparin assay 0.4–0.7 u/mL.

C. Long-term prophylaxis (hereditary defect)
Administer 5000–10,000 U sodium heparin SC* every 12 h. Monitor with heparin level (0.1–0.15 U/mL of plasma) or APTT, upper limits of normal at 4 h post-injection and adjust dose accordingly. Patients require more heparin as pregnancy progresses (relative heparin resistance). When a dosage of $\geq$ 20,000 U/day is required, an 8-h regimen may be preferable. Platelet count should be monitored.

*Note that particular care is required in the instruction of both nursing staff and patients in the use of SC heparin. A tuberculin-type syringe and a 25- or 26-gauge needle, 1/2 inch (1.5 cm) in length, is used. A fold of skin is gently raised on the lateral aspect of the anterior abdominal wall—this is facilitated if the patient bends forward. The skin is cleansed, and the needle is inserted full depth directly at right angles to the skin. The hub of the needle is held firmly between the thumb and index finger as the exact dose of heparin is injected. The needle is slowly removed at the same angle as it was inserted; care should be taken to avoid damaging the skin and SC fat at the injection site. The injection site should not be rubbed or massaged. SC heparin is best avoided in the arms and legs.

Previous Thromboembolic Disease

The management of women without known hereditary defects but with a history of prior venous thromboemboli event is controversial. Certainly, if the suspicion of a familial disorder (undiagnosed) is high or recurrent DVT or prior PE is known, the patient should be placed on prophylaxis throughout pregnancy and for 6 weeks postpartum.

Fibrinolytic Therapy

Thrombolytic therapy during pregnancy is not recommended except for possible trial in life-threatening PE.

Pregnancy after Heart Valve Replacement

This topic has been recently reviewed (Gallus reference). Optimal prophylaxis for heart valve replacement must consider fetal well-being (no warfarin during first trimester) and maternal thrombotic complications (requires therapeutic heparin to prevent; low dose subcutaneous heparin is not totally effective). A less thrombogenic bioprosthesis may be the answer, but concern about durability during pregnancy remains. Currently our recommendations are for subcutaneous heparin throughout pregnancy in a dosage adjusted to maintain heparin effect on APTT at 1.5 to 2 times normal (doses every 8 h may be needed). Treatment should be continued for 1 week after delivery while warfarin therapy is reinstituted.

Anticoagulants and Breast-feeding

Only small amounts of coumarin compounds are found in the breast milk of women receiving these oral anticoagulants; no definite effect on the breast-feeding infant's prothrombin time has been noted. Breast-feeding is not contraindicated if the baby has received adequate neonatal vitamin K prophylaxis.

ORAL CONTRACEPTIVE AGENTS AND RISK OF THROMBOSIS

The major effect of OCA on the hemostatic system is related to the amount of estrogen as ethinyl estradiol contained in the oral contraceptive agent. This dose-dependent rise in coagulation factors includes elevated levels of factors XII, II, VII, X, plasminogen, and fibrinogen. Large doses raise von Willebrand factor, factor VIII, and protein C; factor XIII and V remain normal; decreased levels of AT III and C1-esterase inhibitor are seen. Overall fibrinolytic activity (clot lysis) is normal or enhanced. More importantly, the "hypercoagulable" state noted with even 50 μg estrogen-containing agents (now commonly prescribed) is associated with a threefold relative risk factor for thromboembolism. Postmenopausal estrogen use (usually with Premarin in replacement doses) has not been proven to be a risk factor for venous thrombosis. Women at risk for thrombotic disease (hereditary or acquired disorders) should be advised to use contraceptive methods other than OCA whenever possible; older women with these disorders would be advised to use lower doses of nonoral agents (avoiding first hepatic passage effect of oral estrogens which raise clotting factors) if estrogens are needed.

Medroxyprogesterone acetate therapy for breast cancer is associated with a hypercoagulable state (short APTT, increased factor II and factor IX: increased fibrinolysis; increased AT III).

BIBLIOGRAPHY

Anderson DR et al: Subcutaneous heparin therapy during pregnancy: A need for concern at the time of delivery. *Thromb Haemost* 65:248, 1991.

Andrew M et al: An anticoagulant dermatan sulfate proteoglycan circulates in the pregnant woman and her fetus. *J Clin Invest* 89:321, 1992.

Caine YG et al: Coagulation activation following estrogen administration to postmenopausal women. *Thromb Haemost* 68:392, 1992.

Conard J et al: Thrombosis and pregnancy in congenital deficiencies in AT III, protein C, or protein S: Study of 78 women. *Thromb Haemost* 63:319, 1990.

de Boer K et al: Deep vein thrombosis in obstetric patients: Diagnosis and risk factors. *Thromb Haemost* 67:4, 1992.

Gallus AS: Anticoagulants in the prevention and treatment of thromboembolic problems in pregnancy including cardiac problems. In: Greer IA, Turpie AGG, Forbes CD (eds): *Haemostasis and Thrombosis in Obstetrics and Gynaecology*, London, Chapman and Hall Medical, 1992, pp 319–341.

Ginsberg JS et al: Risks to the fetus of anticoagulant therapy during pregnancy. *Thromb Haemost* 61:197, 1989.

Ginsberg JS et al: Venous thrombosis during pregnancy: Leg and trimester of presentation. *Thromb Haemost* 67:519, 1992.

Hathaway WE, Bonnar J: Thrombotic disorders in pregnancy and the newborn infant. In: *Hemostatic Disorders of the Pregnant Woman and Newborn Infant*, New York, Elsevier, 1987, pp 151–168.

Hathaway WE: Antithrombin III deficiencies. In: Bern MM, Frigoletto FD, Jr (eds): *Hematologic Disorders in Maternal-Fetal Medicine*, New York, Wiley-Liss, 1990, pp 467–476.

Helmrich SP et al: Venous thromboembolism in relation to oral contraceptive use. *Obstet Gynecol* 69:91, 1987.

Le Clerc JR, Roy J: The diagnosis of venous thromboembolism during pregnancy and the postpartum period. In: Greer IA, Turpie AGG, Forbes CD (eds): *Haemostasis and Thrombosis in Obstetrics and Gynaecology*, London, Chapman and Hall Medical, 1992, pp 267–298.

Lobo RA: Estrogen and the risk of coagulopathy. *Am J Med* 92:283, 1992.

Rutherford SE, Phelan JP: Deep venous thrombosis and pulmonary embolism in pregnancy. *Obstet Gynecol Clin North Am* 18:345, 1991.

Whitfield LR et al: Effect of pregnancy on the relationship between concentration and anticoagulant action of heparin. *Clin Pharmacol Ther* 34:23, 1983.

Yamamoto H et al: Changes in hematologic parameters during treatment with medroxyprogesterone acetate for breast cancer. *Jpn J Cancer Res* 82:420, 1991.

Treatment

Modalities

Platelet Transfusions

Platelet transfusions are currently a necessary component in the arrest or prevention of hemorrhage in patients with thrombocytopenia or platelet dysfunction. The most frequent use is in patients with bone marrow failure. Although pharmacologic substances may sometimes help in thrombocytopenic bleeding (DDAVP, antifibrinolytic agents), in most instances there is no substitute for platelet replacement therapy. Bleeding due to low numbers or poorly functioning platelets is characterized by diffuse oozing from trauma sites (punctures, wounds); formation of petechiae and superficial ecchymoses; mucosal hemorrhage such as gingival, oral, epistaxis, hematuria, melena or menorrhagia; and spontaneous CNS hemorrhage.

INDICATIONS FOR PLATELET TRANSFUSION

Even though the platelet count is the single most helpful indicator of the need for platelet transfusion, many other bleeding risk factors must be considered. Associated coagulation factor deficiencies (such as factor VIII level in HIV-induced thrombocytopenia in hemophiliacs and coagulopathy of liver disease), uremia, disseminated intravascular coagulation (DIC), splenomegaly, platelet function-decreasing drugs (ASA, antibiotics), mucosal and vascular integrity (injury or infection), high leukocyte count in acute nonlymphocytic leukemia, fever, and infection can increase the risk of bleeding at any given level of platelet count. In addition, the mechanism for the thrombocytopenia affects what is considered the minimal hemostatic level of platelets in a particular patient. For example, conditions associated with increased turnover of platelets (younger and larger platelets as in immune thrombocytopenic purpura [ITP]) with normal or increased platelet production will have shorter bleeding times and less clinical bleeding than conditions associated with decreased platelet production (like leukemia or aplastic anemia) at the same low platelet count.

Mildly thrombocytopenic patients (platelet count down to 50,000/μL with no additional risk factors) have little risk of spontaneous bleeding and rarely require platelet transfusion except for major surgical events. Patients with a platelet count of 20,000 to 50,000/μL have a low risk of spontaneous bleeding and usually do not require platelets except for trauma (invasive procedures, surgery) or after injury. Platelet transfusions are rarely indicated in hemolytic uremic syndrome (contraindicated in thrombotic thrombocytopenic purpura) or ITP unless for life-threatening hemorrhage. When the platelet count is 20,000 or less in patients with a hypoproliferative marrow, consideration is given to the prophylactic use of platelets.

Studies in hypoproliferative thrombocytopenias indicate (both adults and children) that serious bleeding (gastrointestinal, genitourinary, CNS) is unusual (3 to 10 percent) when the platelet count is 10,000 to 20,000/μL but increases markedly when the platelet count is < 5000/μL. A minimal hemostatic level of 10,000/μL would appear appropriate in those patients with no other risk factors. When a patient has bleeding at a platelet count > 10,000/μL, one should consider platelet dysfunction (drugs, infection) or see if the vascular system has been disrupted.

The minimal hemostatic level may be different in newborn infants with thrombocytopenia because the mechanism for decreased platelets is not only increased destruction but is also due to platelet dysfunction in the sick infant. Until better studies are available, the level of 20,000/μL is suggested for minimal hemostasis in the infant; below this level consideration for prophylactic transfusion is indicated.

PLATELET TRANSFUSION PREPARATION

To optimally prepare platelet concentrates for transfusion, the following technical details should be followed. Blood is procured from donors meeting standard selection criteria for disease-causing agents, blood group, Rh, and antibody detection. Single donor concentrates for neonates should be collected from donors not receiving ASA for several days. The blood is typically collected into plastic containers permeable to oxygen and carbon dioxide (polyolefin is better than polyvinylchloride) in CPD, CPA-1, or ACD anticoagulants giving a pH of 7.0. The blood is centrifuged to obtain at least 5.5×10^{10} platelets in a volume of 50 to 70 mL. The platelet concentrate, which can be used as soon as safety testing is done, may be stored at 22°C (room temperature) with agitation for up to 5 to 7 days.

Two general types of platelet preparations are available: (1) random donor platelet concentrate (5.5×10^{10} platelets; 45 to 65 mL volume, shelf life of up to 5 to 7 days); (2) single donor platelet concentrate prepared by apheresis (3×10^{11} platelets minimum, 200 to 500 mL of plasma; shelf life of 1 day unless collected in a closed system). Pretransfusion modification of platelet preparations that may be needed in certain circumstances include volume reduction by centrifugation, resuspension in ABO-compatible plasma or saline (to remove antibody), reduction of leukocyte content by filtration or ultraviolet irradiation (to prevent alloimmunization), and X irradiation (to prevent graft-versus-host reaction, GVHR).

DOSAGE GUIDELINES

Table 53-1 displays dosage guidelines for platelet transfusions. The guidelines assume that 1/3 of transfused platelets are sequestered in the spleen. Since recipients of platelets vary in size and blood volume and number of platelets per unit or bag varies, to assess whether a response was as anticipated, the following formula has been used. Pre- and 1 h postplatelet counts are measured. One can assume a platelet concentrate contains 5.5 $\times$ 10^{10} platelets.

$$\text{Correct count increment (CCI)} = \frac{(\text{Post} - \text{Pre count})(\text{Body surface area})}{\text{Number platelets transfused} (\times 10^{10})}$$

The CCI at the beginning of a course of platelet transfusions can be compared with a CCI later in the treatment course to determine the presence of accelerated platelet destruction. (A 10 to 15 min posttransfusion platelet count gives comparable results to 1-h post.) The CCI (using the dosage guideline) usually falls to $< 10,000/\mu L$ when antibody is present in platelet alloimmunization. Practically, hemostasis in a severely thrombocytopenic patient should be achieved by about 6 platelet concentrates in an adult (CCI will be $20,000/\mu L$) or 10 mL/kg of platelet concentrate in an infant.

COMPLICATIONS

Complications of platelet transfusion include alloimmunization, transfusion-transmitted diseases (especially bacterial contamination of stored platelets), circulatory overload, transfusion reactions (allergic, febrile), and GVHR in

TABLE 53-1 Dosage Guidelines for Platelet Transfusions

Newborn Infant
  10 mL/kg platelet concentrate should raise platelet count 75,000–100,000/μL

Older child and adult
  1U/10 kg body weight (or) 4 U/m² body surface area
  should raise platelet count (1 h) by 50,000/μL.

*U, platelet concentrate; assume normal splenic pooling and nonrefractoriness.

susceptible recipients (immunocompromised hosts and nonimmunocompromised hosts receiving blood products from first- and probably second-degree relatives, i.e., those with same HLA haplotypes). Alloimmunization or platelet refractoriness occurs in 40 to 60 percent of patients receiving variable numbers of platelets for hematologic malignancies. The diagnosis of alloimmunization requires demonstration of platelet or lymphocytotoxic antibodies (anti-HLA A or B); however the presence of antibodies does not mean that a poor response to platelet therapy is due to immunization. Platelet refractoriness (defined as failure to increase the platelet count at least $5000/\mu L$ on two sequential occasions after 4 to 6 U of random donor platelets) may also be due to an enlarged spleen, prior bone marrow transplant, DIC, amphotericin B therapy and stored platelets (response may be much better to "fresh" platelets at times). The median time for alloimmunization is 3 to 4 weeks (range 2 to 56 weeks) which may be delayed in acute lymphocytic leukemia patients on steroids (i.e., most children during induction therapy). Alloimmunization is more common in aplastic anemia than in leukemias. Alloantibodies tend to disappear with time and may not recur with subsequent platelet transfusions.

Table 53-2 outlines an approach to management of alloimmunization. This approach requires a sophisticated blood transfusion service, and if not available, the protocol will need to be modified. Empiric trials of apheresis platelets (single donor) may result in a regimen for prolonged support in the refractory patient. Other adjunctive treatments which may be tried singly and in combination in such a patient include intravenous immunoglobulin administration, possible cyclosporine A therapy, antifibrinolytic therapy, and DDAVP plus increased dose and frequency of platelets.

TABLE 53-2 Management of Alloimmunization During Platelet Transfusion Therapy

Prevention
Limit number of blood transfusions
Limit number of platelet product donors; use random single donor platelets or single donor apheresis platelets
Use leukocyte-poor blood components
Inactivation of antigen presenting cells with UV irradiation

Treatment of Refractoriness
Determine antibody specificity (HLA or platelet-specific alloantibodies)
Select compatible donors (for apheresis)
  ABO compatibility
  HLA-matched donors (A, B1, B2)
  Platelet-specific antigen matching
  Platelet crossmatch testing

BIBLIOGRAPHY

Castle V et al: Frequency and mechanism of neonatal thrombocytopenia. *J Pediatr* 108:749, 1986.

Daly PA et al: Platelet transfusion therapy. One hour posttransfusion increments are valuable in predicting the need for HLA-matched preparations. *JAMA* 243:435, 1980.

Gmur J et al: Safety of stringent prophylactic platelet transfusion policy for patients with acute leukaemia. *Lancet* 338:1223, 1991.

Herman JH, Kamel HT: Platelet transfusion: Current techniques, remaining problems, and future prospects. *Am J Pediatr Hematol/Oncol* 9:272, 1987.

Kanter MH: Transfusion-associated graft-versus-host disease: Do transfusions from second-degree relatives pose a greater risk than those from first-degree relatives? *Transfusion* 32:323, 1992.

Lee VS et al: Platelet transfusion therapy: Platelet concentrate preparation and storage. *J Lab Clin Med* 111:371, 1988.

Mintz PD: Febrile reactions to platelet transfusions. *Am J Clin Pathol* 95:609, 1991.

Moroff G et al: Reduction of the volume of stored platelet concentrates for use in neonatal patients. *Transfusion* 24:144, 1984.

O'Connell B et al: The value of 10-minute posttransfusion platelet counts. *Transfusion* 28:66, 1988.

Schiffer CA: Prophylactic platelet transfusion. *Transfusion* 32:295, 1992.

Slichter SJ: Platelet transfusions a constantly evolving therapy. *Thromb Haemost* 66:178, 1991.

Fresh Frozen Plasma

Fresh frozen plasma (FFP) is defined as the fluid portion of 1 U of human blood that has been centrifuged, separated, and frozen solid at $-18°C$ or colder within 6 h of collection. The product contains all of the procoagulant and anticoagulant plasma proteins in concentrations about 80 to 100 percent of normal and is usually stored at temperatures $< 18°C$ for up to 1 year. Other single donor plasma units prepared from whole blood at various ages and either frozen or liquid may have lower levels of the labile clotting factors, V and VIII ("liquid plasma," "source plasma"). One unit of FFP contains 200 to 280 mL and is thawed at $37°C$ just prior to transfusion.

INDICATIONS FOR USE

In general, the major indication for the use of FFP is for replacement of specific clotting factors (both procoagulant and anticoagulant) in patients for whom a specific factor concentrate is not available or is considered less safe or otherwise undesirable. Other less specific uses are for multiple clotting factor replacement in patients with severe coagulopathies such as disseminated intravascular coagulation (DIC), massive blood transfusion, vitamin K deficiency (reversal of warfarin effect), and severe liver disease. The practice of using FFP as a volume expander in patients with shock or routinely in patients requiring large amounts of packed red blood cells should be discouraged because other colloids (albumin) and crystalloids may be used without exposing the patient to additional viral risks. However, in these clinical situations FFP may be specifically indicated to obtain hemostasis (DIC, liver disease, massive blood transfusion with microvascular bleeding) by clotting factor replacement. Thus, a bleeding patient in shock could require packed red blood cells, albumin, crystalloids, *and* FFP (see Chap. 27). Sometimes whole blood may be used instead of packed red blood cells and FFP in these cases. FFP is also used with packed erythrocytes for "reconstituted" blood to be used for exchange transfusion in infants or alone to replace "washed out" clotting factors during plasmapheresis in adults (see Chap. 57).

Specific indications for the use of FFP are listed in Table 54-1 and are

TABLE 54-1 Indications for Clinical Use of Fresh Frozen Plasma

---

Replacement of isolated procoagulant factor deficiencies, particularly factor II, V, VII, X, XI, XIII (sometimes IX and VIII)

Emergent reversal of warfarin effect or vitamin K deficiency in bleeding patients

Replacement of anticoagulants in certain hereditary or severe acquired deficiencies
    Antithrombin III deficiency (surgery, perinatal)
    Protein C deficiency (homozygous state, warfarin skin necrosis, sick newborn)
    Protein S deficiency (homozygous state)
    Plasminogen deficiency (sick newborn during fibrinolytic therapy)

Massive blood transfusion

Liver disease

Thrombotic thrombocytopenia purpura–hemolytic uremic syndrome (plasma exchange)

Disseminated intravascular coagulation

---

discussed below. Whenever a specific coagulation factor concentrate has been safety tested and shown to be essentially "viral free" and otherwise safe, it is more efficient to use it instead of FFP because higher levels can be achieved without overloading the circulation. The best example is for treatment of factor VIII and IX deficiencies where essentially only coagulation factor concentrate is used in the United States.

In most instances, parenteral vitamin K administration is effective for rapid correction of vitamin K deficiency or warfarin effect; however, in an emergency (potential or actual serious bleeding) FFP or single donor plasma may be used.

Although few studies support the routine use of FFP in massive blood transfusion (either prophylactically or to "correct" clotting studies), in certain individuals with severe bleeding, FFP, and even more often, platelet concentrates may be helpful in arresting bleeding. The use of FFP to correct screening tests (PT, PTT) in patients with severe liver disease correlates poorly with bleeding tendency unless the defect is very severe; DDAVP use appears more helpful to prevent bleeding. In DIC, low fibrinogen levels are best repaired with cryoprecipitate administration rather than FFP.

DOSAGE RECOMMENDATIONS

One unit or bag of FFP contains 200 to 280 mL with 0.7 to 1.0 U/mL of clotting activity of each coagulation factor and 1 to 2 mg/mL of fibrinogen. The dose of 10 mL/kg body weight will cause a rise in clotting factors of about 15 to 20 percent; if the factor is distributed quickly extravascularly, a dose of 15 mL/kg will be needed to reach 20 percent level (i.e., for factors VII and IX). The

TABLE 54-2 Coagulation Factor Characteristics in Plasma

Coagulation factor	T$_{1/2}$ in vitro	T$_{1/2}$ postinfusion, h
Fibrinogen	—	96
II	Stable	60
V	3–5 days	24
VII	Stable	4
VIII	1–2 weeks	11–12
IX	Stable	22
X	Stable	35
XI	Stable (?)	60
XIII	Stable	6 days
vWf	Stable	8–12

*T$_{1/2}$, half disappearance time; stable, no decrease of activity during blood bank storage; vWf, von Willebrand factor.

dose should be given rapidly (about an hour or less) to produce a peak level. The initial volume administered in an adult is often 600 to 2000 mL to produce a hemostatic effect (level of 15 to 30 percent of most coagulation factors). Additional doses of FFP are repeated at intervals depending on the half-disappearance time of the factor being replaced (Table 54-2). Circulatory overload tends to occur at total dosages $\geq$ 30 mL/kg per 24 h; therefore, it is difficult to safely achieve hemostatic levels for clinical situations like surgery or severe trauma in hereditary deficient patients (hemophilia A or B) with FFP alone. Other maneuvers which help in using large amounts of plasma to achieve hemostatic levels include concomitant diuretics, prolonged administration (start early) for clotting factors with long half-life, and plasma exchange. ABO-compatible plasma should always be used.

COMPLICATIONS

The risks of the use of FFP include disease transmission; risks are the same as for other blood components and with optimal screening tests range from 3/10,000 for hepatitis C to one in a million for HIV (using HIV antibody and antigen screening); 3/1000 for hepatitis B; non A– non B hepatitis risk (after elimination of hepatitis C virus) is not known. The New York Blood Center has developed a solvent/detergent-treated plasma that is essentially virus-free and can be used for treatment of coagulation factor deficiencies for which safe concentrates are not available. Other risks include allergic or anaphylactoid reactions (hives to fatal noncardiac pulmonary edema), hypervolemia and cardiac failure, IgA antibodies leading to anaphylaxis in IgA-deficient patients, and the rare occurrence of Rh sensitization.

With the availability of cryoprecipitate and safe concentrates, practically the only indications for FFP use are hereditary factor II, V, X, XI, XIII, protein C, and protein S deficiency; severe liver disease; massive blood transfusion; and consumption coagulopathies (concentrates for XIII, XI, and protein C are available in some areas).

BIBLIOGRAPHY

Blumberg N et al: A critical survey of fresh-frozen plasma use. *Transfusion* 26:511, 1986.

Braunstein AH, Oberman HA: Transfusion of plasma components. *Transfusion* 24:281, 1984.

Counts RB et al: Hemostasis in massively transfused trauma patients. *Ann Surg* 190:91, 1979.

Dzik WH et al: Refreezing previously thawed fresh-frozen plasma. Stability of coagulation factors V and VIII:C. *Transfusion* 29:600, 1989.

Hondow JA et al: The stability of coagulation factors in stored blood. *Aust NZ J Surg* 52:265, 1982.

Horowitz B et al: Solvent/detergent-treated plasma: A virus inactivated substitute for FFP. *Blood* 79:826, 1992.

Huestis DW et al: *Practical Blood Transfusion*, 3d ed. Boston, Little, Brown, 1981.

Mannucci PM et al: Hemostasis testing during massive blood replacement. A study of 172 cases. *Vox Sang* 42:113, 1982.

National Institutes of Health Consensus Conference: Fresh-frozen plasma, indications and risks. *JAMA* 253:551, 1985.

Cryoprecipitate

Cryoprecipitate (cryo) is the cold-insoluble fraction of plasma protein recovered by centrifugation when fresh frozen plasma is thawed at 4°C. Since the simple procedure using a sterile closed-bag system was described in 1965 by Pool and Shannon, most blood banks have produced cryo for treatment of hemophilia without interfering with the production of other blood components. Cryo is a single donor product and contains about half the original factor VIII activity and 20 to 40 percent of the fibrinogen in < 3 percent of the plasma protein. Table 55-1 lists the clinically important constituents in a single cryo unit or bag. The total amount of each substance varies according to the amount of plasma retained to dissolve the cryoprecipitate (5 to 30 mL); however, to meet standards each bag must contain a minimum of 80 U factor VIII. Cryo is stored frozen (at least −18°C) for up to 1 year. To prepare the product for clinical use, the appropriate number of bags are thawed at 37°C and pooled in a large syringe or another bag after filtering the product through a 40-μ filter.

INDICATIONS FOR CLINICAL USE

In many parts of the world cryo is the main product for treatment of hemophilia A and von Willebrand disease although the latest generation factor VIII concentrates and DDAVP have largely replaced cryo in the

TABLE 55-1 Major Plasma Proteins Contained in a Single Unit of Cryoprecipitate

Constituent	Amount (total)
Factor VIII	average 100 U (must have at least 80 U)
Fibrinogen	100–250 mg
von Willebrand factor	40–70% of original plasma
Fibronectin	50–60 mg
Anti-A and anti-B isohemagglutinins	trace
Other clotting factors (XIII, protein S)	trace

United States, Canada, Japan, and Europe. In addition to its use for treatment of bleeding episodes in hemophilia A and von Willebrand disease, cryo is the main product available for fibrinogen replacement and the treatment of dysfibrinogenemias. Another use for cryo is in the preparation of fibrin glue for local use in arrest of surgical bleeding and for topical use in removal of ureteral stones and stabilization of auditory ossicles.

DOSAGE GUIDELINES

The disadvantages of using cryo for clinical situations in which a concentrate is available are related to the risks of viral transmission. Although cryo cannot be treated with virucidal methods like concentrates, the use of modern donor screening tests and family donors substantially reduces the risk of viral transmission. A recent report indicates that the current risk of posttransfusion hepatitis C is about 3/10,000 U transfused. In addition, the yield of factor VIII and von Willebrand factor in cryo can be increased one- to fivefold by administration of DDAVP to the blood donor prior to plasmapheresis.

Hemophilia A

Use dosage guidelines outline for concentrates (see Chap. 56) assuming 1 bag cryo contains 100 U factor VIII. Alternatively, 1 bag/6 kg will give a hemostatic level of factor VIII of about 35 percent.

von Willebrand Disease

In adults in whom DDAVP is not appropriate, 10 to 12 bags cryo every 12 h will usually ensure hemostasis even though the bleeding time may not always show correction. In children, 1 bag/6 kg is an approximate equivalent dose. One bag of cryo contains about 100 U of vWf with a normal multimeric pattern.

Fibrinogen Replacement

Ten bags of cryo will raise the fibrinogen level by 60 to 100 mg in a 70-kg person. In the term newborn infant a single pack of cryo will increase the fibrinogen level more than 100 mg/dL. The minimal hemostatic level of fibrinogen is 75 to 100 mg/dL and the half-disappearance time is 3.5 days.

COMPLICATIONS

Transfusion reactions and disease transmission risks are the same as for fresh frozen plasma. In addition, the importance of using an administration filter (40 μ) to prevent the infusion of fibrin and particulate matter should be emphasized. Patients receiving large amounts of cryo for hemophilia A over an extended period of time (for surgical procedures) have been subject to increased bleeding manifestations despite adequate factor VIII or vWf ristocetin cofactor levels. This "paradoxical" bleeding has been related to high fibrinogen levels, increased fibrin degradation products, and prolonged bleeding time. Anti-A and anti-B isohemagglutinins may also produce hemolysis in patients receiving large amounts of the product (if the patient becomes anemic and needs erythrocyte transfusion, use O cells): cryo should be type specific when possible (both ABO group and Rh).

BIBLIOGRAPHY

Burka ER et al: A protocol for cryoprecipitate production. *Transfusion* 15:307, 1975.

Chediak JR et al: Platelet function and immunologic parameters in von Willebrand's disease following cryoprecipitate and factor VIII concentrate infusion. *Am J Med* 62:369, 1977.

Donahue JG et al: The declining risk of post-transfusion hepatitis C virus infection. *N Engl J Med* 327:369, 1992.

Hathaway WE et al: Paradoxical bleeding in intensively transfused hemophiliacs: Alteration of platelet function. *Transfusion* 13:6, 1973.

Hoffman M et al: Fibrinogen content of low-volume cryoprecipitate. *Transfusion* 27:356, 1987.

Inwood MJ et al: Filtration of cryoprecipitate: A microscopic assessment of filter deposition. *Transfusion* 18:722, 1978.

Pool JG, Shannon AE: Production of high-potency concentrates of antihemophilic globulin in a closed-bag system. *N Engl J Med* 273:1443, 1965.

Smiley RK et al: Studies on the prolonged bleeding time in von Willebrand's disease. *Thromb Res* 53:417, 1989.

Coagulation Factor
Concentrates

During the past 25 years steady advances have been made in the development and manufacture of coagulation factor concentrates for clinical use (see Roberts reference). Viral complications of concentrate therapy (HIV, hepatitis viruses) have been catastrophic, but in recent years it appears that current methodology has all but eliminated the viral threat; at the present time mostly the parvovirus is known to resist virucidal techniques. The advent of recombinant protein technology (already established for factors VII and VIII) should provide the means for the ultimate pure and safe product. A great deal of the progress is due to systematic safety testing of new products as they become available. Since 1984, guidelines prepared by the International Committee on Thrombosis and Hemostasis (ICTH) have been available for the use of investigators and manufacturers in testing new products. A recent revision of the protocol, which was designed mainly to detect hepatitis, is summarized here.

1. Patients to be enrolled in clinical studies of the safety from hepatitis should be previously untreated with blood or blood product and should be tested for aminotransferase levels at 15-day intervals for at least 4 months after infusion.

2. Patients missing two consecutive laboratory values in the first 4 months and one value in the next 2 months should be excluded from analysis.

3. Studies should include at least 20 analyzable patients treated with 10 batches of concentrate.

4. Studies should be stopped when at least two cases of hepatitis are detected. Routine laboratory tests for hepatitis B virus (HBV), hepatitis C virus (HCV), and HIV are also performed.

Physicians using the commercially available products should be aware of the results of hepatitis safety testing for the product.

CONCENTRATE DESCRIPTION AND PRINCIPLES OF THERAPY

Although it is beyond the scope of this discussion to review methodology for preparation of concentrates, a few general remarks are in order. Current production of clotting factor concentrates requires a large starting pool of carefully screened donor plasma which is processed to produce as pure a clotting factor(s) as practical. Affinity chromatography using monoclonal antibodies currently provides the purest product (Table 56-1). Viral inactivation procedures (pasteurization or solvent-detergent treatment) are effective against HIV and hepatitis viruses. The final product is assayed against international coagulation factor standards and labeled accordingly. A unit is the coagulant activity in 1 mL fresh normal plasma (the standard); for instance, 100 U factor VIII is the amount of clotting activity in 100 mL fresh plasma.

TABLE 56-1 Coagulation Factor Concentrates Available for Treatment of Hemophilia in the United States

Product	Preparation	Viral inactivation	Specific activity μ/mg
Factor VIII replacement			
Profilate OSD (Alpha)	PEG-amino acid ppt	Solvent-detergent	<10
New York Blood Ctr FVIII-SD		Solvent-detergent	<10
Koate-HP (Cutter)	Chromatography	TNBP—Tween 80	9–22
Monoclate (Armour)	Immuno-affinity	Pasteurization	15 (diluted-albumin)
Hemophil M (Baxter)	Immuno-affinity	Solvent-detergent	15 (diluted-albumin)
AHF (Human), Method M (Amer Red Cross)	Immuno-affinity	Solvent-detergent	15 (diluted-albumin)
Factor IX replacement			**Units/mg**
Alpha Nine-SD (Alpha)	Chromatography	Solvent-detergent	50–150
Mononine (Armour)	Immuno-affinity	Na thiocyanate; ultrafiltration	150
von Willebrand factor replacement			
Humate P (Behring)	Glycine and salt precipitation	Pasteurization	3–8

Other PCC products (Konyne, Proplex, Profilnine) have variable bypassing activity and have been used to halt bleeding in inhibitor patients.

Both plasma-derived and recombinant-activated factor VII have been used to treat hemorrhage in inhibitor patients. At present recombinant factor VIIa is available for investigative and compassionate use (Novo Nordisk). The dosage schedule has not been determined but doses of 70 to 90 μg/kg every 3 h have been effective in halting life-threatening surgical bleeding. Under therapy, the PT and APTT shorten and factor VII activity increases greatly; plasminogen levels may fall. No thrombotic complications have been reported.

COMPLICATIONS

The major complications of clotting factor therapy are related to the transmission of viral disease, mainly HIV or hepatitis viruses. As noted above, the current use of donor screening and virucidal techniques (solvent-detergent, pasteurization) and the insistence on safety testing when the product is first used has led to a generation of products which have been proven at extremely low risk of viral transmission (comparable to albumin products). A nonlipid envelope virus (B19 parvovirus) is currently the exception to elimination by dry, wet, and steam-heated methods. Parvovirus has been transmitted to hemophiliacs in factor VIII concentrates and has even caused mild hypoplastic anemia in a solvent–detergent-treated concentrate recipient.

Several studies have suggested that alloantigen exposure to repeated administration of factor concentrates (intermediate purity) can alter the immune response in HIV-negative hemophiliacs (decreased CD4 cells, elevated immunoglobulins, and decreased delayed-type immunity). Whether ultrapure products (monoclonally derived, recombinant) may influence the progression of decreased immunity in HIV-positive hemophiliacs remains controversial. So far no harm is apparent from the use of the purer products which, with the foregoing data, suggest that "pure is better" when choice of products is made. Additional evidence for this concept comes from the observations that high-purity factor IX products have distinctly fewer thrombogenic properties than previous intermediate-purity material.

The major obstacles to the widespread use of the more pure products are related to availability (Food and Drug Administration approval) and cost.

CONCENTRATES OF ANTICOAGULANT FACTORS

At present, two anticoagulant proteins are available in concentrate form, antithrombin III (AT III) and protein C. At least four manufacturers have

AT III concentrates available or soon to be available in Europe or the United States (Behringwerke, Cutter, Kabi Vitrum, Hyland-Baxter). Viral inactivation has usually been by pasteurization or wet heat and has not been associated with transmission of hepatitis or HIV agents. The composition of the final product is > 95 percent AT III. Vials of the lyophilized product are labeled in international units (IU). A dose of 1 U/kg will produce a rise of approximately 2 percent with a half-disappearance time of approximately 60 h. In patients with heterozygous AT III deficiency requiring surgery (in whom heparinization increases hemorrhagic risk), a dose of 25 U/kg should increase base levels by 50 percent (AT III activity assay).

However, in ill patients, in pregnancy, and in preeclampsia only a 1 percent rise per international unit per kilogram may be seen (use 50 U/kg); the half-disappearance time may also be less (29 h) so that a daily dose may be required.

Other clinical situations where AT III concentrates have shown efficacy include fulminant hepatic failure (patients with liver failure requiring hemodialysis need less heparin and platelets when supplemented with AT III concentrate), posttrauma shock and DIC; acute fatty liver of pregnancy, and HELLP (hemolysis, elevated liver enzymes, low platelet count) syndrome in preeclampsia.

Protein C concentrate has been produced by Immuno; it has been used with success in cases of homozygous protein C deficiency (see Chap. 40) and in the perinatal period. Future uses may include prophylaxis for thrombotic episodes in heterozygous protein C deficiency at time of surgery.

BIBLIOGRAPHY

Abildgaard CF et al: Anti-inhibitor coagulant complex (Autoplex) for treatment of factor VIII inhibitors in hemophilia. *Blood* 56:978, 1980.

Aronstam A et al: Double-blind controlled trial of three dosage regimens in treatment of haemarthroses in haemophilia A. *Lancet* i:169, 1980.

Bloom AL: Progress in the clinical management of haemophilia. *Thromb Haemost* 66:166, 1991.

Bjorkman S et al: Pharmacokinetics of factor VIII in humans; obtaining clinically relevant data from comparative studies. *Clin Pharmacokinet* 22:385-395, 1992.

Bolton-Maggs PHB et al: Production and therapeutic use of a factor XI concentrate from plasma. *Thromb Haemost* 67:314, 1992.

Brettler DB et al: The use of porcine factor VIII concentrate (Hyate:C) in the treatment of patients with inhibitor antibodies to factor VIII. A multicenter US experience. *Arch Intern Med* 149:1381, 1989.

Cuthbert RJ et al: Immunological studies in HIV seronegative haemophiliacs: Relationships to blood product therapy. *Br J Haematol* 80:364, 1992.

Goudemand J et al: Clinical and biological evaluation in von Willebrand's disease of a von Willebrand factor concentrate with low factor VIII activity. *Br J Haematol* 80:214, 1992.

Hathaway WE et al: Comparison of continuous and intermittent factor VIII concentrate therapy in hemophilia A. *Am J Hematol* 17:85, 1984.

Hedner U et al: Successful use of recombinant factor VIIa in a patient with severe haemophilia A during synovectomy. *Lancet* 2:1193, 1988.

Hilgartner MW, Knatterud GL, FEIBA Study Group: The use of factor eight inhibitor by-passing activity (FEIBA Immuno) product for treatment of bleeding episodes in hemophiliacs with inhibitors. *Blood* 61:36, 1983.

Horowitz B: Blood protein derivative viral safety: Observations and analysis. *Yale J Biol Med* 63:361, 1990.

Kim HC et al: Purified factor IX using monoclonal immunoaffinity technique: Clinical trials in hemophilia B and comparison to prothrombin complex concentrates. *Blood* 79:568, 1992.

Lusher JM et al: Recombinant factor VIII for the treatment of previously untreated patients with hemophilia A. Safety, efficacy, and development of inhibitors. *N Engl J Med* 328:453, 1993.

Manno CS et al: Low recovery in vivo of highly purified factor VIII in patients with hemophilia. *J Pediatr* 121:814, 1992.

Mannucci PM, Colombo M: Revision of the protocol recommended for studies of safety from hepatitis of clotting factor concentrates. *Thromb Haemost* 61:532, 1989.

Mannucci PM et al: Comparison of four virus-inactivated plasma concentrates for treatment of severe von Willebrand disease: A cross-over randomized trial. *Blood* 79:3130, 1992.

Menache D et al: Evaluation of the safety, recovery, half-life, and clinical efficacy of antithrombin III (human) in patients with hereditary antithrombin III deficiency, Cooperative Group Study. *Blood* 75:33, 1990.

Morfini M et al: Hypoplastic anemia in a hemophiliac first infused with a solvent/detergent treated factor VIII concentrate: The role of human B19 Parvovirus. *Am J Hematol* 39:149, 1992.

Pierce GF et al: The use of purified clotting factor concentrates in hemophilia. Influence of viral safety, cost and supply on therapy. *JAMA* 261:3434, 1989.

Roberts HR: Factor VIII replacement therapy; issues and future prospects. *Ann N Y Acad Sci* 614:106, 1991.

Rodeqhiero F et al: Clinical pharmacokinetics of a placenta-derived factor XIII concentrate in type I and type II factor XIII deficiency. *Am J Hematol* 36:30, 1991.

Apheresis and

Exchange Transfusion

Apheresis and exchange transfusion are treatment procedures whose purpose is to remove certain pathologic substances from the circulation and to replace missing or defective components. Apheresis is used widely by transfusion services to obtain necessary products (platelet pheresis, leukapheresis, plasmapheresis) such as platelet packs, granulocyte transfusions, fresh frozen plasma, and packed red blood cells. Exchange transfusion using whole blood or blood components is mostly limited to the neonatal and infancy period. The use of plasmapheresis and exchange transfusion are sometimes life-saving in the hemostatically deficient patient. Clinical situations where these and closely related techniques (protein A-antibody immunoadsorption) have proven useful are listed in Table 57-1 and discussed below.

PLASMAPHERESIS

Plasmapheresis or plasma exchange is performed by automated apheresis instruments which use microprocessor technology to draw and anticoagulate blood, separate plasma by centrifugation or filtration, and recombine cells with volume replacement for return to the patient. Anticoagulant is citrate with or without heparin and the volume replacement is 5 percent albumin in isotonic saline, plasma expanders, or donor plasma. The procedure is performed from peripheral venous access or multilumen central venous catheters at flow rates of 30 to 80 mL/min. Potential mechanisms for positive effects of the procedure include removal of antigen, antibody, immune complex, and protein degradation products; enhancement of splenic clearance of immune complexes; and replacement (when plasma is used) of normal plasma components which may be deficient in the disease state. About 40 mL/kg (plasma volume) of plasma removed results in a reduction of IgG antibody to slightly less than half; however, a rebound rise is expected because of equilibration of extravascular antibody. A 4-L plasma exchange in an adult removed more

TABLE 57-1 Hemostatic and Thrombotic Disorders in which Plasmapheresis and Exchange Transfusion Have Been Helpful

Disorder	Rationale
Plasmapheresis	
Coagulation factor inhibitors	Remove antibody
ITP	Remove antibody and CIC
ITP/hemolytic uremic syndrome	Remove platelet aggregating substances and replace protective substances (antibody, enzymes?)
Severe liver disease (acute fatty liver of pregnancy)	Remove degradation products; replace clotting factors
Post transfusion purpura	Remove antibody, CIC
Macroglobulinemia	Remove paraprotein
Platelet apheresis	
Thrombocythemia, myeloproliferative disorder	Remove excess platelets
Exchange transfusion	
Severe erythroblastosis fetalis, fetal hydrops	Remove antibody; replace clotting factors
Severe liver disease; disseminated intravascular coagulation	Remove clotting factor degradation products; replace clotting factors
Immunoadsorption	
Hemophilia A, B, with alloantibody	Remove antibody
ITP	Remove antibody and CIC (Immune modulation)

*CIC, circulating immune complexes; ITP, immune thrombocytopenia purpura.

than 50 percent of a factor VIII antibody (intensive plasma exchange). Other experience with plasma exchange in both auto- and alloantibodies against factor VIII has indicated the procedure to be helpful in lowering the antibody titer to levels where hemostatic treatment could be effective. One series indicated that 45 ± 7 mL/kg plasma exchanged resulted in an average antibody decrease of 61 ± 8 percent.

In the treatment of thrombotic thrombocytopenia purpura (TTP), a daily plasma exchange using fresh frozen plasma, 65 to 140 mL/kg was performed (see Chap. 29). This intensive regimen using cryoprecipitate-poor plasma or fresh frozen plasma is considered necessary because of the possibility of replacing a platelet-aggregating factor inhibitor. If the plasma exchange is primarily being performed to treat a severe coagulopathy such as acute fatty liver of pregnancy or prepare a severe liver disease patient for biopsy or surgery, fresh frozen plasma should be used as a replacement therapy. In the other uses of plasmapheresis to reduce antibody levels, albumin-saline or mixtures of albumin-saline and plasma are effective replacement fluids.

On-line immunoadsorption with staphylococcal protein A sepharose and silica columns have been used in conjunction with plasmapheresis to lower antibody titers and immune complexes in patients with factor VIII antibodies, refractory immune thrombocytopenic purpura, and cancer-related TTP.

Complications

With therapeutic plasmapheresis, the main function of the replacement fluid is to maintain intravascular volume, colloid osmotic pressure, and electrolyte balance. In most well-nourished patients, homeostatic mechanisms obviate the need for precise plasma replacement. When 5 percent albumin or plasma protein fraction is used, the APTT, PT, and TCT are prolonged and fibrinogen, plasminogen, and antithrombin III are reduced as are factors V, VII, IX, X, and the contact factors. These changes, especially of decreased platelets, can be marked down to 20 to 30 percent after repeated pheresis, but return to normal in 24 to 36 h. These alterations have rarely caused a bleeding episode; however, an occasional thrombotic complication has been noted.

EXCHANGE TRANSFUSION

Although plasmapheresis is feasible in children, the small size of young infants and newborn babies preclude the use of the procedure in them. A similar physiologic effect (removal of antibody, replacement of coagulation factors) can be achieved by a double blood volume exchange transfusion. Exchange transfusions have been used in severely ill infants with marked derangements of coagulation (severe sepsis or liver disease and disseminated intravascular coagulation). Our preference for blood for neonatal exchange transfusion is CPD-anticoagulated blood less than 48 h old or fresh frozen plasma-reconstituted packed red blood cells; use of heparinized blood has been associated with increased bleeding manifestations. Because neither 48-h CPD blood nor reconstituted blood has adequate platelets, supplemental platelet concentrates are necessary at the end of the procedure to correct significant thrombocytopenia.

Complications

Most of the complications listed in Table 57-2 are related to use of umbilical vessels, inexperienced operators, and improper choice of blood for exchange (blood too old or overheated).

TABLE 57-2 Complications of Neonatal Exchange Transfusion

Complication	Cause
Liver necrosis	Improper umbilical vessel catheter
Hemoperitoneum	placement and manipulation
Necrotizing enterocolitis	
Air embolism	
Tetany	Hypocalcemia (citrated blood)
Cardiac arrest	Electrolyte imbalance, hyperkalemia
Hyperviscosity	Use of packed red blood cells
Infection	Portal of entry
Thrombosis	Catheter-vessel damage
Graft-versus-host reaction	Failure to irradiate donor blood

BIBLIOGRAPHY

Barnard DR et al: Blood for use in exchange transfusion in the newborn. *Transfusion* 20:401, 1980.

Chudwin DS et al: Posttransfusion syndrome: Rash, eosinophilia, and thrombocytopenia following intrauterine and exchange transfusions. *Am J Dis Child* 136:612, 1982.

Flaum MA et al: The hemostatic imbalance of plasma-exchange transfusion. *Blood* 54:694, 1979.

Francesconi M et al: Plasmapheresis: Its value in the management of patients with antibodies to factor VIII. *Haemostasis* 11:79, 1982.

Rao AK et al: The hemostatic system in children undergoing intensive plasma exchange. *J Pediatr* 100:69, 1982.

Rosen MS, Reich SB: Umbilical venous catheterization in the newborn: Identification of correct positioning. *Radiology* 95:335, 1970.

Slocombe GW et al: The role of intensive plasma exchange in the prevention and management of haemorrhage in patients with inhibitors to factor VIII. *Br J Haematol* 47:577, 1981.

Snyder HW et al: Experience with protein A-immunoadsorption in treatment-resistant adult immune thrombocytopenic purpura. *Blood* 79:2237, 1992.

CHAPTER 58

Intravenous

Immunoglobulin

Intravenous immunoglobulin (IVIG) was introduced over a decade ago for the treatment of immunodeficiency diseases. Since that time several refined products have been developed and the indications for its therapeutic use have been expanded to include infectious complications of disease and autoimmune disorders. It is in the latter category that IVIG has become an important therapeutic tool in hemostatic disorders such as immune thrombocytopenias and acquired coagulation inhibitors.

As discussed by Dietrich and others, several mechanisms of action have been proposed to explain the efficacy of IVIG in autoimmune disease. These include reversible blockade of Fc receptors on cells of the reticuloendothelial system by Fc fragments of injected IVIG, inhibition of autoantibody synthesis through Fc-dependent or anticlass II-dependent modulation of T-cell and B-cell function, interference of IVIG with complement (C3)-mediated damage or cytokine secretion, and the presence in IVIG of anti-idiotypic activity against disease-associated autoantibodies.

The evidence that IVIG contains anti-idiotypic antibodies can be summarized: F (ab')2 fragments from IVIG inhibit autoantibody activity and the fragments can be retained on affinity columns of the autoantibody; IVIG and heterologous anti-idiotypic reagents recognize the same idiotypes on autoantibodies. IVIG interacts with constitutive elements of the physiologic antibody network and alters the regulatory function of the network in vivo; this alteration may help to restore control of autoimmunity.

INDICATION FOR USE IN HEMOSTATIC DISORDERS

In addition to indications for the use of IVIG in many autoimmune and inflammatory disorders (myasthenia gravis, multiple sclerosis, Grave's disease, autoimmune cytopenias, systemic lupus erythematosus [SLE], rheumatoid arthritis, and Kawasaki disease) and immunodeficiency syndromes, several hemostatic disorders have benefited from its use (Table 58-1). The better established of these indications are discussed below.

Immune Thrombocytopenia

Intravenous immunoglobulin is an acceptable form of therapy for severe thrombocytopenia in immune thrombocytopenia purpura (ITP), especially in children where the majority of cases are self-limited and only one course of therapy is needed. The major use in adult ITP is for rapid control of acute bleeding episodes, preparation of patient for surgery, and when steroids or splenectomy is contraindicated (elderly, pregnancy, diabetes mellitus). Its use has proven efficacious in both acute and chronic ITP (to delay or be used instead of splenectomy) and in passively transferred autoantibody-induced thrombocytopenia in offspring of mothers with ITP or SLE. The advantages for using IVIG include rapidity of action (1 to 2 days) and general absence of side effects; disadvantages include need for multiple intravenous infusions and significant cost. IVIG is also effective in the treatment of thrombocytopenia in HIV-infected individuals.

Intravenous immunoglobulin has been demonstrated to be effective in a preliminary fashion in neonatal alloimmune thrombocytopenia, both as a treatment for the severely thrombocytopenic newborn and as a prevention for intracranial bleeding by raising the platelet count in the fetus when the IVIG is administered to the mother weeks before delivery. Controlled studies are in progress to substantiate these findings. Platelet alloimmunization after repeated platelet transfusions has also shown partial responses to IVIG in refractory cases.

TABLE 58-1   Uses of Intravenous Immunoglobulin in Disorders of Hemostasis

Established benefit
   Immune thrombocytopenia purpura (childhood and adult)
   Neonatal alloimmune thrombocytopenia
   Wiscott-Aldrich syndrome

Potential benefit
   Factor VIII acquired autoantibodies
   Anticardiolipin antibodies and recurrent abortions
   Acquired von Willebrand disease
   HIV-induced thrombocytopenia
   Immune tolerance treatment—hemophilia
   Thrombotic thrombocytopenia purpura

Acquired Factor VIII Autoantibodies

Administration of IVIG has reduced the level of factor VIII autoantibody in association with recovery of factor VIII levels in patients with the acquired or spontaneous factor VIII autoantibody syndrome. This effect was considered due to suppression of the autoantibodies by the anti-idiotypic antibodies contained in the IVIG. In contrast, IVIG has had little effect in suppression of antibody in hemophilia patients with inhibitors, although IVIG is included in the immune tolerance regimen of the Malmo group (see Chap. 21).

DOSAGE GUIDELINES

Intravenous immunoglobulin is a therapeutic preparation of polyspecific IgG obtained from plasma pools of 8000 to over 20,000 healthy blood donors. Current preparations (Sando-globin, Gammagard, Gamimmune, Endobulin) are made of intact IgG with low amounts (2 to 610 μg/mL) of IgA and a normal distribution of IgG subclasses. Fragments and aggregates are < 10 percent but up to 30 percent of F(ab')2 dimers are present. The lyophilized product is reconstituted (3 to 6 percent solution) and given slowly intravenously. IVIG has a half-life of approximately 3 weeks.

The standard dose for the hemostatic disorders is 400 mg/kg per day for 5 days (infants, children, and adults). In ITP or neonatal alloimmune thrombocytopenia a prompt rise in platelet count is expected in the first few days; if the count is > 50,000 by day 3, the remainder of the course may be omitted. Alternatively, in ITP 1 g/kg may be given on day 1 and 2 (total of 2 g/kg). Maintenance doses for ITP in children are the single 400-mg/kg dose at appropriate intervals. Maintenance therapy with 60 g IVIG administered when platelet count falls below 20,000/μL has been used in adults.

Complications

Reactions to present IVIG preparations are minimal, generally of the mild discomfort type, and often related to speed of administration. The reactions include pallor, sweating, nausea, chills, low-grade fever, back discomfort, muscle aches, chest tightening, and blood pressure changes. Temporary slowing or stopping of the infusion leads to decreased or disappearance of symptoms. Rarely, a true anaphylactic reaction will occur due to anti-IgA antibodies. Serum sickness can occur. Direct Coombs' test may become positive. Rapid hemolysis due to anti-A and anti-B antibody with fever and disseminated intravascular coagulation has been reported after IVIG in a patient with Kawasaki's disease.

INTRAVENOUS ANTI-D TREATMENT

An intravenous preparation of anti-D immunoglobulin (Winrho) has been used successfully in Rh positive ITP patients to produce reticuloendothelial cell blockade and to increase the platelet count. Toxicity was minimal and the infusions can be completed in < 5 min. Preliminary studies indicated that children respond better than adults; HIV-infected patients respond as well as ITP patients; and platelet counts could be maintained at adequate levels at a mean interval of 24 days between infusions.

BIBLIOGRAPHY

Blanchette VS et al: Role of intravenous immunoglobulin G in autoimmune hematologic disorders. *Sem Hematol* 29:72, 1992.

Bussel JB et al: Antenatal treatment of neonatal alloimmune thrombocytopenia. *N Engl J Med* 319:1374, 1988.

Bussel JB et al: Intravenous anti-D treatment of immune thrombocytopenic purpura; analysis of efficacy, toxicity, and mechanism of effect. *Blood* 77:1884, 1991.

Comenzo RL et al: Immune hemolysis, disseminated intravascular coagulation, and serum sickness after large doses of immune globulin given intravenously for Kawasaki disease. *J Pediatr* 120:926, 1992.

Dietrich G et al: Modulation of autoimmunity by intravenous immune globulin through interaction with the function of the immune/idiotypic network. *Clin Immunol Immunopathol* 62:S73, 1992.

Gordon DS (Guest editor): Symposium on innovative uses of intravenous immune globulins in clinical hematology. *Am J Med* 83(4A):1–52, 1987.

Green D, Kwaan HC: An acquired factor VIII inhibitor responsive to high-dose gamma globulin. *Thromb Haemost* 58:1005, 1987.

Kaveri SV et al: Intravenous immunoglobulins (IVIg) in the treatment of autoimmune diseases. *Clin Exp Immunol* 86:192, 1991.

Lee EJ et al: Intravenous immune globulin for patients alloimmunized to random donor platelet transfusion. *Transfusion* 27:245, 1987.

Pietz J et al: High-dose intravenous gamma globulin for neonatal alloimmune thrombocytopenia in twins. *Acta Paediatr Scand* 80:129, 1991.

Pirofsky B, Kinzey DM: Intravenous immune globulins. A review of their uses in selected immunodeficiency and autoimmune diseases. *Drugs* 43:6, 1992.

Suarez CR, Anderson C: High-dose intravenous gamma globulin (IVG) in neonatal immune thrombocytopenia. *Am J Hematol* 26:247, 1987.

Sultan Y et al: Anti-idiotypic suppression of autoantibodies to factor VIII (anti-haemophilic factor) by high-dose intravenous gamma globulin. *Lancet* i:765, 1984.

Desmopressin (DDAVP)

Desmopressin (1-desamino-8-D-arginine vasopressin; DDAVP) is a synthetic analogue of the antidiuretic hormone L-arginine vasopressin, AVP. Following earlier observations that adrenaline and strenuous exercise raised factor VIII levels in man, Cash and colleagues in Scotland and Mannucci and colleagues in Italy found that DDAVP increased factor VIII levels when infused into healthy volunteers. Soon it was established that DDAVP, like adrenaline, induced a threefold rise of factor VIII, von Willebrand factor, and tissue plasminogen activator (t-PA) with a slightly shorter half-disappearance time than homologous proteins. Since the early 1980s, DDAVP has been the standard hemostatic treatment for bleeding episodes in mild hemophilia A and most patients with von Willebrand disease.

MECHANISM OF ACTION

As shown in Fig. 59-1, DDAVP differs from AVP by two structural changes. These changes increase the antidiuretic effect which is mediated through the V_2 receptor and a calcium-independent cyclic adenosine monophosphate (AMP)-dependent second messenger; factor VIII and von Willebrand factor release is also apparently mediated by the V_2 receptor mechanism. The V_1 receptor, by means of a calcium-dependent, cyclic AMP-independent second messenger, mediates vascular smooth muscle and is responsible for the pressor effects of AVP. This oxytocic activity is decreased to 0.013 to 0.25 of that of AVP in the altered molecule, DDAVP. Thus, DDAVP exhibits superior antidiuretic effects without the undesirable pressor and uterotonic side effects and is responsible for the release through the V_2 receptor mechanism of factor VIII, von Willebrand factor and t-PA from endothelial cells without increasing plasma levels of other endothelial cell constituents (fibronectin, antithrombin III, platelet factor-4). In fact, no other clotting factor levels are raised by DDAVP administration except perhaps factor VII and XII activity. DDAVP does not increase factor VIII and von Willebrand factor release when incubated with cultured or perfused endothelial cells; this observation and others suggest that a "second messenger" is involved in the raised plasma

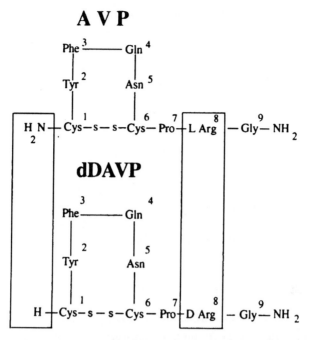

Figure 59-1 Comparison of the structure of arginine vasopressin (AVP) with the synthetic analogue (DDAVP). The boxes enclose the differences between the two peptide molecules: deamination of hemicysteine at position 1 and substitution of the D-isomer of arginine for L Arg at position 8. (Used with permission from Richardson DW, Robinson AG: Desmopressin. Ann Intern Med 103:228, 1985.)

levels of clotting factors after DDAVP. The concept that desmopressin exerts its effects directly through its strong V_2 agonist effect is supported by the finding that patients with nephrogenic diabetes insipidus (who lack V_2 receptors) had no increase factor VIII and von Willebrand factor levels after DDAVP.

Several studies in normal adults have indicated that pharmacologic doses of DDAVP (0.3 to 0.4 μg/kg intravenously) produce slight shortening of the bleeding time, a three- to fivefold increase in factor VIII and von Willebrand factor (antigen and activity), and a three- to fourfold increase in t-PA without significant changes in fibrinogen, plasminogen, and a_2-antiplasmin (a_2-AP). However, plasmin a_2-AP inhibitor complex increases and fibrin degradation products have been normal or slightly increased. Plasminogen activator inhibitor (PAI) decreases. Although clinically significant fibrinolysis with bleeding is not produced, the relevance of these findings to a thrombotic situation remains to be investigated. Of interest is the observation that patients with type III von Willebrand disease do not release t-PA (even though it is stored in endothelial cells) after DDAVP or venous occlusion.

Administration of DDAVP results in an increased concentration of high molecular weight multimers as well as the appearance of UL von Willebrand factor forms in normal individuals and type I von Willebrand disease. In type IIA the larger multimers do not appear; however, all multimers appear transiently in type IIB von Willebrand disease.

CLINICAL USE

In addition to the therapeutic uses of DDAVP (Table 59-1), several diagnostic uses are known which have included detection of hemophilia A carriers (using a post-DDAVP instead of the standard factor VIII/von Willebrand factor ratio increases the accuracy of carrier detection to 95 percent) and for detection of acquired and hereditary defects in t-PA release (DDAVP in a standard dose can be used instead of venous occlusion). Test doses of DDAVP are

TABLE 59-1 Hemostatic Uses of Desmopressin (DDAVP)

Hemophilia (factor VIII deficiency)
    Hereditary, mild
    Carriers
    Acquired

von Willebrand disease (see Table 12-2)
    (not types IIB and III)

Acquired von Willebrand disease

Hereditary platelet function defects
    Storage pool deficiencies
    Secretion defects
    Bernard-Soulier syndrome

Acquired platelet function defects
    Uremia
    Liver disease
    Cardiovascular surgery
    Plastic surgery
    ASA-induced defects
    Myeloproliferative disorders
    Vascular defects
    Glycogen storage diseases
    Unexplained prolonged bleeding time

Other disorders
    Heparin-induced bleeding
    Thrombocytopenic bleeding

frequently used to confirm responses in von Willebrand disease and detect subtypes; that is, type IA and IB with low platelet von Willebrand factor as well as IIC and IID have poor bleeding time responses to DDAVP.

Desmopressin is the major hemostatic therapy for bleeding episodes and for surgical procedures in mild hemophilia A, hemophilia A carriers with low levels, and most patients with von Willebrand disease. Test doses are used in hemophilia A when the baseline level is < 10 percent. Responses in a given patient are reasonably consistent on different occasions. The expected factor VIII rise (from two- to sixfold, mean of threefold) will produce a hemostatic level of at least 20 percent in almost all mild hemophilia A patients (base level of 6 percent or above) and an occasional moderately severe (4 to 5 percent) patient. In general, if the base level is at least 10 percent, adequate hemostasis is ensured; patients with levels of 4 to 9 percent may also respond but should be monitored for effect. The factor VIII level may also be raised to hemostatic levels (if only briefly) in some patients with acquired factor VIII inhibitors.

As noted in Table 12-2, DDAVP is usually effective in the common type of von Willebrand disease (IA), type IC, and some variants; is sometimes not effective in type II and "platelet low" types of IA, IB; is ineffective in type III and Normandy variant; and is contraindicated in type IIB and platelet-type disease. Factor VIII and ristocetin cofactor levels increase with variable bleeding time correction (up to 6 h) in patients responding with good clinical hemostasis; however, hemostasis may be adequate even though only partial or little correction of the bleeding time occurs.

Bleeding episodes in most hereditary platelet function defects also respond to DDAVP; the notable exceptions are thrombasthenia, cyclooxygenase deficiency, and some cases of Bernard-Soulier syndrome. The responses are not related to correction of the platelet aggregation defects (usually they do not correct) but rather to improvement in the bleeding time. Bleeding times and clinical hemostasis are improved in many acquired disorders of platelet function, in particular in uremia and liver disease (cirrhosis, biliary atresia, Alagille's syndrome) despite the presence of elevated baseline levels of factor VIII and von Willebrand factor. Other acquired platelet function defects where DDAVP has been effective in shortening the bleeding time or decreasing bleeding include myeloproliferative syndromes (see Chap. 44); some forms of acquired von Willebrand disease; after drugs like aspirin, dextran, and heparin; and glycogen storage disease, type 1. Uncontrolled bleeding in surgical procedures like cardiovascular surgery, scoliosis surgery, and skin flap procedures, frequently respond to DDAVP. Several reports have indicated the usefulness of DDAVP in shortening the bleeding time and controlling hemostasis in patients with isolated prolongation of the bleeding time.

Although tranexamic acid or ε-aminocaproic acid has been used with DDAVP (to prevent excess fibrinolysis), our experience is that the hemostatic effect is good without the need for antifibrinolytic agents in most instances. The exceptions are oral bleeding or dental surgery in von Willebrand disease or mild hemophilia A where antifibrinolytic agents are used.

DOSAGE GUIDELINES

Desmopressin causes a transient increase in the factor VIII-von Willebrand factor complex and t-PA, which is dose dependent within ranges of 0.2 to 0.6 μg/kg when given intravenously. An optimal response (all ages) occurs with the dose of 0.3μg/kg (up to 28 μg total dose) in 15 to 30 mL isotonic saline given by slow intravenous push or drip over 15 to 30 min. The peak effect is in 30 to 60 min and the duration of raised clotting factors is similar to that seen in administered cryoprecipitate. DDAVP or desmopressin is available in vials containing 4 μg/mL (DDAVP injection, 1-mL ampules and 10-mL multidose vials, Rhone-Poulenc Rorer Pharmaceuticals). A more concentrated (40 μg/mL) form is available for use by subcutaneous route (Ferring, Malmo, Sweden). The intranasal form of DDAVP, widely used for diabetes insipidus, has also been used in the treatment of bleeding in mild factor VIII deficiency and von Willebrand disease.

The response to repeated doses of DDAVP is of four patterns: equally good responses to doses every 12 h, gradually less response with each dose, essentially no response after the first dose, and reduced but steady responses after first dose. About half the responses to repeated doses will show resistance or tachyphylaxis; thus, when higher factor levels are needed for longer periods of time (i.e., major surgery), von Willebrand factor concentrate therapy may be needed. Often only one or two doses are needed for surgical procedures in patients with mild hemophilia or von Willebrand disease. The initial dose should be timed so that the procedure is started within 30 to 60 min after administration of the DDAVP. DDAVP has been used effectively at all ages and immediately following delivery; the response in small infants is sometimes less than optimal.

COMPLICATIONS

For a drug with such wide use in difficult clinical situations, only a few adverse effects have been observed with desmopressin. Probably the most frequent side effect is facial flushing due to mild skin vasodilation. A few patients complain of headache; some patients show slight increases in heart rate and minor alterations in blood pressure; the concomitant use of pressor agents should be avoided. The most serious complication is hyponatremia which occurs in a few patients (over a dozen instances have been reported) usually after repeated doses of intravenous DDAVP in conjunction with excessive intakes of hypotonic fluids (intravenous fluids with surgical procedures). The hyponatremia (serum sodium 114 to 123 meq/L) was usually associated with tonic-clonic convulsions and altered mental status; the lowest sodium level occurred 6 to 21 h after multiple doses of DDAVP. Most of the patients were infants, children, or young adults. Young children, especially those under the age of 2 years, are especially prone to develop symptomatic hyponatremia and should be monitored carefully. Serum sodium concentration should be checked every 12 h or more frequently if the level is falling, and total fluid intake should be restricted by 1/3. Avoid repeated doses of DDAVP if the serum sodium level is decreasing. Elderly patients with evidence of athero-sclerosis may be at increased risk for acute thrombotic vascular occlusion after DDAVP therapy.

BIBLIOGRAPHY

Byrnes JJ et al: Thrombosis following desmopressin for uremic bleeding. *Am J Hematol* 28:63, 1988.

Chistolini A et al: Intranasal DDAVP: Biological and clinical evaluation in mild factor VIII deficiency. *Hemostasis* 21:273, 1991.

de la Fuente B et al: Response of patients with mild and moderate hemophilia A and von Willebrand's disease to treatment with desmopressin. *Ann Intern Med* 103:6, 1985.

Di Michele DM, Hathaway WE: Use of DDAVP in inherited and acquired platelet dysfunction. *Am J Hematol* 33:39, 1990.

Gralnick HR et al: DDAVP in type IIa von Willebrand's disease. *Blood* 67:465, 1988.

Jeanneau CH et al: Absence of functional activity of tissue plasminogen activator in patients with severe forms of von Willebrand's disease. *Br J Haematol* 67:79, 1987.

Kim HC et al: Patients with prolonged bleeding time of undefined etiology, and their response to desmopressin. *Thromb Haemost* 59:221, 1988.

Kobrinsky NL et al: Absent factor VIII response to synthetic vasopressin analogue (DDAVP) in nephrogenic diabetes insipidus. *Lancet* i:1293, 1985

Mannucci PM: Desmopressin: A nontransfusional form of treatment for congenital and acquired bleeding disorders. *Blood* 72:1449, 1988.

Mannucci PM et al: Patterns of development of tachphylaxis in patients with haemophilia and von Willebrand disease after repeated doses of desmopressin (DDAVP). *Br J Haematol* 82:87, 1992.

Schulman S et al: DDAVP-induced correction of prolonged bleeding time in patients with congenital platelet function defects. *Thromb Res* 45:165, 1987.

Smith TJ et al: Hyponatremia and seizures in young children given DDAVP. *Am J Hematol* 31:199, 1989.

Waldenstrom E et al: Bernard-Soulier syndrome in two Swedish families: Effect of DDAVP on bleeding time. *Eur J Haematol* 46:182, 1991.

Weinstein M et al: Changes in von Willebrand factor during cardiac surgery: Effect of desmopressin acetate. *Blood* 71:1648, 1988.

Antifibrinolytic Agents

Antifibrinolytic agents are used for treatment or prevention of bleeding in two clinical settings: to block systemic fibrinolysis or to inhibit local fibrinolysis at sites of vascular injury. Two drugs are available for use in the United States, ε-aminocaproic acid (EACA) and tranexamic acid (TA). Both inhibit the fibrinolytic enzymes tissue plasminogen activator (t-PA) and plasmin. A third preparation is available in Europe. Aprotinin inhibits plasmin as well as other proteases such as trypsin or kallikrein.

PHARMACOLOGY

Both EACA and TA are similar in structure to the amino acid lysine (Fig. 60-1). Since lysine binding sites are required for binding of plasminogen and

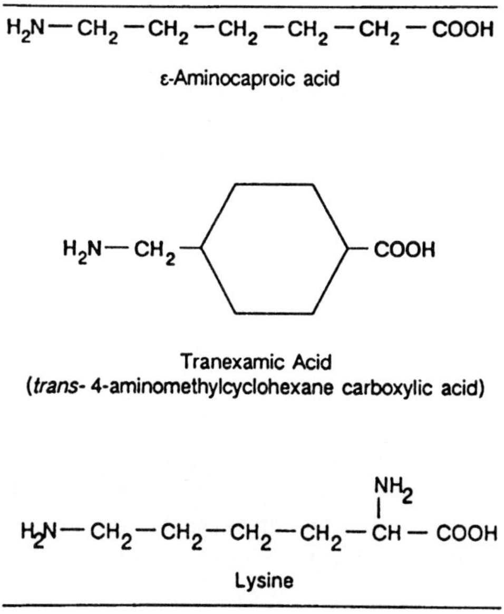

$$H_2N - CH_2 - CH_2 - CH_2 - CH_2 - CH_2 - COOH$$

ε-Aminocaproic acid

$$H_2N - CH_2 \langle \bigcirc \rangle COOH$$

Tranexamic Acid
(*trans-* 4-aminomethylcyclohexane carboxylic acid)

$$H_2N - CH_2 - CH_2 - CH_2 - CH_2 - \overset{\overset{\displaystyle NH_2}{|}}{CH} - COOH$$

Lysine

Figure 60-1 Lysine and the lysine analogue antifibrinolytic drugs. (Reprinted with permission from International Anesthesiology Clinics 28:230, 1990.)

TABLE 60-1 Dosage and Administration of the Antifibrinolytic Agents

	Loading Dose	Maintenance Dose
EACA*	100 mg/kg IV or PO	500–1000 mg/h IV or PO
Tranexamic acid	10 mg/kg IV	10 mg/kg IV q 6–8 h
		25 mg/kg PO q 6–8 h

* In children, a loading dose of 200 mg/kg of EACA is given followed by 100 mg/kg q 6 h (orally) up to a total of 6 g/6 h.

t-PA to fibrin, these agents competitively inhibit these interactions and thereby effectively block fibrinolysis. In contrast, aprotinin blocks the serine site within the active center of the plasmin molecule.

Both drugs are very small molecules (Mr 131 and 157 d) and are readily absorbed with peak blood concentrations at 2 (EACA) and 4 (TA) h after oral ingestion. Both agents have short plasma half-lifes and are rapidly cleared from the plasma and concentrated in the urine; EACA urinary levels are 100 times higher than those in plasma. Moreover, because of their small size, they cross the blood-brain barrier and enter most tissues and body cavities. Both can be given intravenously, used topically, or administered orally. TA differs from EACA in at least two respects, both of which have therapeutic implications. TA provides equivalent anti-fibrinolytic therapy at only one tenth the concentration and has a slower renal clearance (6 to 8 h compared to < 3 h for EACA). Therefore, TA is used in lower doses and given at less frequent intervals than EACA (Table 60-1).

Aprotinin (Mr 6512) is not adsorbed from the gastrointestinal tract, is cleared from the plasma in two phases (half-life of 2 and 7 h), and undergoes degradation to small polypeptides or amino acids before excretion into the urine. It is administered only by intravenous injection or used topically.

LABORATORY MONITORING

Laboratory tests are not used to moniter the clinical effects of the anti-fibrinolytic agents. Instead, cessation of bleeding is the best therapeutic end point. Evidence of circulating fibrinolytic activity (e.g., shortened euglobulin lysis time) should be sought and disseminated intravascular coagulation (DIC) excluded before EACA or TA are used to treat bleeding in patients with systemic fibrinolysis.

CLINICAL USE

Treatment of Systemic Fibrinolysis

Antifibrinolytic agents are used to treat or prevent bleeding due to systemic fibrinolysis. Although the primary fibrinolytic syndromes are distinctly uncommon, hemorrhage can be severe and refractory to clotting factor replacement therapy. Listed below are several fibrinolytic disorders in which treatment may be useful.

Hereditary a_2-Antiplasmin or Plasminogen Activator Inhibitor Deficiencies. Deficiencies of the natural fibrinoloytic inhibitors result in bleeding due to excessive fibrinolysis (see Chap. 20). Chronic or intermittent therapy with EACA or TA are effective for treatment of bleeding episodes in these patients.

Bleeding Following Thrombolytic Therapy.   Antifibrinolytic agents are seldom needed because of the very short half-life of most of the thrombolytic agents (e.g., 5 to 30 min). Consequently, continued bleeding is more likely to be due to clotting factor depletion, platelet function defects, or structural lesions rather than persistent systemic fibrinolysis. Occasionally, however, infusions of EACA and TA are warranted for treatment of acute catastrophic bleeding that develops during or shortly after thrombolysis, particularly if immediate surgery is required.

Acute Promyelocytic Leukemia.   Recently it has been appreciated that a subset of these patients have systemic fibrinolysis with or without DIC. Antifibrinolytic agents are used for treatment of isolated primary fibrinolysis or can be administered in conjunction with heparin when patients have concurrent DIC and systemic fibrinolysis.

Anhepatic Phase of Liver Transplantation.   A rapid rise in plasma levels of t-PA frequently occurs during liver transplantation surgery after the removal of the diseased liver (anhepatic phase). In some instances, severe systemic fibrinolysis produces massive hemorrhage. Intravenous EACA or TA (or aprotinin) can reduce bleeding, especially if therapy is combined with aggressive clotting factor and platelet replacement.

Systemic Amyloidosis with Primary Fibrinolysis.   Some patients with widespread amyloidosis have severe and recurrent fibrinolytic bleeding which responds to chronic oral antifibrinolytic therapy.

Rare Catastrophic Events Associated with Systemic Fibrinolysis.   Examples include heat stroke and amniotic fluid embolism. Often these syndromes involve DIC with rapid changes in the character of the hemostatic defects from hour to hour. Laboratory tests must be performed to implicate systemic fibrinolysis and exclude DIC before treatment with antifibrinolytic agents is instituted (see Chap. 26).

Cardiopulmonary Bypass. All three antifibrinolytic agents, EACA, TA, and aprotinin, have been effective in the reduction of bleeding and transfusion requirements in patients undergoing cardiac surgery with cardiopulmonary bypass. However, it has not been established whether benefit is due to inhibition of fibrinolysis or preservation of platelet function (see Chap. 32). Many surgeons and cardiovascular anesthesiologists reserve antifibrinolytic therapy for patients who require complicated and prolonged surgical procedures or who bleed following termination of bypass.

Prevention of Local Fibrinolysis

A normal and usually appropriate physiologic response to thrombosis is local fibrinolysis. This process often occurs slowly and hemorrhage does not occur. However, the presence of an associated hemostatic defect (e.g., hemophilia) or excessive local fibrinolysis (e.g., release of plasminogen activators in the genitourinary tract) can accentuate bleeding from sites of injury. Local fibrinolysis can be blocked by the systemic administration of the antifibrinolytic agents and occasionally by direct topical application to an injury site (particularly for dental surgery). Examples are listed below.

Bleeding from the Mouth and Upper Respiratory Tract. The antifibrinolytic agents effectively control bleeding from the mouth in patients with hereditary or acquired hemostatic defects. Controlled clinical trials have shown that the oral administration of EACA can substitute for continued infusions of clotting factor concentrates in children or adults undergoing dental extractions. Patients with severe hemophilia who require dental surgery are usually given a single dose of clotting factor concentrate along with EACA or TA which is continued for 4 to 7 days. Patients with mild or moderate hemophilia A and many patients with von Willebrand disease can be managed with antifibrinolytic agents with or without the addition of DDAVP.

Antifibrinolytic agents have been successfully used for dental surgery in patients with artificial cardiac valves on chronic warfarin therapy (see Sindet-Pedersen reference). TA was applied topically at dental extraction sites for 2 min every 6 h. Bleeding was controlled without systemic administration of the drug, a route of administration that could promote cardiac valvular thrombosis. EACA and TA can often control bleeding from the nose and mouth in patients with other hemostatic defects, such as chronic epistaxis in patients with thrombocytopenia due to myelodysplasia. If there are no contraindications to systemic use, an effective strategy for management of oral bleeding is to combine topical applications with systemic therapy, that is, "swish and swallow."

Subarachnoid Hemorrhage and Hyphema. Patients who survive a subarachnoid hemorrhage due to rupture of a cerebral artery aneurysm often have recurrent bleeding before surgical repair can be safely attempted. Since EACA and TA diffuse rapidly into vascular tissues and cerebrospinal fluid, clinical trials have been conducted to determine if antifibrinolytic therapy lowers the rate of recurrent hemorrhage in this clinical setting. Although late bleeding was reduced by 40 percent, disability from thrombosis and cerebral infarction was increased, so that overall complication rates were unchanged. Ophthalmologists have used antifibrinolytic agents for the prevention of persistent bleeding in patients with traumatic hyphema, but randomized clinical trials are needed to prove benefit.

Bleeding from the Gastrointestinal Tract. Antifibrinolytic therapy has occasionally been used for treatment of patients with persistent bleeding from the upper gastrointestinal tract (e.g., diffuse gastritis, peptic ulcer disease, and esophageal varices). In general, these drugs are not effective in the control of massive bleeding, but may be helpful for chronic low-grade oozing in patients with associated hemostatic defects (e.g., severe von Willebrand's disease or thrombocytopenia), or in individuals who are not candidates for surgery or other invasive procedures. Intractable lower gastrointestinal bleeding due to ulcerative colitis (often with associated hemostatic defects) has also been treated with possible benefit, although the development of thrombosis in patients with inflammatory bowel disease is a major concern.

Bleeding from the Urinary Tract. Antifibrinolytic agents have been advocated for treatment of patients who have persistent bleeding from the kidney. Subjects at risk include patients with hemophilia or sickle cell disease, or following renal biopsy. A major problem is the formation and retention of large blood clots in the renal collecting system, which require surgical removal to preserve renal function. Because of this, antifibrinolytic drugs are rarely indicated in upper urinary tract bleeding. However, if the bleeding is intractable and no other alternatives are available, then these risks may be acceptable in selected patients.

Prolonged severe bleeding from the prostatic bed can occur following prostate resection. Because the operative site is bathed in plasminogen activator (e.g., urokinase in the urine and prostatic tissues), antifibrinolytic therapy has been used to control hemorrhage. Most urologists reserve treatment for patients in whom standard approaches such as cystoscopy and cautery have failed. Randomized clinical trials have suggested that prophylactic administration of EACA reduces blood loss in patients with transurethral prostatectomy, although postoperative venous thrombosis remains a concern. One additional complication of antifibrinolytic therapy in lower urinary tract bleeding is retention of large clots in the bladder that are resistent to fibrinolysis.

Uterine Bleeding.   Excessive bleeding from the uterine cervix following cone biopsy or refractory hemorrhage in women with intrauterine contraceptive devices has responded to antifibrinolytic drugs. Occasionally patients with refractory menorrhagia may also benefit. In general, however, more standard approaches to control bleeding should be tried before antifibrinolytic agents are considered.

COMPLICATIONS AND SIDE EFFECTS

Thrombosis

Pharmacologic blockade of the fibrinolytic system can accelerate thrombus growth or allow clots to persist in an unwelcome location. The possibility of thrombosis should be weighed each time the use of antifibrinolytic agents is considered. If, for example, a patient with carcinoma has DIC, then antifibrinolytic therapy can precipitate glomerular thrombosis and acute renal failure. Deep venous thrombosis is always a concern in patients who are bedridden or those who have had recent abdominal or pelvic surgery. As previously mentioned, clots may persist in body cavities such as the renal pelvis and require surgical removal. Although only isolated reports are available, a few patients with atherosclerosis have developed acute coronary insufficiency following antifibrinolytic therapy.

Orthostatic Hypertension

Patients given large oral doses or rapid intravenous infusions of EACA have developed symptomatic orthostatic hypotension. This complication is more frequent in older individuals and can persist for several hours. Symptoms are relieved by recumbency and a reduction in dose. Outpatients who are treated with antifibrinolytic agents should be warned of this potential side effect.

Rhabdomyolysis

Severe myopathy that develops several weeks after the start of long-term antifibrinolytic therapy has been described. The myopathy targets the proximal musculature of the legs and occasionally the muscles surrounding the shoulder girdle. Symptoms slowly regress after therapy has been stopped.

Other Problems

Nausea, vomiting, diarrhea, headache, conjunctival suffusion, skin rash, and stuffy nose have all been reported. Rarely, visual symptoms can occur; these agents are not recommended for persons with impaired color vision. Other patients have developed significant liver damage. Importantly, because EACA and TA are largely excreted by the kidney, high plasma levels can occur in patients with renal insufficiency. Doses must be reduced in this setting.

BIBLIOGRAPHY

Avvisati G et al: Tranexamic acid for control of haemorrhage in acute promyelocytic leukaemia. *Lancet* 2:122, 1989.

Bartholomew JR et al: Control of bleeding in patients with immune and nonimmune thrombocytopenia with aminocaproic acid. *Arch Intern Med* 149:1959, 1989.

Curry SC et al: Drug- and toxin-induced rhabdomyolysis. *Ann Emerg Med* 18:1068, 1989.

Fricke W et al: Lack of efficacy of tranexamic acid in thrombocytopenic bleeding. *Transfusion* 31:345, 1991.

Gardner FH, Helmer RC: Aminocaproic acid. Use in control of hemorrhage in patients with amegakaryocytic thrombocytopenia. *JAMA* 243:35, 1980.

Horrow JC: Desmopressin and antifibrinolytics. *Int Anesthesiol Clin* 28:230, 1990.

Kane MJ et al: Myonecrosis as a complication of the use of epsilon amino-caproic acid: A case report and review of the literature. *Am J Med* 85:861, 1988.

Kang Y et al: ε-aminocaproic acid for treatment of fibrinolysis during liver transplantation. *Anesthesiology* 66:766, 1987.

Pitts TO et al: Acute renal failure due to high-grade obstruction following therapy with ε-aminocaproic acid. *Am J Kid Dis* 8:441, 1986.

Sindet-Pedersen S et al: Hemostatic effect of tranexamic acid mouthwash in anticoagulant-treated patients undergoing oral surgery. *N Engl J Med* 320:840, 1989.

Stefanini M et al: Safe and effective, prolonged administration of epsilon amino-caproic acid in bleeding from the urinary tract. *J Urol* 143:559, 1990.

Verstraete M: Clinical application of inhibitors of fibrinolysis. *Drugs* 29:236, 1985.

Walsh PN et al: Epsilon-aminocaproic acid therapy for dental extractions in haemophilia and Christmas disease: A double blind controlled trial. *Br J Haematol* 20:463, 1971.

Williamson R, Eggleston, DJ: DDAVP and EACA used for minor oral surgery in von Willebrand disease. *Austr Dent J* 33:32, 1988.

Heparins

For over 30 years heparin has been standard therapy for the initial treatment of vascular thrombosis. When used skillfully, heparin prevents recurrent thromboembolism without major risks of bleeding. Recently however, the dominance of standard heparin (SH) in our therapeutic armamentarium is being challenged by low molecular weight heparins (LMWH) and heparinoids. The data from current clinical trials suggest that LMWH are at least as effective, are easier to administer, and may be safer than SH.

PHARMACOLOGY

Standard heparin is a complex glycosaminoglycan isolated and purified from animal tissues (porcine intestinal mucosa or bovine lung). It functions as an anticoagulant by inducing a conformational change in the structure of antithrombin III (AT III) that dramatically augments the ability of AT III to neutralize thrombin, and to a lesser extent, factor Xa and other serine proteases that participate in the formation of fibrin. The higher molecular weight fractions of SH also accelerate the neutralization of thrombin by heparin cofactor II. Heparin binds to endothelial cells and macrophages as well as to several plasma proteins (e.g., platelet factor 4, vitronectin, fibronectin, von Willebrand factor, histidine-rich glycoprotein), which explains the substantial variability in plasma heparin activity observed after parenteral injection. Platelet function is also impaired by heparin due to inhibition of platelet aggregation mediated by collagen and von Willebrand factor.

The LMWH are prepared from SH by enzymatic or chemical hydrolysis, procedures that substantially alter the biologic properties and clinical attributes of the anticoagulant (Table 61-1). For example, the LMWH inhibit factor Xa more potently than thrombin. A major stimulus for the development of these new heparins has been the hope that the low molecular weight preparations will provide equal or greater antithrombotic effects but less bleeding than SH. At least in part, these expectations have been realized; LMWH have more predictable biologic availability and are administered in a fixed subcutaneous dose once or twice daily without the need for laboratory

TABLE 61-1 Comparisons Between Standard Heparin and Low Molecular Weight Heparins (LMWH)

	Standard Unfractionated Heparin	LMWH
Mean molecular weight	12,000–15,000	4000–6500
Saccharide units (mean)	40–50	13–22
Anti-Xa; anti-IIa activity	1:1	2:1–4:1
Inactivates factor Xa on platelet surface	Weak	Strong
Inhibitable by platelet factor 4 (PF4)	Yes	No
Inhibits thrombin generation in platelet-rich plasma	++	++++
Main action through inhibition of factor IIa	Yes	Yes
Protein binding	Histidine-rich glycoprotein, fibronectin, vitronectin, PF4, von Willebrand factor	vitronectin
Binds to endothelium	Yes	No (weak)
Dose-dependent clearance	Yes	No
Bioavailability at low doses	Poor	Good
Inhibits platelet function	++++	++
Increases vascular permeability	Yes	No
Augments microvascular bleeding	++++	++

*Used with permission from Hirsh J, Levine MN: *Blood* 79:1, 1992.

monitoring. Because of these attributes, some patients with uncomplicated venous thrombosis may ultimately be treated at home rather than in the hospital.

Two other heparin-like agents are now being used in clinical trials. Low molecular weight heparinoid is composed of 80 percent heparan and a mixture of dermatan sulfate and chondroitin sulfate. This product has similar efficacy and safety as LMWH, but has a much longer plasma half-life (e.g., 16 h). A third preparation, purified dermatan sulfate, interacts with heparin cofactor II to produce an anticoagulant effect.

CLINICAL USE

Standard heparin has been rigorously tested in a large number of clinical trials and is an effective anticoagulant. Fewer studies have been conducted with the LMWH, but most of the trials have been of high quality. LMWH are equal to or superior to SH for treatment and prophylaxis of deep venous thrombosis (DVT; Fig. 61-1). At least five preparations of LMWH are now being produced throughout the world. Recommended doses vary and depend on the methods of manufacture and the results of human clinical trials.

Deep Venous Thrombosis and Pulmonary Embolus

An important principle in the management of venous thrombosis is that sufficient heparin should be given to prolong the APTT into the therapeutic range (e.g., 1.5 to 2 times control) as quickly as possible (Table 61-2). Rates of major bleeding are low during the early hours of therapy, but the risk of recurrent thromboembolism is substantial if APTTs remain suboptimal during the first 24 h of treatment. Rates of recurrent thromboembolism approaching 25 to 30 percent have been reported over the next 3 months when insufficient heparin has been administered. The McMaster group has devised a simple and convenient protocol for adjustments in heparin doses which has

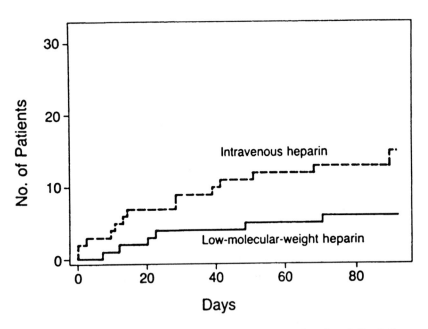

Figure 61-1 Frequency of objectively documented recurrent venous thromboembolism in the treatment groups. This outcome occurred in 6 of the 213 patients receiving low molecular weight heparin (2.8 percent), as compared with 15 of the 219 patients receiving intravenous heparin (6.9 percent) (P = 0.049). (Reprinted with permission of The New England Journal of Medicine, 326:975, 1992.)

TABLE 61-2 Use of Heparin for Deep Vein Thrombosis or Pulmonary Embolism

Tests ordered before heparin is given	PT, APTT, platelet count
Loading dose	5000 U (may increase to 10,000 U if massive thromboembolism)
Mean daily dose for continuous infusion	40,000 U/day—low risk of bleeding
	30,000 U/day—high risk of bleeding
Optimal therapeutic range: APTT	1.5–2.0 times control
anti-Xa assay	0.35–0.7 U/mL
First APTT	6 h
Monitor platelet count, hematocrit	daily
Approximate duration of therapy:	
Proximal DVT	5 days
Iliofemoral DVT or pulmonary emboli	5–10 days

been shown to shorten the time to full anticoagulation by several hours (Cruickshank reference).

In patients with proximal (or distal) DVT, oral anticoagulants should be started on the first day of heparin therapy, so that the total duration of intravenous heparin is only 4 to 5 days. The PT should be prolonged into the therapeutic range by the warfarin (e.g., INR 2 to 3) for at least 24 h before discontinuing the heparin. If the heparin is stopped prematurely, risks of recurrent thrombosis may be increased because of lower levels of AT III (due to the heparin), reduced protein C (due to the warfarin), and the persistence of a highly thrombogenic clot. Warfarin causes a rapid fall in factor VII ($T_{1/2}$ 5 h) which prolongs the PT, but reductions in clotting factors II, IX, and X ($T_{1/2}$ 24 to 48 h) are necessary for optimal anticoagulation.

Other Venous Thromboses

Although controlled clinical trials are not available, SH appears effective for treatment of thromboses in sites other than the extremities, which include the hepatic, mesenteric, and portal veins. Heparin has recently been shown to be safe and effective in the treatment of patients with acute cerebral vein thrombosis. Dural sinus vein thromboses regressed without evidence of CNS bleeding.

Cardiac Disorders

Clinical trials have shown convincingly that heparin is equal to or even more effective than aspirin for reduction of chest pain, subsequent myocardial infarction, and mortality in patients with unstable angina. Heparin is also used routinely following thrombolytic therapy for acute coronary artery thrombosis in an attempt to maintain arterial patency following resolution of the clot. Lastly, heparin in doses of at least 7500 U twice daily are recommended for patients with transmural anterior myocardial infarctions to prevent the formation of mural thrombi in the left ventricle.

Cardioembolic Stroke

Following an embolic stroke, the rate of recurrent cerebral embolization has been estimated to be as high as 1 percent per day for the next 2 weeks. Because a feared complication of heparin therapy is CNS bleeding, anticoagulants should be withheld for 24 to 48 h and a CT scan obtained. If the cerebral infarct is not large (e.g., > 4 to 5 cm) and there is no evidence of hemorrhagic transformation, intravenous heparin can be begun at that time at a rate of 1000 U/h without a loading dose.

Prophylaxis for Venous Thromboembolism in Surgical and Medical Patients

Low doses of SH prevent DVT in surgical and medical patients without excessive risks of bleeding. Regimens used include fixed amounts (e.g., 5000 U bid or tid) or doses of heparin adjusted to maintain the APTT or heparin assay in a target range. For example, heparin prevents proximal DVT following orthopedic surgery when given subcutaneously every 8 h in sufficient doses to maintain the APTT in the upper range of normal or sometimes slightly higher (at 6 h postinjection). A small study of antithrombotic prophylaxis in pregnancy used heparin concentrations in the range of 0.08 to 0.15 U/mL as measured by an anti-Xa assay with apparent success.

In general, when standard heparin is used for prophylaxis in surgical patients, adjusted dose regimens are more effective than fixed doses and are equally safe. One possible reason for this observation is that heparin requirements almost always increase postoperatively (and also in the second or early third trimesters of pregnancy). The LMWH has been shown to be very effective for prophylaxis of postoperative thrombosis in orthopedic and general surgery and medical patients when administered by daily subcutaneous injection without laboratory monitoring.

Heparin in Infants and Children

Venous thrombosis is uncommon in infants, but arterial occlusion is relatively frequent (1 to 5 percent or more) in newborns who require umbilical catheters. Optimal heparin therapy is difficult due to its large volume of distribution in neonates (compared to adults) and its accelerated clearance from the blood. Other problems include low levels of AT III (as low as 25 percent in premature infants), difficulties in obtaining accurate blood samples for laboratory monitoring, and the risk of intraventricular hemorrhage; nevertheless, when necessary, heparinization can be effectively accomplished. A protocol for the administration of heparin to infants and children is described in Chap. 39.

Pregnancy

See also Chaps. 38 and 52.

Therapy for Acute Venous Thrombosis

Heparin is used for two reasons during pregnancy: therapeutic anticoagulation in women following an acute DVT and prophylactic anticoagulation in patients with a history of a previous thrombosis. After initial intravenous heparin for acute thrombosis, therapeutic doses of heparin are usually given every 12 h as subcutaneous injections with monitoring 4 h later to keep the APTT in the therapeutic range (for details see Chap. 52). Available data suggest that this approach is effective, has a low rate of bleeding, and is not harmful to the fetus. If possible, the heparin should be stopped at least 24 h before delivery to allow adequate time for its clearance from the blood and tissues. If desired, prophylactic doses of heparin can be given during labor, delivery, and immediately postpartum (see below). Oral anticoagulants (warfarin) are started following delivery and continued for 4 to 6 weeks.

Prophylaxis

Prophylactic heparin schedules for women with a past history of venous thromboembolism are more controversial. Studies have shown that 5000 U subcutaneously twice daily may not be fully protective, whereas full-dose (APTT 1.5 to 2 times control) therapy for prophylactic use incurs a substantial risk of heparin-induced osteopenia (see later). An intermediate approach that has experimental support is to administer heparin subcutaneously at 12-hourly intervals at doses regulated to keep the 4-h APTT in the upper normal range or the heparin assay (using an anti-Xa method) between 0.10 and 0.15 U/mL. Alternatively, a fixed dose of heparin of about 7500 U twice daily can be used.

LABORATORY MONITORING

Activated Partial Thromboplastin Time

The APTT is used to monitor the therapeutic effects of SH although recently heparin assays are being used more frequently, particularly in complicated patients (see below). It is important to recall that heparin also prolongs the TCT and PT. With low doses of heparin, the dilute thrombin time (normal, 20 to 25 s) is prolonged and may reach clotting times of > 200 s; with larger doses of heparin the APTT increases, followed thereafter by prolongation of the PT. As a rule, when sufficient heparin is given to increase the APTT to 1.5 to 2 times control (i.e., the therapeutic range), the PT is prolonged by only 1 or 2 s.

An APTT of 1.5 to 2 times control is an appropriate target for heparin treatment of venous thrombosis. However, as of yet, there is no conversion factor for normalizing the APTT similar to the INR for oral anticoagulant therapy. Various APTT reagents and instruments may be more or less sensitive to a standard concentration of plasma heparin. Some have recommended calibrating the APTT used in hospital laboratories to a heparin concentration of 0.35 to 0.7 U/mL by the Xa inhibition assay.

During treatment for venous thromboembolism, the dose of heparin required to prolong the APTT into the therapeutic range often falls by the second to fourth day, which is due in part to shorter heparin survival immediately after a large thromboembolism and because cellular and protein binding sites are saturated with heparin. If heparin requirements should suddenly increase after 4 to 5 days of therapy, the possibility of heparin-associated thrombocytopenia (HAT) should be considered, because platelet factor 4 released from activated platelets neutralizes circulating heparin. Recent data suggest that the response of the APTT to a constant infusion of heparin is subject to diurnal variations, so that laboratory monitoring is best performed at the same time each day in stable patients. The LMWH and heparinoids do not always prolong the APTT; heparin assays are required if monitoring is desired (see below).

Heparin Assays

Heparin assays such as the Xa inhibition test are increasingly used to monitor heparin therapy in patients with complex hemostatic disorders that can independently alter the APTT. In this assay, a known quantity of purified factor Xa (and an excess of AT III) is added to patient plasma containing heparin or to normal plasmas that contain heparin standards. The ability of heparin-AT III to inhibit cleavage of a chromogenic substrate by factor Xa is then measured in a spectrophotometer. Heparin standards are tailored to the clinical situation; for example, SH or various LMWH. The provisional therapeutic range for SH is 0.35 to 0.7 U/mL of anti-Xa activity for treatment of venous thrombosis. Other heparin preparations have different therapeutic ranges.

Heparin assays are extremely useful for monitoring heparin therapy in difficult clinical situations in which the APTT may be unreliable such as in patients with a lupus anticoagulant. Other conditions include concomitant warfarin therapy, associated intrinsic coagulation system defects, and in infants who often have prolonged APTTs for various reasons.

Platelet Counts

Daily platelet counts are recommended in patients receiving therapeutic doses of heparin for early recognition and treatment of HAT. Hematocrits should be obtained at the same time to detect occult bleeding.

SIDE EFFECTS AND COMPLICATIONS

Bleeding

Rates of serious hemorrhage with heparin therapy are low and average 3 to 5 percent in most clinical trials. Bleeding has been shown to be higher in patients with one or more risk factors such as low performance status, recent trauma or surgery, or a history of a bleeding diathesis (Table 61-3). If bleeding is severe, protamine sulfate can be used for immediate neutralization of the anticoagulant. When the heparin has been given very recently, then 1 mg protamine sulfate neutralizes approximately 100 U heparin. However, lesser doses of protamine (e.g., 10 to 20 mg) are often effective, particularly when several hours have elapsed since heparin was administered. The relative prolongations of the PT and APTT and heparin assays are useful for estimating the quantity of circulating heparin and the need for protamine. If extremely large doses of heparin have been given in error, repeated infusions of protamine sulfate may be required because the survival of heparin in the plasma is dose related; that is, the $T_{1/2}$ is longer with larger doses of heparin.

TABLE 61-3   Clinical Conditions That Increase the Risk of Bleeding with Heparin Therapy

Advanced age (women > 60, men > 70)
Surgery within 10 days
Elevated serum creatinine
Recent intracranial hemorrhage or stroke
Active peptic ulcer disease
Hypertension (diastolic pressure >120 mm Hg)
Recent CPR
History of bleeding diathesis
Multiple comorbid conditions
APTT > 2 times control

The efficacy of protamine neutralization of heparin is assessed by repeated measurement of the APTT.

Heparin-Associated Thrombocytopenia

This important clinical problem is discussed in detail in Chap. 46.

Osteopenia

Long-term full-dose heparin has been reported to cause osteopenia. In one series of pregnant women treated with heparin, 17 percent had measurable bone loss and 3 percent developed overt fractures. Fortunately, the osteopenia was reversible in 6 to 12 months. Recent studies have suggested lower doses of heparin (< 20,000 U daily) may be safer. It is not known as yet whether LMWH also cause bone loss.

Reduction in Antithrombin III Levels

The concentration of circulating AT III often falls acutely after a large thrombosis, but then drops further as a result of heparin therapy (by as much as 20 to 30 percent). Although usually of little consequence, lowered levels of AT III could predispose to recurrent thrombosis if heparin is stopped prematurely before oral anticoagulants are fully effective.

Heparin Resistance

Some patients are resistant to the anticoagulant effects of heparin and require large doses of the anticoagulant to prolong the APTT into the therapeutic range. Possible explanations include shortened heparin survival associated with large thrombi, short preheparin APTTs due to elevated levels of factor VIII or circulating activated clotting factors, hereditary or acquired AT III deficiency, and HAT (due to heparin neutralization by platelet factor 4 released from aggregating platelets). Frequent APTTs during the first 24 h of therapy may be necessary, and in complex situations, heparin assays, HAT tests, and AT III measurements can be useful.

BIBLIOGRAPHY

Collins R et al: Reduction in fatal pulmonary embolism and venous thrombosis by perioperative administration of subcutaneous heparin. *N Engl J Med* 318:1162, 1988.

Cruickshank MK et al: A standard heparin nomogram for the management of heparin therapy. *Arch Intern Med* 151:333, 1991.

Dahlman TC et al: Thrombosis prophylaxis in pregnancy with use of subcutaneous heparin adjusted by monitoring heparin concentration in plasma. *Am J Obstet Gynecol* 161:420, 1989.

Dahlman T et al: Osteopenia in pregnancy during long-term heparin treatment: A radiological study post partum. *Br J Obstet Gynaecol* 97:221, 1990.

Einhaupl KM et al: Heparin treatment in sinus venous thrombosis. *Lancet* 338:597, 1991.

Gallus AS: Anticoagulants in the prevention of venous thromboembolism. *Baillieres Clin Haematol* 3:651, 1990.

Ginsberg JS et al: Heparin therapy during pregnancy. Risks to the fetus and mother. *Arch Intern Med* 149:2233, 1989.

Hirsh J: Heparin. *N Engl J Med* 324:1565, 1991.

Hirsh J, Levine MN: Low molecular weight heparin. *Blood* 79:1, 1992.

Hommes DW et al: Subcutaneous heparin compared with continuous intravenous heparin administration in the initial treatment of deep vein thrombosis. A meta-analysis. *Ann Intern Med* 116:279, 1992.

Hull RD et al: Subcutaneous low-molecular-weight heparin compared with continuous intravenous heparin in the treatment of proximal-vein thrombosis. *N Engl J Med* 326:975, 1992.

Landefeld CS et al: A bleeding risk index for estimating the probability of major bleeding in hospitalized patients starting anticoagulant therapy. *Am J Med* 89:569, 1990.

McDonald MM, Hathaway WE: Anticoagulant therapy by continuous heparinization in newborn and older infants. *J Pediatr* 101:451, 1982.

Nieuwenhuis HK et al: Identification of risk factors for bleeding during treatment of acute venous thromboembolism with heparin or low molecular weight heparin. *Blood* 78:2337, 1991.

Nurmohamed MT et al: Low-molecular-weight heparin versus standard heparin in general and orthopaedic surgery: A meta-analysis. *Lancet* 340:152, 1992.

CHAPTER
62

Oral Anticoagulants

Coumarin oral anticoagulants are highly effective antithrombotic agents with relatively low risks of serious bleeding. Although available for decades, clinical uses and applications have evolved over the years. Recent changes include:

1. Lower doses are used to treat most patients with thrombosis.

2. Laboratory monitoring has been standardized so that intensities of anti-coagulation are equivalent around the world.

3. New indications for treatment have emerged from prospective con-trolled clinical trials; for example, prophylaxis of embolic stroke in pa-tients with chronic nonrheumatic atrial fibrillation.

PHARMACOLOGY

Warfarin is a 4-hydroxycoumarin derivative that exerts an antithrombotic effect by blocking the regeneration of vitamin K from its epoxide (Fig. 62-1). Vitamin K is necessary for the addition of γ-carboxyglutamic acid (Gla) residues to clotting factors II, VII, IX, and X (and also protein C and protein S). Gla residues bind metal ions such as calcium and undergo a conformational change that is necessary for the protein to bind to their cofactors on phospholipid surfaces and participate in coagulation. Warfarin treatment reduces the number of Gla residues (normal 10 to 13) per clotting factor molecule with a concomitant fall in coagulant activity. When the number of residues decreases to 9, only 70 percent of the activity of the clotting factor remains; when there are 6, only 2 percent activity is present.

Warfarin is rapidly absorbed from the gastrointestinal tract in 1.5 to 2 h, is 99 percent bound to albumin, and has prolonged survival (half-life, 40 h) in the circulation. The effects of warfarin on coagulation are dependent on the half-life of the vitamin K clotting factors in plasma. Thus, factor VII activity (half-life, 5 h) falls quickly following initiation of therapy and prolongs the PT. The remaining three vitamin K-dependent coagulation

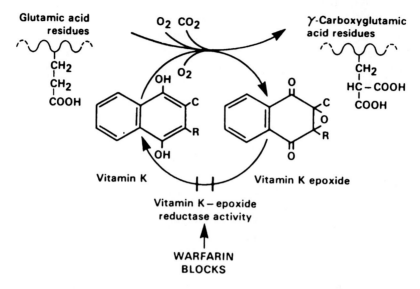

Figure 62-1 Interactions of warfarin and vitamin K. (Reprinted with permission from Seminars in Thrombosis and Hemostasis 12:1, 1986.)

factors (II, IX, X) have half-lives ranging from 24 to 48 h and therefore fall more slowly and only gradually contribute to the lengthening of the PT and APTT. The reductions in these longer-lived clotting factors are most likely responsible for the antithrombotic effects of warfarin. The relationships between oral doses of warfarin and the prolongation of the PT are complex and sometimes unpredictable. Variables include patient compliance, vitamin K content of the diet, concurrent illness, and liver function. The effects of warfarin are also significantly modified by the use of many pharmaceutical agents. Drug interactions can be caused by displacement of warfarin from albumin-binding sites (dilantin), inhibition or acceleration of drug clearance (trimethoprim-sulfamethoxazole, barbiturates), or reduced absorption (cholestyramine).

LABORATORY TESTING

Prothrombin Time

Both the PT and the APTT are prolonged in patients who are treated with long-term oral anticoagulants. Shortly after the initiation of therapy, the PT is the first to lengthen due to the rapid fall in factor VII activity, followed in several days by an increase in the APTT as factors II, IX, and X are reduced. The TCT and concentrations of fibrinogen are not altered by warfarin treatment.

Traditionally, the PT has been used to monitor the antithrombotic affects of the oral anticoagulants. The test is performed by the addition of a thromboplastin (a combination of tissue factor and phospholipid from an organ such as rabbit brain) to recalcified plasma. The sensitivity of the thromboplastin to warfarin-induced reductions in clotting factor activity is a critical variable in the assay. Some thromboplastins are very sensitive, (i.e., produce long PTs for a given intensity of anticoagulation), whereas others are insensitive. Consequently, patients can receive substantially different doses of an oral anticoagulant depending on the thromboplastin used in the PT test.

To address this important clinical problem, the PT ratio (patient PT/control PT) is now modified by a factor (the International Sensitivity Index or ISI) that reflects the "sensitivity" of the thromboplastin used in the assay. Highly sensitive thromboplastins are assigned a low ISI (e.g., 1.0 to 1.8), whereas insensitive reagents have high ISIs (e.g., 2.8). After correction of the PT ratio by the ISI assigned to the thromboplastin, the result is termed the *International Normalized Ratio* (INR). The calculation is performed as follows:

$$INR = (PT\ ratio)^{ISI}$$

Thus, a patient taking warfarin who has a PT of 18 s (with a control PT performed in the same laboratory of 12 s) would have an PT ratio of 1.5. If the ISI of the thromboplastin being used for the assay is 2.0, then the INR is 2.25; that is, $(1.5)^2 = 2.25$.

Large controlled clinical trials have shown that an INR ranging between 2 and 3 (low intensity) provides effective treatment for most patients with deep venous thrombosis or pulmonary embolism. High-intensity anticoagulation (used for some patients with mechanical heart valves or recurrent thrombosis) is defined as an INR of 3 to 4.5. Because the ISI of the many thromboplastins used around the world varies from 1 to 3, clinicians and laboratories must change their practice and report and interpret PT results in the INR format. Otherwise, some patients may receive insufficient warfarin with potential recurrent thromboembolism, whereas others will be at increased risk for hemorrhage.

Native Prothrombin Antigen

Efforts have been made to devise other tests that more accurately reflect the antithrombotic and hemorrhagic risks of oral anticoagulant therapy. One test is for "native prothrombin antigen," an assay that measures fully carboxylated prothrombin, so that a fall in concentration of the clotting factor reflects the intensity of anticoagulation. One study suggested that bleeding risks were reduced when warfarin administration was regulated with this assay. Additional trials are underway to more fully evaluate this test in larger cohorts of patients. Another assay that is being studied measures des-carboxy prothrombin (prothrombin molecules with reduced numbers of Gla residues).

Whole Blood Prothrombin Time Instruments

Small portable instruments that have been designed to measure a PT on finger-stick blood samples are now available for use in the hospital or patients' homes. A special cartridge is used that allows a drop of blood to move by capillary attraction through a small-caliber tube. After the column of blood encounters PT reagents, the formation of a fibrin clot halts blood flow, which is detected by a laser beam. The machine calculates the PT, PT ratio, and INR. Clinical trials have suggested that these instruments give results comparable to those obtained in hospital laboratories. They are particularly useful in infants and children or for homebound patients who are unable to travel to the hospital.

CLINICAL USE

Institution of Therapy

Warfarin is usually started with a dose of 10 mg daily for the first 2 days in hospitalized adult patients who have been treated with heparin for an acute thrombosis. Daily PTs are obtained and subsequent warfarin orders are based on the results with a goal of attaining an INR of 2 to 3. The heparin infusion should not be stopped until the INR has remained in the therapeutic range for 24 h, which allows clotting factors II, IX, and X to reach antithrombotic levels.

Most clinicians order oral anticoagulants for the evening and obtain the PT in the morning; this practice allows time for absorption of the prior dose of warfarin and the return of laboratory test results. Each dose should be ordered daily and only after the results of the laboratory tests and the clinical status of the patient have been reviewed. When patients are electively anticoagulated as outpatients (e.g., for atrial fibrillation), loading doses of warfarin are usually omitted; 5 to 7.5 mg is given daily with adjustments as needed.

The administration of anticoagulants to children is difficult because of their variable responses to therapy. One approach is to give a warfarin loading dose of 0.4 mg/kg per day for the first 2 days, and then modify future orders as indicated by the INR.

Therapeutic Ranges

Most patients with thromboembolism require low-intensity anticoagulation which corresponds to an INR of 2 to 3. Examples are patients with deep venous thrombosis and pulmonary embolism, atrial fibrillation, and tissue valves. High-intensity therapy (INR 3 to 4.5) has been recommended for patients with mechanical valve prostheses. However, a recent study suggested that lower intensities of anticoagulation (e.g., INR of 2.5 to 3.5), may be adequate (and safer) for patients with artificial valves. High-intensity therapy may be appropriate for treatment of infants and children with homozygous protein C or protein S deficiency.

"Mini-intensity" oral anticoagulation therapy that uses either 1 mg warfarin daily without laboratory monitoring or aims for INRs in the range of 1.5 is under active investigation. One study showed that INRs of < 2 are associated with suppression of F1.2 levels (i.e., inhibition of thrombin formation) at these ranges. Large clinical trials will be necessary to determine efficacy of oral anticoagulants in these low ranges.

Maintenance Therapy

Because of the long half-life of warfarin, changes in therapy should be based on a percent of the total weekly dose in patients on chronic anticoagulants rather than an alteration in each daily dose. An effective strategy is to make an initial adjustment to bring the PT rapidly into the therapeutic range, and then alter the weekly dose as necessary. A protocol for management of outpatient anticoagulation therapy is shown in Table 62-1.

Problems in Management

Unstable Prothrombin Times

The great majority of patients on long-term anticoagulants require only minor adjustments in dose. However, some patients have widely fluctuating PTs which pose major challenges in management. Changes in the vitamin K content of the diet can sometimes be responsible (salads in the summer) or intercurrent illness can be a problem. Heart failure, liver disease, and diarrhea all lower anticoagulant requirements. Viral illnesses are a particular challenge in infants and children who often have a dramatic increase in INR a day or two following an upper respiratory infection or gastrointestinal upset. Drug interactions as a cause of instability are common (especially antibiotics) and excessive use of alcohol can alter dietary patterns as well as compliance. Older or mentally impaired patients can become confused about

TABLE 62-1   Protocol for Warfarin Dosage Adjustment in Outpatients with a Target INR of 2 to 3

INR	Adjustment
1.1–1.4	*Day 1*: Add 10–20% of TWD* *Weekly*: Increase TWD by 10–20% *Return*: 1 wk
1.5–1.9	*Day 1*: Add 5–10% of TWD *Weekly*: Increase TWD by 5–10% *Return*: 2 wks
2–3	No change *Return:* 4 wks
3.1–3.9	*Day 1*: Subtract 5–10% of TWD *Weekly*: Reduce TWD by 5–10% *Return*: 2 wks
4.0–5.0	*Day 1*: No warfarin *Weekly*: Reduce TWD by 10–20% *Return*: 1 wk
> 5	Stop warfarin; monitor INR until 3.0, reinstitute at lower TWD—e.g., decrease by 20–50%. *Return*: daily

*TWD, Total weekly dose of warfarin. A patient taking 5 mg on Monday, Wednesday, and Friday, with 7.5 on the remaining days would have a TWD of 45 mg.

tablet size or therapeutic regimen. Finally, if no other cause for instability is identified, patient compliance is often less than optimal.

Intercurrent Surgical Procedures

Surgical or invasive diagnostic procedures such as dental extractions, biopsies, or gastrointestinal endoscopy are often necessary in patients on oral anticoagulants. Relatively minor procedures can often be safely performed by allowing the PT to drift toward normal with subsequent replacement of missing warfarin doses (Table 62-2). Major surgical procedures in patients at high risk for thrombosis pose a bigger problem. Withholding anticoagulants for several days in a patient with a stable mechanical heart valve is not associated with a major risk of embolization. However, prophylactic antithrombotic measures should be used during surgery (e.g., intermittent pneumatic compression devices, prophylactic heparin), and oral anticoagulants should be reinstituted as soon as possible. Individuals at extremely high risk of thrombosis require a more complicated (and expensive) protocol (Table 62-3).

TABLE 62-2 Management of Warfarin for Minor Surgical Procedures

Step 1: Obtain INR 5–7 days before procedure

Step 2: Stop warfarin 1–4 days before the procedure depending on INR (e.g., INR 2–3 = 2 days; INR 3–4 = 3–4 days; INR > 4 = 5 days)

Step 3: On the evening following the surgical procedure, reinstitute warfarin if no bleeding.

Replace missing doses of warfarin on a day to day basis; e.g.,

Th	F	Sa	S	M	T	W	Th	F	Sa
5 mg	5 mg	5 mg	5 mg	0	0	10 mg	10 mg	5 mg	5 mg
(INR 2.5)						↑ (procedure)			

Step 4: Check INR 5–7 days after procedure.

Pregnancy and Lactation

Oral anticoagulants are not recommended during pregnancy because of the risks of warfarin-induced embryonopathy particularly during weeks 6 to 12, fetal neural deformities in the mid trimester, and bleeding that can occur in the neonate at time of delivery. Maternal warfarin therapy does not pose a

TABLE 62-3 Protocol for the Very High-Risk Patient Scheduled for Major Surgery

Day −7: Stop warfarin; begin SC heparin (q 12 h) at a dose sufficient to prolong the APTT to 1.5–2 times control

Day −6 to −1: Continue SC heparin; frequent APTT and platelet count

Day −1: Hospital admission; stop SC heparin; begin IV heparin without loading dose at 400–500 U/h. APTT target upper limit of normal (e.g., 33–35 s).

Day of surgery: Continue heparin before, during, and after surgery (APTT upper limit of normal). Apply intermittent pneumatic compression devices preoperatively (if applicable).

Postop day 2–3: Increase heparin infusion gradually to APTT 1.5–2 times control. Start warfarin when PO fluids are given.

Postop day 7–8: When INR reaches 2–3, heparin is discontinued.

problem for nursing infants as long as they are not vitamin K deficient (i.e., the infant should have had parenteral or repeated oral neonatal prophylaxis, see Chap. 23).

Refractory Patients

Most recurrent thrombosis occurs when the INR is allowed to fall to < 2.0. However, some patients develop thromboembolism despite an adequate intensity of anticoagulation which mandates a change in therapy. One approach is to re-treat with heparin followed by warfarin at a high-intensity level (INR 3 to 4.5). An alternative strategy is to add low doses of aspirin (e.g., 75 to 160 mg daily) to low-intensity warfarin, although sufficient data are not yet available to assess the risks of bleeding. Finally, some refractory patients (particularly those with cancer) require outpatient heparin therapy (given subcutaneously at 12-h intervals).

SIDE EFFECTS AND COMPLICATIONS

Hemorrhage

Bleeding is directly related to increases in the INR, so that low-intensity anticoagulation has a lower rate of both major and minor hemorrhages than high-intensity therapy. Most studies in unselected groups of patients suggest that the risk of major bleeding (as defined by need to discontinue warfarin, hospitalization, or blood transfusion) is approximately 3 percent a year (3 of 100 patients treated for 1 year) and that CNS hemorrhage occurs at a rate of about 0.1 percent per year. Risk factors include female sex, concurrent use of multiple drugs, and associated serious illness such as renal failure or congestive heart failure and intercurrent illnesses in small children. Advanced age does not appear to increase bleeding, but elderly patients require less warfarin to maintain a target INR.

The management of excessively anticoagulated patients who are not bleeding depends in part on the prolongation of the PT. Mild elevations are simply treated with appropriate dose adjustments, whereas moderately increased PTs (e.g., 25 to 35 s) require discontinuation of the anticoagulant for 1 to 2 days. More marked PT prolongations can be corrected with small oral doses of vitamin K (e.g., 2 to 3 mg). In each case, frequent PT determinations are essential, so that anticoagulants can be restarted at an appropriate time.

Minor bleeding (e.g., epistaxis) in patients with INRs in the low-intensity range can usually be managed with local measures alone. However, more serious bleeding associated with an excessively prolonged PT requires parenteral vitamin K (e.g., 5 to 10 mg subcutaneously or intravenously) or infusions of fresh frozen plasma if bleeding is life-threatening. Prothrombin-complex concentrates are rarely necessary, except perhaps in the unusual patient with CNS hemorrhage and neurologic deterioration.

Poisoning or surreptitious ingestion of coumarins are treated as indicated above. However, long-acting agents such as those found in some rodenticides usually require multiple doses of vitamin K to avoid a rebound rise in the PT at a later date.

Warfarin Skin Necrosis

Most, but not all, episodes of warfarin skin necrosis have occurred in patients with hereditary protein C (and occasionally protein S) deficiency. The pathogenesis of this often devastating complication involves a warfarin-induced rapid fall in protein C activity from levels of about 50 percent to < 5 percent, which is a consequence of the short plasma half-life of protein C. Infants with homozygous protein C deficiency also have extremely low levels of protein C activity and develop a similar syndrome termed neonatal purpura fulminans (see Chap. 40). Concurrent inflammation or other prothrombotic states such as surgery or cancer may predispose patients to this syndrome, via cytokine-induced down-regulation of thrombomodulin on the surface of vascular endothelium with impaired activation of any remaining protein C. Because of the risks of warfarin skin necrosis, patients who have a history of venous thrombosis should be tested for deficiencies of protein C and protein S before oral anticoagulants are given electively (i.e., without heparin pretreatment).

Anticoagulation of patients with protein C deficiency or a history of warfarin skin necrosis can be accomplished by the use of concomitant heparin therapy, or by the administration of markedly low doses of warfarin with gradual increases to slow the fall in protein C relative to other vitamin K-dependent clotting factors. One strategy involves starting warfarin at 0.5 mg/day for 3 days and then sequentially increasing the dose at 3-day intervals (e.g., 0.5 mg/day for 3 days, 1 mg/day for 3 days, 2 mg, 4 mg, etc.) until therapeutic anticoagulation has been achieved. Both approaches can be used in high-risk patients.

Other Complications

Other side effects of warfarin therapy include alopecia, skin rash, and diarrhea. One rare but striking complication is the purple toe syndrome, which is thought to be due to warfarin-induced embolization of cholesterol particles from atherosclerotic plaques in the aorta or other major artery to the microvasculature of the toes.

BIBLIOGRAPHY

Braun PJ, Szewczyk KM: Relationship between total prothrombin, native prothrombin, and the international normalized ratio (INR). *Thromb Haemost* 68:160, 1992.

Dalen JE, Hirsh J: Third ACCP Consensus Conference on Antithrombotic Therapy. *Chest* 102:303S, 1992.

Doyle JJ et al: Anticoagulation with sodium warfarin in children: Effect of a loading regimen. *J Pediatr* 113:1095, 1988.

Fredriksson K et al: Emergency reversal of anticoagulation after intracerebral hemorrhage. *Stroke* 23:972, 1992.

Furie B et al: Randomized prospective trial comparing the native prothrombin antigen with the prothrombin time for monitoring oral anticoagulant therapy. *Blood* 75:344, 1990.

Hirsh J: Oral anticoagulant drugs. *N Engl J Med* 324:1865, 1991.

Hirsh J: Substandard monitoring of warfarin in North America. Time for change. *Arch Intern Med* 152:257, 1992.

Kumar S et al: Poor compliance is a major factor in unstable outpatient control of anticoagulant therapy. *Thromb Haemost* 62:729, 1989.

Kumar S et al: Effect of warfarin on plasma concentrations of vitamin K dependent coagulation factors in patients with stable control and monitored compliance. *Br J Haematol* 74:82, 1990.

Millenson MM et al: Monitoring "mini-intensity" anticoagulation with warfarin: Comparison of the prothrombin time using a sensitive thromboplastin with prothrombin fragment F_{1+2} levels. *Blood* 79:2034, 1992.

Saour JN et al: Trial of different intensities of anticoagulation in patients with prosthetic heart valves. *N Engl J Med* 322:428, 1990.

Weiss P et al: Decline of proteins C and S and factors II, VII, IX, and X during the initiation of warfarin therapy. *Thromb Res* 45:783, 1987.

White RH et al: Home prothrombin time monitoring after the initiation of warfarin therapy. A randomized, prospective study. *Ann Intern Med* 111:730, 1989.

Thrombolytic Agents

Acute coronary artery thrombosis, venous thromboembolism, and peripheral artery occlusion have all been successfully treated with infusions of fibrinolytic agents. Although thrombolysis is an attractive therapeutic modality, potential problems include a risk of serious bleeding and recurrent thrombosis of newly reperfused vessels. Streptokinase (SK), urokinase (UK), and tissue plasminogen activator (t-PA) are currently available for clinical use. New generations of thrombolytic agents are being developed to try to maximize clot lysis with lower rates of hemorrhage.

PHARMACOLOGY

Thrombolytic agents are plasminogen activators that promote clot lysis by converting plasminogen, which is adsorbed onto the strands of fibrin within a thrombus, to the fibrinolytic enzyme plasmin. Plasmin cleaves fibrin, breaks down the clot, and generates soluble fibrin degradation products (FDP) which are subsequently cleared by the kidney and reticuloendothelial system. The various fibrinolytic drugs differ as to mechanisms of plasminogen activation, their survival time in the circulation, and specificity for fibrin (Table 63-1).

TABLE 63-1 Thrombolytic Agents

Agent	Abbreviation	Source	$T_{1/2}$
Streptokinase	SK	Streptococcal culture	20–30 min
Urokinase	UK	Renal cell culture	15–30 min
Tissue plasminogen activator	t-PA	Recombinant technology	5 min
Anisolated plasminogen: streptokinase activator complex	APSAC	Streptococcal culture	75–90 min
Single-chain urokinase plasminogen activator	SCU-PA	Renal cell culture	5 min

Unfortunately, all currently available thrombolytic agents can produce marked impairment of hemostasis and bleeding (Fig. 63-1):

1. Fibrinolytic enzymes cannot distinguish pathologic thromboses (e.g., obstructing a coronary artery) from hemostatic plugs that prevent bleeding from a critical vascular defect (e.g., a small injury to a cerebral ves-

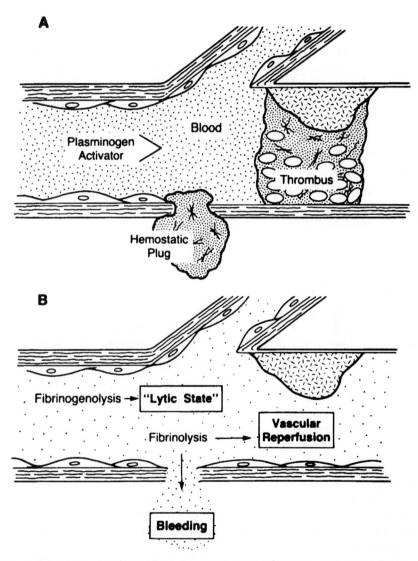

Figure 63-1 The three principal sites of action of plasminogen activators on intravascular substrates: the pathologic thrombus, the hemostatic plug, and the circulating blood. (Reprinted by permission of The New England Journal of Medicine 318:1512, 1988.)

sel). Effective clot lysis leads to potentially lifesaving vascular reperfusion in the former instance, but to catastrophic bleeding in the latter.

2. Plasminogen activators not only act on plasminogen bound to fibrin but also on circulating plasminogen which generates plasmin and produces subsequent systemic fibrinolysis. Circulating plasmin destroys fibrinogen, factor V, and factor VIII.

3. Platelet function is compromised because of inhibition of platelet aggregation by FDP and to impaired platelet adhesion by plasmin-induced proteolysis of glycoprotein Ib and von Willebrand factor.

Thrombolytic agents must be administered by intravenous or intra-arterial routes. Protocols for clinical use include intravenous bolus (for acute coronary artery thrombosis), continuous long-term intravenous infusion (for deep venous thrombosis [DVT]), and site-directed arterial infusions (peripheral artery thrombosis). Although fibrinolytic agents are usually administered in large amounts designed to produce rapid clot lysis, lower doses are sometimes administered directly into the clot in an attempt to destroy thrombi without producing a systemic fibrinolytic state. Dosage and schedules of administration for SK, UK, and t-PA differ depending on the fibrinolytic agent and its intended use; pharmaceutical product information should be consulted for details of therapy.

LABORATORY MONITORING

Fibrinolytic therapy alters most laboratory measurements of hemostatic function, but few tests predict either efficacy of thrombolysis or the risks of bleeding (Table 63-2). Most of the assays reflect a systemic fibrinolytic state, for example, a short euglobulin lysis time (ELT); hypofibrinogenemia; and a long TCT, PT, and APTT. Impaired platelet function is suggested by prolongation of the bleeding time. FDP tests that measure both fibrinogen and fibrin degradation products are markedly elevated, whereas those that detect only fibrin degradation products (such as the D-dimer test) are more nearly normal (see below).

The bleeding time may help to identify patients at increased risk of bleeding. In one study, bleeding times obtained 90 min following the completion of fibrinolytic therapy for acute coronary artery occlusion were longer in patients who subsequently hemorrhaged than those who did not. Other studies have suggested that lower platelet counts are also associated with bleeding.

Most short-term infusions of thrombolytic agents do not require laboratory monitoring. However, the dilute thrombin time (normal range of 20 to 30 s) is sometimes used to ensure continued fibrinolysis in patients treated

TABLE 63-2 Laboratory Tests in Thrombolytic Therapy

Test	Primary Use	Comments
Thrombin time	Identify persistent lytic state	Heparin also prolongs
Partial thromboplastin time	Identify persistent lytic state	Alternative to thrombin time; heparin also prolongs
Reptilase time	Identify persistent lytic state in heparinized patients	
Fibrinogen	Guide therapy with cryoprecipitate	Check to ensure adequate repletion; clotting rate assay (Clauss) method preferred
Bleeding time	Persistent bleeding despite cryoprecipitate and fresh frozen plasma	Useful when considering platelet transfusion
Factors V and VIII	Identify specific factor deficiencies	Not generally useful
Fibrinogen degradation products	Elevation confirms lytic state	Not useful in therapy
a_2-Antiplasmin	Depletion confirms lytic state	Not useful in therapy

*Reproduced with permission from Sane DC et al: Bleeding during thrombolytic therapy for acute myocardial infarction: Mechanisms and management. *Ann Intern Med* 111:1010, 1989.

with long-term SK (e.g., 3 days) for DVT. Tests that can be used to document the presence of a systemic fibrinolytic state in children and adults include shortening of the ELT, prolongation of the TCT, and a fall in the concentration of fibrinogen. Unfortunately, levels of D-dimer (a FDP), have not been helpful as a marker of reperfusion success because lysis of circulating soluble fibrin complexes can also elevate D-dimer.

CLINICAL USE

Coronary Thrombolysis

Angiographic and pathologic studies have shown that up to 90 percent of acute transmural myocardial infarctions are caused by a thrombus located on the surface of a ruptured atherosclerotic plaque in a stenotic coronary artery. Intra-arterial or intravenous fibrinolytic therapy produces vascular reperfusion in 55 to 90 percent of patients, particularly if treatment is administered within 6 h of the onset of symptoms. The intravenous route is now preferred because patients can be treated rapidly with less bleeding although reperfusion rates are slightly lower. Clinical studies have convincingly shown that early thrombolytic therapy is of benefit for acute coronary artery occlusion; salvage of myocardium, improved left ventricular function, and most importantly, reduction in both short-term and 1-year mortality rates have all been documented. A major problem is rethrombosis, an event that occurs in 5 to 15 percent of patients. Because of this, most patients are treated with aspirin and heparin; some may also require coronary artery revascularization procedures following thrombolysis.

Controversy persists as to the optimal fibrinolytic agent for coronary thrombolysis and debate centers on rates of reperfusion or rethrombosis, hemorrhage, and cost. However, most would agree that thrombolytic therapy is the treatment of choice for patients with acute myocardial infarction.

Peripheral Arterial Thrombosis

Acute occlusion of peripheral arteries (usually in the lower extremities) is most often due to emboli from the heart or more proximal vessels, or to thrombosis at sites of advanced atherosclerotic disease. Thrombolytic therapy in these patients has been only moderately successful; substantial lysis occurs in only 20 percent of patients. In general, response rates are higher with embolic vascular occlusion than in situ thrombosis. Early therapy is most successful although later treatment may occasionally be of benefit. Most patients are treated within a week of the onset of acute ischemic symptoms.

Indications for fibrinolytic therapy in peripheral vascular disease include acute embolic occlusion of a major artery, patients with contraindications to surgical revascularization, and treatment of very peripheral arterial occlusions that are not amenable to surgical correction. Most clinical studies in peripheral artery disease have used catheter-directed regional fibrinolysis in hopes of maximizing local thrombolysis and minimizing bleeding. However, systemic fibrinolysis still occurs and bleeding rates remain high especially at the insertion sites of arterial catheters. Most patients ultimately require definitive correction of their vascular lesions by transluminal angioplasty or, in many cases, surgical bypass.

Deep Venous Thrombosis

Fibrinolytic therapy produces substantial thrombolysis in approximately 50 percent of patients with DVT of the extremities (compared to only 5 percent of patients treated with heparin). Results are improved if fibrinolytic therapy is administered within 2 days of the onset of symptoms; thrombus resolution is decreased with delays in treatment of up to 7 days. The fibrinolytic agents are usually administered by continuous intravenous infusion for 3 or more days in an attempt to maximize clot lysis. However, most thrombolysis occurs during the early phases of therapy, so that the ratio of benefit to bleeding risk decreases after 24 to 48 h of treatment.

The long-term benefit of thrombolytic therapy for DVT remains controversial. Although it is clear that treatment improves the appearance of both early and late venograms, the data are less certain that symptoms due to the postphlebitic syndrome are reduced. Additional long-term controlled clinical trials will be required to settle the issue and to compare functional improvement with the risks of serious (e.g., intracranial) bleeding.

Pulmonary Embolism

Thrombolytic agents are effective in the treatment of acute massive pulmonary embolism with systemic hypotension and occasionally produce dramatic improvement in cardiopulmonary status. Patients with less extensive emboli have significant improvements in early pulmonary angiograms and perfusion lung scans. However, clinical trials have not shown a reduction in mortality rates 14 or more days after therapy. Sufficient data are not yet available to determine whether early thrombolytic treatment of patients with pulmonary embolism produces clinically significant long-term improvements in pulmonary function or decreased rates of chronic pulmonary hypertension.

Successful lysis of pulmonary emboli has been observed with SK, UK, and t-PA. Earlier trials with SK and UK used infusions (either intravenous or via pulmonary artery catheters) that lasted for 12 to 24 h or more. More recently, investigators have tried short-term high-dose infusion regimens in attempts to induce brisk fibrinolysis with lower risks of bleeding.

Acute Stroke

Enthusiasm has been mounting for the use of fibrinolytic agents in patients with acute thrombotic stroke. Studies in animals (including primates) have suggested that neurologic function can be spared if reperfusion occurs within 3 h of acute middle cerebral artery occlusion. Clinical trials are now underway to evaluate the efficacy and safety of thrombolytic therapy (particularly with t-PA) in patients who are treated soon after cerebral vascular thrombosis. In preliminary trials, the relatively low risk of hemorrhagic transformation of cerebral infarcts may prove to be acceptable if permanent neurologic dysfunction or death can be reduced with treatment.

Other Indications

A myriad of individual case reports or small clinical series have appeared in the medical literature that describe thrombolytic therapy for a wide range of vascular occlusions, including thrombosis of cerebral, retinal, and abdominal veins. Prompt catheter-directed thrombolytic therapy has also been reported to preserve vision in patients with central retinal artery occlusion. Acute aortic thrombosis (often due to umbilical catheters) has resolved in infants and children after fibrinolytic therapy, although concerns about CNS hemorrhage may limit its use.

SIDE EFFECTS AND COMPLICATIONS

Hemorrhage has occurred in virtually all clinical trials in which large doses of fibrinolytic agents have been used. Most bleeding occurs at sites of vascular injury (e.g., in vessels punctured for diagnostic procedures) or in surgical wounds and may be severe. Rates of major bleeding in large clinical trials vary from 5 to 20 percent or more, and depend on patient selection, duration of therapy, and dose of thrombolytic agents. In general, the risk of serious hemorrhage is at least two to three times greater than that of heparin for the same indication. Because of the risks of bleeding, careful patient selection is important. Table 63-3 lists some commonly accepted absolute and relative contraindications to fibrinolytic therapy.

One of the most feared complications of thrombolytic therapy is intracranial hemorrhage, which occurs in 0.5 to 1 percent of patients and is fatal at least two-thirds of the time. Bleeding risks must be carefully considered before decisions are made about the use of fibrinolytic agents in clinical practice. In

TABLE 63-3 Contraindications to Thrombolytic Therapy

Absolute Contraindications
Recent neurosurgery, head trauma, or CNS hemorrhage
Intracranial neoplasm or aneurysm
Stroke within 6 months
Active or recent internal bleeding
Uncontrolled hypertension (diastolic pressure > 120 mm Hg)

Relative Contraindications
Surgery or organ biopsy in prior 2 weeks
Recent trauma (including CPR)
Puncture of major noncompressible vessel within 10 days
Infective endocarditis
Pregnancy or recent delivery
Hemostatic defects

some cases, the potential benefit may be substantial (e.g., the treatment of acute coronary artery occlusion), so that the risks of CNS bleeding are clearly acceptable. However, the risk/benefit ratio does not seem reasonable in a patient with a venous thrombosis limited to the popliteal vein in the leg. Prospective controlled clinical trials will help provide the information needed for physicians and patients to make accurate and informed decisions about the risks and benefits of thrombolytic therapy.

Treatment of serious bleeding associated with fibrinolytic therapy requires

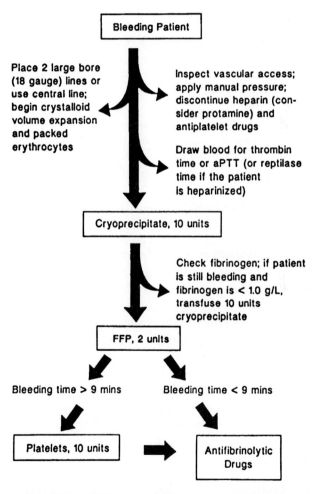

Figure 63-2 A typical strategy for the management of major bleeding produced by thrombolytic therapy and causing hemodynamic compromise that is not immediately life-threatening. APTT, activated partial thromboplastin time; FFP, fresh frozen plasma. (Reproduced with permission from Sane DC et al: Bleeding during thrombolytic therapy for acute myocardial infarction: Mechanisms and management. Ann Intern Med 111:1010, 1989.)

immediate cessation of the infusion and rapid correction of residual hemostatic defects. The management of systemic fibrinolysis is discussed in Chap. 26, and a therapeutic strategy for major hemorrhage that complicates thrombolytic therapy of coronary artery occlusion is shown in Fig. 63-2.

BIBLIOGRAPHY

Bovill EG et al: Monitoring thrombolytic therapy. *Prog Cardiovasc Dis* 34:279, 1992.

Califf RM et al: Clinical risks of thrombolytic therapy. *Am J Cardiol* 69:12A, 1992.

Collen D, Lijnen HR: Basic and clinical aspects of fibrinolysis and thrombolysis. *Blood* 78:3114, 1991.

Coller BS: Platelets and thrombolytic therapy. *N Engl J Med* 322:33, 1990.

De Jaegere PP et al: Intracranial hemorrhage in association with thrombolytic therapy: Incidence and clinical predictive factors. *J Am Coll Cardiol* 19:289, 1992.

Gill JB, Massel D, Cairns J: Fibrinolytic therapy in coronary artery disease. *Baillieres Clin Haematol* 3:745, 1990.

Gimple LW et al: Correlation between template bleeding times and spontaneous bleeding during treatment of acute myocardial infarction with recombinant tissue-type plasminogen activator. *Circulation* 80:581, 1989.

Goldhaber SZ: Thrombolytic therapy for venous thromboembolism. *Baillieres Clin Haematol* 3:693, 1990.

Goldhaber SZ: Managing pulmonary embolism. *Hosp Pract* 26:37, 1991.

ISIS-2 (Second International Study of Infarct Survival) Collaborative Group: Randomised trial of intravenous streptokinase, oral aspirin, both, or neither among 17,187 cases of suspected acute myocardial infarction: ISIS-2. *Lancet* 2:349, 1988.

Levine SR, Brott TG: Thrombolytic therapy in cerebrovascular disorders. *Prog Cardiovas Dis* 34:235, 1992.

Maggioni AP et al: The risk of stroke in patients with acute myocardial infarction after thrombolytic and antithrombotic treatment. *N Engl J Med* 327:1, 1992.

Marder VJ, Sherry S: Thrombolytic therapy: Current status. *N Engl J Med* 318:1512, 1988.

Marder VJ: Bleeding complications of thrombolytic treatment. *Am J Hosp Pharm* 47:S15, 1990.

Sane DC et al: Bleeding during thrombolytic therapy for acute myocardial infarction: Mechanisms and management. *Ann Intern Med* 111:1010, 1989.

Verstraete M: Advances in thrombolytic therapy. *Cardiovasc Drugs Ther* 6:111, 1992.

Antiplatelet Agents

A major goal of antiplatelet therapy is to block platelet deposition on the surface of disrupted atherosclerotic plaques to prevent acute vascular occlusion or embolization of thrombotic debris. Clinical trials have now clearly shown that antiplatelet therapy significantly reduces arterial thrombosis in patients suffering from coronary, cerebral, or peripheral vascular disease. Aspirin is the most commonly used antiplatelet agent because it is cheap, widely available, relatively safe, and demonstrably effective. An alternative to aspirin, ticlopidine, is also an effective platelet inhibitor that has recently been tested in clinical trials for cerebral vascular disease and unstable angina. The use of sulfinpyrazone and dipyridamole has diminished substantially because they are less effective and more costly than aspirin.

PHARMACOLOGY

Aspirin's antithrombotic effects are due to inhibition of platelet aggregation (but not platelet adhesion). A key platelet enzyme, cyclooxygenase, is permanently acetylated by aspirin, which impairs the synthesis of thromboxane A_2, a prostanoid with potent platelet aggregating properties. Aspirin also inhibits the cyclooxygenase of endothelial cells, and therefore reduces the synthesis of prostacyclin (PGI_2), a prostaglandin that inhibits platelet function. In contrast to platelets, however, endothelial cell cyclooxygenase is renewable, so that PGI_2 synthesis recovers in 24 to 48 h (see Fig. 64-1). Platelet cyclooxygenase may also be more sensitive than the endothelial cell enzyme to the inhibitory affects of aspirin. Efforts have been made to exploit these differences between platelets and endothelial cells by the use of very low doses of aspirin or by prolonging the interval between aspirin doses to allow time for recovery of prostacyclin synthesis.

Since aspirin permanently inhibits platelet cyclooxygenase, abnormalities in laboratory tests of platelet function (platelet aggregation) persist for a week or more after a single dose of the drug. The bleeding time, however, is less sensitive, returning to normal in most people within 2 to 3 days.

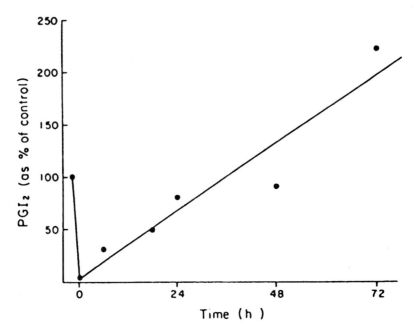

Figure 64-1 Using human vascular cell cultures, prostacyclin synthesis is inhibited temporarily by low-dose aspirin, but synthetic ability is quickly restored. Time course of recovery of endothelial prostacyclin is shown. (Reproduced from the Journal of Clinical Investigation, 1979, 63:532, by copyright permission of the American Society for Clinical Investigation.)

Substantial controversy surrounds the dose of aspirin that provides an optimal antithrombotic effect. Studies using the renal excretion of thromboxane and prostacyclin metabolites as surrogate markers of aspirin's antithrombotic effects have suggested that low doses, (e.g., 60 to 325 mg daily) of the drug are more effective than higher amounts, and that less frequent administration (e.g., daily or every other day) is better than multiple daily doses. Based on these data and the results of recent clinical trials, current recommendations are for the use of 60 to 325 mg aspirin daily or 325 mg every other day.

Recently, a new formulation of aspirin has been developed that effectively inhibits platelet thromboxane and spares prostacyclin synthesis. A sustained-release preparation of low-dose aspirin has been formulated that allows gastrointestinal adsorption at a near constant rate of 10 mg/h. Presumably, platelets are inhibited when the drug is present in the prehepatic circulation, but after the aspirin passes through the liver, it is de-acetylated and loses its ability to inhibit systemic prostacyclin synthesis. Clinical trials will be necessary to show that this new aspirin preparation is superior to other low-dose aspirin regimens.

Ticlopidine is a thienopyridine derivative that blocks platelet aggregation possibly by inhibition of the fibrinogen binding site, glycoprotein IIb/IIIa, on the platelet membrane. This agent has been approved for use in the United States for treatment of patients with transient ischemic attacks (TIAs) who cannot tolerate aspirin.

CLINICAL USE

Aspirin is used for prevention of thrombosis in patients with atherosclerosis. Antiplatelet therapy does not seem to be of benefit for treatment of deep venous thrombosis or pulmonary embolism. However, low-dose aspirin has recently been shown to provide effective prophylaxis against embolic stroke in some patients with chronic nonrheumatic atrial fibrillation.

As discussed above, the most appropriate dose of aspirin for management of patients with atherosclerosis is a matter of controversy. Aspirin has proven successful in therapeutic trials in doses ranging from as low as 30 mg once daily to as high as 650 mg twice a day. A reasonable clinical practice is to treat most patients with a single standard low dose of aspirin (e.g., 325 mg once daily).

Myocardial Infarction

Primary Prevention

Two large prospective clinical trials of low-dose aspirin in male physicians showed that first attacks of fatal or nonfatal myocardial infarction were significantly reduced by at least 1/3, although overall mortality was unchanged (Fig. 64-2). A similar reduction in risk was found in a prospective but nonrandomized trial of aspirin in nurses. Based on these data, males (and most likely females) over 50 years of age with a predisposition to coronary atherosclerosis, such as a family history of coronary heart disease, hyperlipidemia or diabetes, should be treated with aspirin. However, aspirin therapy should not substitute for effective management of coronary risk factors such as smoking, hyperlipidemia, lack of exercise, or hypertension.

Secondary Prevention

A meta-analysis was recently published that included 25 trials of antiplatelet therapy in patients with a history of coronary artery disease. This study showed that aspirin significantly reduced all cause mortality, vascular mortality, and stroke or myocardial infarction. In each instance, event rates were reduced by 15 to 30 percent. Low doses of aspirin were as effective as higher doses. Accordingly, long-term low-dose aspirin therapy is now recommended for all patients who have had an acute myocardial infarction.

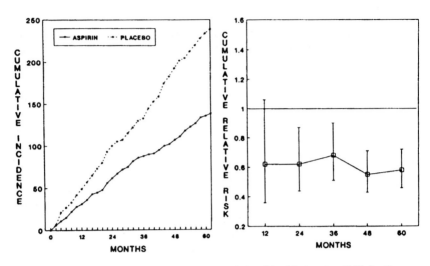

Figure 64-2 Cumulative incidence and cumulative relative risk of first myocardial infarction among subjects randomized in the Physicians' Health Study, by month of followup. (Reproduced with permission. Ridker PM et al: Am Heart J 122:1588, 1991. Copyright 1991 American Heart Association.)

Unstable and Chronic Stable Angina

Aspirin prevents myocardial infarction and death in patients with unstable angina with benefits that persist for at least a year. Ticlopidine is also effective (in a dose of 250 mg twice daily) for reduction of a combination end point of vascular death and nonfatal myocardial infarction. Although aspirin has been beneficial, many cardiologists recommend the use of heparin when a patient presents with acute chest pain until the ultimate diagnosis (unstable angina, myocardial infarction) becomes more clear and future therapy (thrombolysis, percutaneous coronary angioplasty, coronary artery bypass grafting) is selected.

The risk of subsequent myocardial infarction in patients with chronic stable angina is significantly reduced with aspirin (by up to 70 percent or more) as noted in the Physicians' Health Study. The relative risk of stroke increased in these patients, although no stroke was fatal. However, aspirin did not prevent the onset of angina pectoris in previously asymptomatic men.

Coronary Artery Thrombolysis, Angioplasty, and Saphenous Vein Bypass Grafts

An extensive multicenter trial (ISIS-2) clearly showed that 160 mg aspirin given concurrently with streptokinase for treatment of acute myocardial infarction produced a 42 percent decline in vascular deaths by 5 weeks, a benefit that persisted for the next 15 months. Other studies have substantiated these findings. Daily low-dose aspirin has also been shown to reduce saphenous vein graft occlusion in patients undergoing coronary artery bypass surgery. In contrast, aspirin has not reduced late restenosis following coronary angioplasty. Long-term aspirin can be recommended in each of these clinical situations for the prevention of future coronary artery occlusion.

Stroke

Primary Prevention

Most cerebral vascular accidents are caused by thrombotic or embolic occlusion of cerebral vessels. The benefit of aspirin in the primary prevention of stroke is a matter of some controversy. At the present time, most would recommend low-dose aspirin for the prevention of stroke in patients who are known to have coronary artery disease, based on a meta-analysis of reported trials showing a subsequent reduction of nonfatal stroke of 40 percent. Nevertheless, patients with risk factors for atherosclerosis such as hypertension or diabetes should probably receive aspirin to prevent coronary artery disease.

Secondary Prevention

A series of individual studies as well as a meta-analysis of a large number of clinical trials have suggested that low-dose aspirin therapy reduces subsequent stroke and death in patients with TIAs. The data are not as strong but still favor the use of antiplatelet therapy following a completed stroke. Two trials have suggested that very low doses of aspirin (e.g., 30 mg and 75 mg daily) are as effective as 325 mg in preventing future vascular events. Ticlopidine has also been shown to be effective in patients with either TIAs or completed stroke.

Carotid Endarterectomy

A recent clinical trial suggested that antiplatelet therapy with aspirin does not prevent restenosis following carotid endarterectomy. However, because most patients with carotid atherosclerosis have coronary artery disease, aspirin therapy is recommended for prevention of myocardial infarction.

Atrial Fibrillation

Patients with chronic nonrheumatic atrial fibrillation have a risk of cerebral vascular accident that ranges from 2 to 8 percent per year. A large randomized clinical trial performed in the United States (SPAF) suggested that aspirin (325 mg/day) reduced ischemic stroke and systemic embolization by 42 percent. However, since oral anticoagulant therapy with warfarin has also been shown to be at least as effective, a new trial is underway that directly compares aspirin and warfarin (SPAF II). Until the results of this and other trials are reported, aspirin therapy should be considered for use in patients with chronic nonrheumatic atrial fibrillation if warfarin is contraindicated, and in younger patients without advanced cardiac disease.

Chronic Lower Extremity Ischemia

The efficacy of antiplatelet therapy for prevention of thrombotic vascular occlusion in patients with lower extremity atherosclerosis or to prevent occlusion of saphenous vein or prosthetic vascular grafts following surgery is not established. Limited data suggest that antiplatelet therapy with aspirin is of benefit if it is started preoperatively in patients undergoing infrainguinal bypass surgery and also in patients with chronic lower extremity ischemia who are treated nonoperatively. Recently, low-dose aspirin significantly reduced the need for peripheral artery surgery over the next 5 years in healthy middle-aged physicians enrolled in the Physicians' Health Study (relative risk 0.54, P = 0.03). An additional indication for antiplatelet therapy is for the prevention of cardiovascular thrombosis, which is exceedingly common in patients with peripheral artery disease.

Other Indications for Antiplatelet Therapy of Vascular Disease

Aspirin has been used in a wide variety of other vascular disorders. Examples include Kawasaki disease, myeloproliferative disorders (particularly erythromelalgia), prophylaxis of venous thrombosis in hip fracture patients, and preeclampsia.

COMPLICATIONS AND SIDE EFFECTS

Although often considered a harmless drug, aspirin can cause gastrointestinal symptoms and hemorrhagic events. Gastrointestinal symptoms are related to the dose of aspirin; higher event rates are observed with doses of aspirin > 3 tablets daily.

Bruising, gastrointestinal bleeding, postoperative hemorrhage, and epistaxis are also more common in patients taking aspirin and have been reported with all doses. Rates of bleeding may be greater when aspirin is combined with alcohol. Template bleeding times were greatly prolonged (> 30 min) in 40 percent of a group of normal subjects given both drugs. When aspirin was given at a dose of 325 mg every other day in the Physicians' Health Study, bleeding occurred in 27 percent of patients, compared to 20 percent of patients who received placebo. A small but not statistically significant increase in CNS hemorrhage has been reported in two large trials of low-dose aspirin in asymptomatic men.

Ticlopidine has been associated with side effects that include severe neutropenia (which is usually reversible) in 1 percent, diarrhea in up to 20 percent, and elevations of plasma cholesterol in 10 percent of patients. A few subjects treated with ticlopidine have developed a severe thrombotic thrombocytopenia purpura-like syndrome, which is often fatal.

Aspirin should be stopped 7 to 10 days before elective surgical procedures, particularly those where small amounts of bleeding could cause major complications (e.g., cataract extraction). In the rare instance when the antiplatelet effect of aspirin is thought to contribute to severe bleeding, DDAVP can be used followed by platelet transfusions, if necessary.

BIBLIOGRAPHY

Albers GW: Role of ticlopidine for prevention of stroke. *Stroke* 23:912, 1992.

Antiplatelet Trialists' Collaboration: Secondary prevention of vascular disease by prolonged antiplatelet treatment. *Br Med J* 296:320, 1988.

Clarke RJ et al: Suppression of thromboxane A_2 but not of systemic prostacyclin by controlled-release aspirin. *N Engl J Med* 325:1137, 1991.

Easton JD: Antiplatelet therapy in the prevention of stroke. *Drugs* 42:39, 1991.

Goldhaber SZ et al: Low-dose aspirin and subsequent peripheral arterial surgery in the Physicians' Health Study. *Lancet* 340:143, 1992.

Goodnight SH et al: Recommendations for the use of antiplatelet therapy in cardiac, cerebral and peripheral vascular disease. Parts 1 and 2. *West J Med*, 1993.

Harker LA et al: Failure of aspirin plus dipyridamole to prevent restenosis after carotid endarterectomy. *Ann Intern Med* 116:731, 1992.

Miller KP, Frishman WH: Platelets and antiplatelet therapy in ischemic heart disease. *Med Clin North Am* 72:117, 1988.

Oczkowski WJ, Turpie AGG: Antithrombotic treatment of cerebrovascular disease. *Ballieres Clin Haematol* 3:781, 1990.

Page Y et al: Thrombotic thrombocytopenic purpura related to ticlopidine. *Lancet* 337:774, 1991.

Peto R et al: Randomised trial of prophylactic daily aspirin in British male doctors. *Br Med J* 296:313, 1988.

Ridker PM et al: The effect of chronic platelet inhibition with low-dose aspirin on atherosclerotic progression and acute thrombosis: Clinical evidence from the Physicians' Health Study. *Am Heart J* 122:1588, 1991.

Steering Committee on the Physicians' Health Study Research Group: Final report on the aspirin component of the ongoing Physicians' Health Study. *N Engl J Med* 321:129, 1989.

Stein B et al: Antithrombotic therapy in cardiac disease. An emerging approach based on pathogenesis and risk. *Circulation* 80:1501, 1989.

Willard JE et al: The use of aspirin in ischemic heart disease. *N Engl J Med* 327:175, 1992.

Other Measures

for Treatment

or Prevention

of Thrombosis

INFERIOR VENA CAVAL FILTERS

Inferior vena caval (IVC) filters are usually inserted just below the renal veins
to stop emboli from the pelvis and lower extremities before they produce
pulmonary artery occlusion. Recent generations of filters have been improved in design. Filters that are currently available include the titanium
Greenfield filter, the "bird's nest" filter, the Nitinol filter, and the Venatech
filter (Fig. 65-1). Randomized clinical trials to directly compare the efficacy
and safety of the various filters are not yet available. The Greenfield filter
has had the widest clinical use.

Clinical indications for placement of IVC filters are in flux, but they are
most frequently used:

1. In patients with thromboembolism who have contraindications to anticoagulants
2. In patients who develop pulmonary emboli despite adequate anticoagulation
3. For prophylaxis in patients with extremely high risk of pulmonary embolism

The filters can be successfully inserted by a percutaneous route in almost
all patients (> 97 percent) by an experienced operator in only 20 to 30 min.

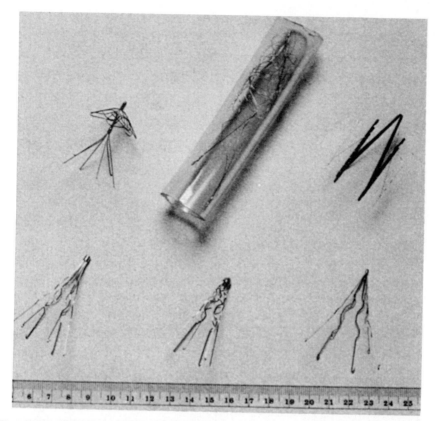

Figure 65-1 Currently available IVC filters, clockwise from above left: Nitinol filter, bird's nest filter in a plastic tube, Venatech filter, titanium Greenfield filter, stainless steel original Greenfield filter, and percutaneous modified-hook stainless steel Greenfield filter. (Used with permission from Greenfield LJ: Arch Surg 127:662, 1992. Copyright 1992, American Medical Association.)

Most often, the right femoral vein is used, followed in frequency by the left femoral vein and the internal jugular veins. The filters are typically placed in an infrarenal position (95 percent), but they can also be positioned above the renal veins and even in the superior vena cava. Although anticoagulants are usually temporarily stopped, they can be restarted shortly after insertion. Long-term anticoagulation is not required to inhibit clotting of the filter, but is often indicated to prevent recurrence of lower extremity venous thrombi with worsening of chronic venous insufficiency.

The complications and risks of IVC filters are listed in Table 65-1. Major morbidity or mortality caused by the filters is relatively low; in most centers it is < 5 percent. Displacement of the filter is usually minimal, but rarely may be serious with migration to the right atrium which necessitates retrieval by catheter or surgery. Thrombi occasionally form on the proximal surface of

TABLE 65-1 Complications of Inferior Vena Caval Filters

Complication	Estimated Risk, %
Bleeding	<1
Migration (>9 mm)	10
Pulmonary embolism	3
Thrombosis at insertion site	9
New onset lower extremity edema	10
Misplacement of filter	5
IVC perforation	<1
Infection	<1

the filter, so that protection from pulmonary emboli is not guaranteed. Obstruction of venous return as a result of in situ thrombosis or from emboli lodging in the filter can also occur. The risks of filter occlusion are higher in patients with extensive thrombosis of the pelvis and legs.

INTERMITTENT PNEUMATIC LEG COMPRESSION

Inflatable pneumatic devices are now widely available for controlled intermittent or sequential compression of the lower extremities to prevent thrombosis in patients undergoing general, pelvic, or orthopedic surgery (Fig. 65-2). Intermittent leg compression has been shown to augment venous blood flow during periods of immobility and to reduce rates of deep venous thrombosis. Of interest, the compression devices enhance systemic fibrinolytic activity and reduce levels of fibrinopeptide A in patients who undergo neurosurgical procedures.

Pneumatic boots have gained in popularity in large part because they provide a measure of antithrombotic prophylaxis but do not cause bleeding, and therefore can be used in patients in whom anticoagulants are risky or contraindicated. The devices should be applied at least 2 h before surgery, maintained throughout the operation, and then continued postoperatively until the patient is fully ambulatory.

Several controlled clinical trials have assessed the benefits of intermittent pneumatic leg compression for thrombotic prophylaxis. In one study of patients with elective hip replacement, the rate of lower extremity thrombosis was reduced from 52 to 25 percent, with proximal venous thrombosis decreasing from 28 to 15 percent (Hull reference). Although these reductions are statistically significant, comparable studies using standard heparin or low molecular weight heparin have produced rates of proximal venous thrombosis as low as 3 to 5 percent. Another study in orthopedic patients suggested

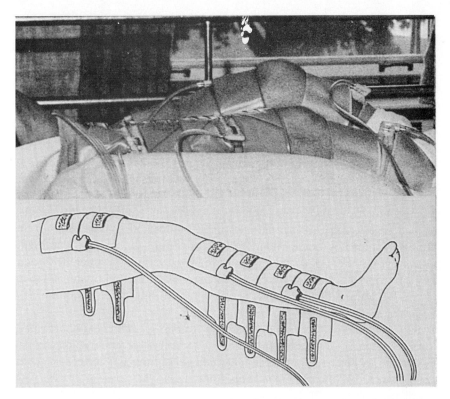

Figure 65-2 Calf and thigh compression cuffs in place on a patient. The calf and thigh cuffs are applied circumferentially around the leg and secured by a Velcro strip on each cuff. (Used with permission from Hull RD et al: JAMA 263:2313, 1990. Copyright 1990, American Medical Association.)

that the compression devices were more effective in the reduction of calf vein than more proximal venous thrombi.

Although intermittent leg compression is a valuable method of prophylaxis for venous thrombosis in surgical patients, sufficient data have not yet been collected to determine if rates of pulmonary embolism or death from pulmonary embolism are also lowered. The devices are clearly indicated in surgery patients in whom anticoagulants cannot be used, and they may also be useful as an adjunct to other methods of prophylaxis.

NEW ANTITHROMBOTIC AGENTS

Novel antithrombotic agents are being developed and tested at a rapid pace. Some of these new drugs were originally isolated from biologic sources such as the saliva of leeches, ticks, or bats. Others have been synthesized in the laboratory to inhibit a specific reaction required for thrombosis such as platelet aggregation. Examples of some of the new platelet inhibitors, anti-coagulants, and fibrinolytic agents are described below.

Platelet Inhibitors

Almost all of the major functions of platelets have been targets for pharmaceutical manipulation. Fibrinogen binding to platelets can be blocked by inhibition of glycoprotein IIb/IIIa using a mouse/human monoclonal antibody, which effectively inhibits platelet aggregation. The antibody is now being tested in human subjects. An alternative approach has been to create small peptides containing an RGDX sequence that recognize and inhibit platelet adhesion molecules such as glycoprotein IIb/IIIa. These agents, termed *disintegrins*, are synthesized in the laboratory or prepared from biologic sources by recombinant DNA technology. One example is Echistatin, a component of a snake venom which prevents experimental thrombosis in primates. Platelet adhesion has also been inhibited by interference of von Willebrand factor binding to glycoprotein Ib using monoclonal antibodies or synthetic peptides.

Finally, a series of compounds that block platelet endoperoxides, thromboxane A_2, or platelet thromboxane receptors are undergoing clinical evaluation. Stable analogs of prostacyclin (e.g., iloprost) have also been developed, some of which have been tested in human subjects.

Anticoagulants

Pharmacologic agents have been used to block fibrin formation at several points along the coagulation pathway. Thrombin activity can be inhibited by hirudin, an extract of leeches (used for centuries for therapeutic purposes), which is a small protein (65 amino acids) that has been cloned and is now available for clinical research (Fig. 65-3). Hirudin forms a nearly irreversible 1:1 complex with thrombin and inhibits its action on platelets as well as fibrinogen, so that thrombin-induced platelet aggregation can be blocked. Hirudin is now being studied in patients with coronary artery thrombosis in hopes of preventing rethrombosis following thrombolysis. Other potent antithrombins such as argatroban and chloromethylketone (PPACK) have been studied in primate thrombosis models.

Potent inhibitors of factor X_a have also been discovered. One of these, tick anticoagulant peptide (TAP) has been cloned; recombinant TAP prevents thrombosis in dogs and rabbits. Antistasin is another factor X_a inhibitor that was originally isolated from the Mexican leech.

Recombinant protein C concentrates have been treated with thrombin to produce activated protein C, which has been used as an antithrombotic agent

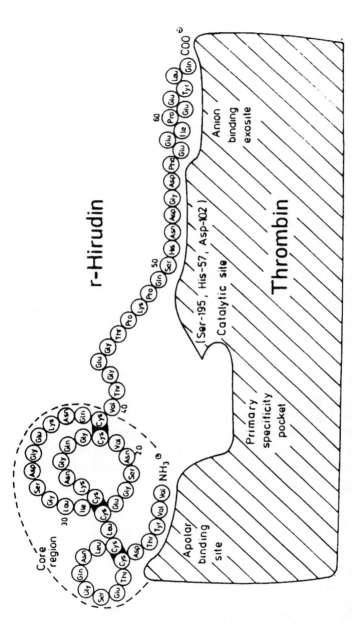

Figure 65-3 Scheme of the hirudin-thrombin interaction. Hirudin interacts simultaneously with the fibrinogen binding exosite and the catalytic site of thrombin. (Used with permission from Markwardt F: Thromb Haemost 66:141, 1991.)

in a baboon thrombosis model, alone or in combination with urokinase. Lastly, a venom from the Malayan pit viper, ancrod, produces therapeutic defibrination by cleaving fibrinopeptide A from fibrinogen which then polymerizes to form loosely knit fibrin that is rapidly lysed and cleared from the circulation. Although ancrod has been available for many years, renewed interest has developed in its potential as an alternative treatment of patients with heparin-associated thrombocytopenia and perhaps also for therapy of patients with acute thrombotic stroke.

Fibrinolytic Agents

New fibrinolytic agents have been developed to increase fibrin specificity, accelerate thrombolysis, and prolong survival of the drugs in the circulation. Mutants of existing fibrinolytic agents have been created using molecular biologic techniques, along with the synthesis of molecular chimeras that combine properties of increased fibrin specificity and more potent fibrinolysis in a single protein. Plasminogen activators have been attached to monoclonal antibodies that are specific for antigens on platelets or fibrin to help target the fibrinolytic agents to thrombi. Unfortunately, it may not be possible to eliminate risks of bleeding with thrombolytic therapy even if systemic fibrinolysis is prevented. Pathologic arterial or venous thrombi are likely to be indistinguishable from normal hemostatic plugs formed to prevent bleeding.

Other Agents

The n-3 fatty acids are long chain polyunsaturated fatty acids from marine and some terrestrial sources that are readily incorporated into platelet and vascular cell membranes. These fatty acids inhibit platelet-mediated thrombosis, and perhaps more importantly, vascular responses to biochemical or physical injury. Clinical trials of dietary fish oil or purified n-3 fatty acids in human beings have shown a modest but significant (26 percent) reduction in arterial restenosis following coronary angioplasty. Mechanisms responsible for these clinical effects may involve inhibition of platelet prostaglandin synthesis or inhibition of vascular proliferative responses mediated by macrophages or cytokines.

Combination Therapies

Innovative combinations of new or traditional antithrombotic agents might increase therapeutic efficacy and yet keep side effects relatively low. An example would be the use of a fibrinolytic agent to produce thrombolysis followed by a potent antithrombin (e.g., hirudin) to maintain vascular patency. In other experimental animal studies, activated protein C has been combined with urokinase; and a thrombin inhibitor, argatroban, has been used with aspirin to provide more effective platelet inhibition. New protocols for "combination chemotherapy" for treatment or prevention of thrombosis are likely to emerge in the near future.

BIBLIOGRAPHY

Bang NU: Leeches, snakes, ticks, and vampire bats in today's cardiovascular drug development. *Circulation* 84:436, 1991.

Coller BS et al: Inhibition of human platelet function in vivo with a monoclonal antibody. With observations on the newly dead as experimental subjects. *Ann Intern Med* 108:635, 1988.

Goodnight SH et al: Assessment of the therapeutic use of N-3 fatty acids in vascular disease and thrombosis. *Chest* 102:374S, 1992.

Greenfield LJ et al: Results of a multicenter study of the modified hook-titanium Greenfield filter. *J Vasc Surg* 14:253, 1991.

Gruber A et al: Antithrombotic effects of combining activated protein C and urokinase in nonhuman primates. *Circulation* 84:2454, 1991.

Hanson SR, Harker LA: Interruption of acute platelet-dependent thrombosis by the synthetic antithrombin D-phenylalanyl-L-prolyl-L-arginyl chloromethylketone. *Proc Natl Acad Sci USA* 85:3184, 1988.

Hull RD et al: Effectiveness of intermittent pneumatic leg compression for preventing deep vein thrombosis after total hip replacement. *JAMA* 263:2313, 1990.

Kanter B, Moser KM: The Greenfield vena cava filter. *Chest* 93:170, 1988.

Kelly AB et al: Hirudin interruption of heparin-resistant arterial thrombus formation in baboons. *Blood* 77:1006, 1991.

Lijnen HR, Collen D: Strategies for the improvement of thrombolytic agents. *Thromb Haemost* 66:88, 1991.

Markwardt F: Hirudin and derivatives as anticoagulant agents. *Thromb Haemost* 66:141, 1991.

Pollak VE et al: Ancrod causes rapid thrombolysis in patients with acute stroke. *Am J Med Sci* 299:319, 1990.

Ruggeri ZM et al: Inhibition of platelet function with synthetic peptides designed to be high-affinity antagonists of fibrinogen binding to platelets. *Proc Natl Acad Sci USA* 83:5708, 1986.

Schaffer LW et al: Antithrombotic efficacy of recombinant tick anticoagulant peptide. A potent inhibitor of coagulation factor Xa in a primate model of arterial thrombosis. *Circulation* 84:1741, 1991.

Weitz J et al: Effects of intermittent pneumatic calf compression on postoperative thrombin and plasmin activity. *Thromb Haemost* 56:198, 1986.

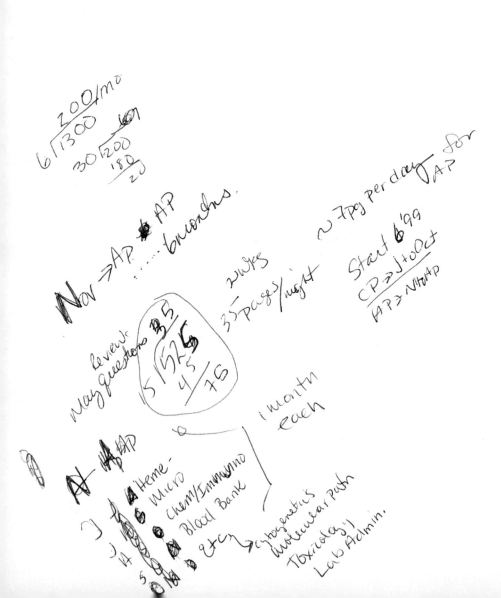

Index